Traumatic Memories of the Second World War and After

Peter Leese • Jason Crouthamel
Editors

Traumatic Memories of the Second World War and After

palgrave
macmillan

Editors
Peter Leese
University of Copenhagen
Copenhagen, Denmark

Jason Crouthamel
Grand Valley State University
Allendale, USA

ISBN 978-3-319-33469-1 ISBN 978-3-319-33470-7 (eBook)
DOI 10.1007/978-3-319-33470-7

Library of Congress Control Number: 2016954176

Printed on acid-free paper

This Palgrave Macmillan imprint is published by Springer Nature
The registered company is Springer International Publishing AG Switzerland

Acknowledgements

This volume has its origins in scholarship presented at the conference "Aftershock: Post-Traumatic Cultures since the Great War" held at the University of Copenhagen in May 2013. The conference and a follow-up event were funded by the Danish Council for Independent Research (FKK) and the Carlsberg Foundation, Denmark. We received additional grants from the Department of English, Germanic and Romance Studies and the Centre for European Studies, both at the University of Copenhagen, and we are most grateful to the University of Copenhagen for its support. We would like to thank Andrew Miller for his herculean work in organizing the conference. At the conference, we received invaluable and stimulating contributions from a wide range of colleagues who shared their expertise. Jay Winter's generosity in offering critical analysis and synthesizing ideas at the conference was an inspiration. Allan Young, Simon Wessely, Edgar Jones, Raya Morag, Mette Bertelsen, Stefan Schilling and Anne Freese posed questions, critiques and observations that helped enrich our thinking and approaches to trauma in the twentieth century. At the last stage of completing the manuscript, we had the tremendous opportunity to present our ideas, joined on a panel with Julia Barbara Köhne and Ville Kivimäki, at a seminar at the Max Planck Institute for Human Development and Research Center on the History of Emotions. We are grateful to Ute Frevert and scholars at the center who formulated illuminating questions about our fundamental arguments that helped us define our approaches to trauma studies and emotions. Ville Kivimäki made that event at the Max Planck Institute possible and we are most grateful to him. We would also like to thank Garry White for his expertise as a translator whose advice and attention to detail is much appreciated. Further, we would like to thank our editor at Palgrave Macmillan, Kristin Purdy, who patiently ushered the project through the process of review and revision, and to Chris Chappell who invited us to submit the manuscript. Thanks also to the anonymous peer reviewers who provided insightful critical comments that helped us revise and improve the essays.

The Center for Scholarly and Creative Excellence, and its director Robert Smart, at Grand Valley State University, kindly provided funding that helped produce this project. We are grateful to the Historical de la Guerre—Peronne (Somme) and Yazid Medmoun/CG80—for permission to reproduce the Amiot Object, and to Sandra Kessler for permission to reproduce her two photographs.

This volume, *Traumatic Memories of the Second World War and After*, is intended to be a companion to our other co-edited collection *Psychological Trauma and the Legacies of the First World War*. Both volumes argue that the traumatic effects of the world wars have been substantially underestimated, and the contributors seek ways to think beyond the strictly medical definitions of what constituted traumatic experience. Further, both volumes search for a broader definition of "mental trauma" by examining wider groups of war victims, including women and children, who were shattered by the experience of total war that engulfed combat and home fronts. By examining varied twentieth-century social, political and cultural sites of trauma, we hope to illuminate the genealogy of trauma at a time when Western societies in the early twenty-first century are asking critical questions about the usefulness of the PTSD (Post-Traumatic Stress Disorder) diagnosis. It is vital that the historical context for the experience, diagnosis and treatment of trauma is fully explored before we can understand the experiences of patients, caregivers and their families today.

Jason Crouthamel (Grand Valley State University)
Peter Leese (University of Copenhagen)

Contents

Notes on Contributors

Joanna Bourke is a Professor of History at Birkbeck, University of London, and a Fellow of the British Academy. She is the author of 12 books, including *What It Means to be Human* (2011), *The Story of Pain: From Prayer to Painkillers* (2014) and *Wounding the World: How Military Violence and War Play are Invading Our Lives* (2015).

Hazel Croft recently finished her PhD dissertation, "War Neurosis and Civilian Mental Health in Second World War Britain" at Birkbeck, University of London. Her research interests include the relationship between war and mental health in the twentieth century, and changing conceptions of "war trauma". These themes are discussed in her chapter 'Emotional Women and Frail Men: Gendered Diagnostics from Shellshock to PTSD, 1914–2010' in Ana Carden-Coyne (ed.), *Gender and Conflict Since 1914*, (Palgrave Macmillan, 2012).

Jason Crouthamel is Associate Professor of History at Grand Valley State University in Michigan. He has written on the history of psychological trauma, memory and masculinity in Germany during the age of total war. He is the author of *An Intimate History of the Front: Masculinity, Sexuality and German Soldiers in the First World War* (New York: Palgrave Macmillan, 2014) and *The Great War and German Memory: Society, Politics and Psychological Trauma, 1914–1945* (2009). Together with Peter Leese, he is the co-editor of Psychological *Trauma and the Legacies of the First World War* (Palgrave Macmillan, 2016).

Mikkel Dack is an adjunct instructor in the Department of History at the University of Calgary. He recently completed his PhD in Modern European History, also at the University of Calgary—his dissertation is entitled "Questioning the Past: The Fragebogen and Everyday Denazification in Occupied Germany". In the past, he has studied at the University of Waterloo, Helmut Schmidt Universität and the Freie Universität Berlin. His research is focused on twentieth-century Germany, especially the Allied occupation and topics of denazification, reeducation, and psychological and social exchanges between "occupier" and "occupied". He has written articles and book chapters on the postwar construction of victim narratives, the expulsion of ethnic Germans from Poland and Czechoslovakia, and transatlantic negative eugenics movements.

Robert Dale is Lecturer in Russian History at Newcastle University. He was awarded a PhD in History from Queen Mary, University of London, in January 2011. His first monograph, *Demobilized Veterans in Late Stalinist Leningrad: Soldiers to Civilians*, was published by Bloomsbury Academic in 2015. His current research builds upon his work on the demobilization and post-war readjustment of Red Army veterans, to explore the post-war reconstruction of Soviet society. This work pays special attention to the Great Patriotic War's painful legacy, and the ways in which the war continued to destabilize and divide post-war society after 1945.

Sophie Delaporte is a historian at the University of Picardie Jules Verne, Amiens. Her work has focused in particular on the trauma of war and its different forms of representations. In February 2012 she submitted her Habilitation thesis on the French director and writer Pierre Schoendoerffer. She is working on "Faces of War from the nineteenth to the twenty-first century": an examination of the thought, treatment and representation of wartime trauma, and an investigation into the testimony of doctors on the battlefields of the Great War.

Susan Derwin is a Professor of German and Comparative Literature and the director of the Interdisciplinary Humanities Center at the University of California, Santa Barbara. Her research examines the relationship between testimonial narrative and healing as it relates to diverse experiences of war. She is the author of *The Ambivalence of Form: Lukács, Freud, and the Novel*, and *Rage is the Subtext: Readings in Holocaust Literature and Film*. She is the founding director of the University of California Student Veterans Writing Workshop.

Sandra Kessler completed her PhD in Social and Cultural Anthropology at the Department of Film, Theater and Cultural Studies at Johannes Gutenberg University in Mainz, Germany. In 2012, she conducted fieldwork in South Korea with a research fellowship as visiting scholar at Hankuk University of Foreign Studies in Seoul; her doctoral thesis analyses biographical memories and life narratives of Korean War veterans in cross-cultural perspective. During her graduate studies in Social and Cultural Anthropology, Economics and American Studies at Johannes Gutenberg University, she undertook research at the Universidad Autónoma de Madrid, Spain, and the Nihon University Tokyo, Japan.

Maria Kobielska completed her PhD in literary studies from the Jagiellonian University (UJ) in Kraków in 2014. She teaches cultural studies, poetics and theory and literature in the Faculty of Polish Studies of the UJ. Her publications include *Nastrajanie pamięci. Artykulacja doświadczenia w poezji Jerzego Ficowskiego* (Universitas, 2010) and, among other articles, "Patterns and Politics. Cultural Memory in Poland after 1989", in *Култура/Culture* 5/2014. She is completing her book on the Polish memory culture after 1989.

Peter Leese is Associate Professor of History at the University of Copenhagen. His publications include *Shell Shock. Traumatic Neurosis and the British Soldiers of the First World War* (2002. Revised paperback, 2014), *Britain Since 1945: aspects of identity* (2006) and, as co-editor, *Migration, Narration, Identity: cross cultural perspectives* (2012). Together with Jason Crouthamel he is also the editor of *Psychological Trauma and the Legacies of the First World War* (2016).

Lisa Pine is Reader in History at the London South Bank University. She obtained her doctorate from the University of London in 1996. Her main research interests are the social history of Nazi Germany and the Holocaust. Her major publications are *Life and Times in Nazi Germany* (London, 2016); *Education in Nazi Germany* (Oxford, 2010); *Hitler's "National Community": Society and Culture in Nazi Germany* (London, 2007); *Nazi Family Policy, 1933–1945* (Oxford, 1997).

Marzena Sokołowska-Paryż is an associate professor at the Institute of English Studies, University of Warsaw, Poland, where she teaches contemporary British and Commonwealth literature, with specific emphasis on the representations of war in relation to history, memory and national identity. She is the author of *Reimagining the War Memorial, Reinterpreting the Great War: The Formats of British Commemorative Fiction* (2012) and *The Myth of War in British and Polish Poetry, 1939–1945* (2002). Together with Martin Löschnigg, she co-edited *The Great War in Post-Memory Literature and Film* (2014).

List of Figures

CHAPTER 1

Introduction

Peter Leese and Jason Crouthamel

The defining event of Jonas Mekas's life was the moment in July 1944 when, to escape arrest for anti-German resistance activities, he was forced to leave his village, his family and his beloved Lithuania. Travelling towards Vienna, he was quickly arrested by a German patrol; the next 5 years he lived in Displaced Person camps before being "dumped" in New York, as he put it, by the United Nations High Commissioner for Refugees. Robert Vas, likewise, was compelled to leave Budapest and his homeland following the failure of the Hungarian Uprising in the autumn of 1956. He travelled to London and found another life, but was unable to forget his departure. The Cold War had hardly begun to thaw when he died in 1978; he never returned home.

Neither Mekas nor Vas was directly involved in Second World War combat, though both became active propagandists against their respective occupiers. Neither was clinically diagnosed with any kind of traumatic condition, although Vas's failure to conform did land him in a Soviet-style mental institution not long after the war. Yet both were undoubtedly damaged by their experiences of forced migration in the aftermath of armed conflict, and their respective careers as filmmakers in New York

P. Leese (✉)
University of Copenhagen, Copenhagen, Denmark

J. Crouthamel
Grand Valley State University, Allendale, MI, USA

P. Leese, J. Crouthamel (eds.), *Traumatic Memories of the Second World War and After*, DOI 10.1007/978-3-319-33470-7_1

and London are, among other things, vivid, artful explorations of traumatic memory played out in film. Their fuller stories are explored later in this collection. Their sufferings, and remarkable achievements, are evoked here to illustrate the elusive, life-changing effects of traumatic experience, to suggest that clinical labels and pension files can hardly do justice to the psychological aftereffects of war. These two lives also raise other historical questions: about who has the right to be called "traumatized", how past and present definitions map accurately onto each other or fall beyond a boundary and whether those whose experiences and psychological reactions are not recognized can be reconciled with their past.[1]

Since the early 1980s, when post-traumatic stress disorder (PTSD) was named, defined, and institutionalized by the American Psychiatric Association, public awareness and academic interest in trauma have dramatically risen. Several related phrases, Gulf War syndrome for instance, circulate widely in public discourse; PTSD is no longer a mere clinical designation, it is widely used as the name of a disease. Soldiers who returned from Afghanistan or Iraq suffering prolonged battlefield exposure are viewed compassionately, but often are misunderstood or feared as irrational and dangerous. Scholars in the humanities, historians among them, know well that those who have experienced violent circumstances and are subsequently troubled by them have often been subjected to this odd mix of curiosity, sympathy and anxiety. Research into the social and cultural histories of trauma can shed much light on the emergence of these present-day responses. Yet, while there has been an extensive discussion of trauma as a theoretical concept, surprisingly little attention has been given to particularities of time or place, to varieties of response beyond the English-language conception of PTSD.

The Second World War and the changing meanings of trauma in the second half of the twentieth century are a particularly rich setting for case studies on the subject, as we discovered when these essays were first presented as research papers in Copenhagen at the "AfterShock: Post-traumatic Cultures since the First World War" conference (May 2013). The extent and variety of recent research and thinking in the field of historical trauma studies led us to a follow-up Copenhagen University meeting on "Comparing Traumatic Cultures" (hosted by Peter Leese, November 2013). On this second occasion, a group of scholars gathered to consider the current state of historical trauma studies: Mark Micale (University of Illinois, Champaign-Urbana), Susan Derwin (University of California, Santa Barbara), Jessica Meyer (University of Leeds), Bill Niven (Nottingham Trent University),

Adam Lowenstein (University of Pittsburgh), Irina Reyn (University of Pittsburgh), Robert Dale (Kings College London), Stefan Schilling (King's College London) and Birthe Hoffmann (University of Copenhagen). We also discussed methodological questions and considered future research directions. Important to our thinking on this occasion were two papers, Susan Derwin's "The Embattled Mind of the Veteran" and Mark Micale's "Historical Trauma Studies: Recent Work, Future Agendas". A group of new themes emerged from these debates, including the ways and extent to which traumatic responses vary, and by implication how we ought to define trauma, the gendered nature of traumatic experience, recognition and diagnosis, and the malleable forms of traumatic memory and traumatic symptoms across time; the distinctions between non-perpetrator and perpetrator trauma also emerged as a subject of particular current interest.

Many of the essays in *Traumatic Memories* incorporate these themes, but this also led to another consideration: the need to place varied methodological approaches from the humanities (historical, literary and visual media readings) in proximity to each other as a way to tackle the complexities of the past.[2] This proximity reflects the remarkable variety of approaches which are now brought to bear on the subject of trauma, but, in our view, also the need to think beyond the various historically bound clinical definitions of what constitutes traumatic experience. Historical documents—medical records, pension appeals and civil service memos—appear as the product of medical, state and financial negotiations. They are defined by the limits of state and bureaucratic interest, and not least by financial liability. While these engagements with the state are themselves of intrinsic interest, they in no way coincide with the human experience of trauma, which historically extends far beyond that which can be recorded in official documentation, or for that matter in family memoirs or intergenerational memory. There is an urgent need, then, for a broader cultural and historical analysis of trauma, which takes account of social dynamics, politics, and medical conceptualization, but which is not confined to them. Hence, the deliberately eclectic approach and choice of subjects, authors and disciplines included in this collection. This is also a question of how trauma is defined. Overwhelmingly, attention to the history of trauma has focussed on male experience, particularly in wartime. This important subject fully deserves the attention it has received, but is possible because soldiers and ex-servicemen leave relatively traceable paper trails, while others caught up in trauma-inducing events and their consequences, non-combatant women, for example, are far less visible in the historical record. Because of selective memories, traumatic war experiences are made predominantly male by definition. Yet, it is equally important that there are limits on what constitutes a traumatic experience, that current media definitions, which incorporate the aftereffects of any mildly disturbing or upsetting "bad event" into the definition of trauma, do not dissipate the usefulness of the term.

Historiography and Methods

Historical trauma studies are today an expanding, urgent subject for scholars and students, yet despite widespread attention in academia and mass media, comparative, interdisciplinary and historically grounded studies remain few. Moreover, discussions of the subject do not often bring together varied approaches in order to examine a particular historical moment. Among the earlier collections that have used this approach, we would cite Mark Micale and Paul Lerner's edited volume *Traumatic Pasts. History, Psychiatry and Trauma in the Modern Age, 1870–1930* (2001) as a rich attempt to contextualize trauma at a particular moment, and within its particular set of social and cultural conditions. Richard Bessel and Dirk Schumann's *Life after Death: Approaches to a Cultural and Social History of Europe During the 1940s and 1950s* (2003) is also an exemplary investigation into many aspects of the human, often mental fallout from the Second World War. A closer attention to specifically psychological aftereffects is explored in *The Politics of War Trauma. The Aftermath of War in Ten European Countries*, edited by Jolande Withuis and Annet Mooij (2010), which was written by an interdisciplinary group of scholars across the humanities and social sciences and which attempts a systematic survey of war-related trauma after 1945.[3] To date, this account remains a rarity in historical trauma studies because it attempts a comparative investigation beyond the borders of Western Europe.

The First World War and the Holocaust have between them been the most sustained subjects of historical trauma studies.[4] A fleshed-out historical and theoretical framework that can link different times and places, interpret the dynamic relations between patients, medics and financial institutions, or understand the interrelationship between memory, representation and ideology remains to be fully developed.[5] There are, of course, already several detailed studies on particular aspects of postwar traumatic experience, among them Ben Shephard's study *A War of Nerves* (2002), which was the first to survey the entire twentieth century and which delineated its subject through a detailed study of patients, but especially their medics. The only comparable volume is Jones and Wessely's *Shell Shock to PTSD: Military Psychiatry from 1900 to the Gulf War*, which takes a more narrowly defined thematic approach, concentrating on the connections between clinical practice, evolving medical conceptualization, and the experience of soldiering.[6] *Traumatic Memories* complements these earlier studies by concentrating in several essays on personal experience, by focussing on a relatively narrow time frame, and by expanding as far as possible the comparative scope. This arrangement captures the present lively state of investigation, with its recently expanded geographies, thematic interests and more radical questioning of the origins and significance of trauma before and after the current post-1980 iteration of PTSD.

There is also an overlap between our collection and the more abstract investigation of "trauma theory", which includes historically oriented work by practitioners, questions about the clinical and ontological status of trauma as well as the broad area incorporating literary and cultural theory.[7] Likewise, there are various investigations into "trauma and culture", which cover more anthropological and sociological themes. These are often related to both recent past and present, including lively debates around cinema, popular literature and the arts as they relate to the cultural conditions which produce traumatic discourse and clinical practice.[8] One methodological puzzle that has yet to be solved is how to research and write a history of trauma which concentrates not on one particular gender experience but on the instability of gender categories. This instability is present in many kinds of traumatic experience, but matters greatly in wartime, when normative roles (nurturer, warrior) assume much greater prominence: when gender roles are patrolled so actively, traumatized men may be either unmanly or heroic, while traumatized women become symbolic or invisible. The question remains as to how these sets of circumstances and representations might be connected. Likewise, we have not yet managed to historicize the wider dynamics of traumatic memory within families and between generations.

Gathered in this collection are essays which begin to address some of these themes, and which together highlight the possibilities of a comparative and interdisciplinary approach to trauma, an approach which is grounded in the local particularity of past attitudes. Our common purpose is to investigate how trauma changes, diagnostically, politically, discursively, according to the social and cultural milieu in which it is manifested. As it turns out, "the return of the soldier", to take one example, is "universal" in that it happens everywhere, but despite this, it is never unproblematically the same. Many soldiers never return, many are very different, and so is the society into which they arrive. In this sense, it is not the "bad event" which makes trauma, but the material, emotional and communal context within which it is remembered. At many times, and in many places, potentially traumatizing events do not result in chronic or acute symptoms. Rather, such symptoms tend to emerge and to persist when there is inadequate clinical consideration, when acknowledgement and recognition are not forthcoming from the receiving community, or when families and employment fail. The ways in which the sick role is sanctioned or censured are also highly variable. It is in the intricacy of particular historical circumstances that the unstable, malleable formation of trauma takes on a certain appearance.

Themes

There is then no straightforward or easily described relationship between culture, trauma, and history; social psychologies are differently inflected according to time and place. This collection tries to explore how these variations change origins and symptomatology as well as medical and social responses. Within this research area, there are a number of sub-questions, among them: whose traumatic experiences gain attention and why? By implication, whose experiences are ignored? What are the particular, localized mechanisms of recognition or non-acknowledgement? How do collaborations and antagonisms between doctors, patients and social institutions vary and with what consequences? How do different groups such as doctors, patients or the public define and claim the authority to understand traumatic conditions? How and why does collective memory and representation of traumatic experience change?

That such questions are only now beginning to be asked is no surprise given the very gradual acknowledgement of trauma, which is still stigmatized as "mental illness" or "disorder" even in the late twentieth and early twenty-first centuries rather than understood as legitimate responses to extreme circumstances. Some of these questions have already been raised in relation to the First World War and the Holocaust. These two particular instances continue to provoke new questions, to be explored from new angles, as the essays by Sophie Delaporte and Lisa Pine in this collection show. But there are now also several specialist studies in various European countries, and attention is increasingly turning to the wider history of the

Second World War and to other, later wars, precisely because they provide such instructive contrasts.

The Second World War is a critical moment because its trauma cases become more recognizably connected to present-day definitions of PTSD, historical sources are greater in number as well as more varied in type, and the possibilities to compare military, medical or social aspects are all greater. Predating current definitions of PTSD, the trauma cases of the Second World War and after are viewed very differently than in current medical aetiology. These past definitions of trauma are less driven by medical, insurance, or pharmaceutical industry profits, or the recent medicalization of emotional states.[9] In short, the Second World War and its aftermath constitute a formative moment in the social, cultural, and political history of trauma. A focussed examination makes it possible to investigate anew given concepts, diagnoses, and moral assumptions. Comparing specific, localized instances, this collection of essays rethinks the history of war trauma at an interim moment: after its first large-scale appearance during the First World War, but before the current socio-medical paradigm of PTSD.

The terms of the reinvestigation, to give three examples, include looking beyond existing studies of male experience among active combatants, considering varieties of personal experience and their wide-ranging implications for the medicalization and social positioning of psychological conditions, and examining various cultural inflections of traumatic experience and diagnosis. Finally, taken together, the essays in this collection ask critical questions about what we now call PTSD. They do so at a time when the usefulness and legitimacy of the diagnosis are increasingly questioned. The issues here include the diagnostic, gender and institutional biases of trauma definition—the ellipses, blind spots and taboos on describing certain forms of traumatic experience (rape, non-compassionate responses, forgetfulness); the requirements and methods by which perpetrators and victims are identified and categorized; the trauma archive: witness, testimony and the erasure of "inconvenient" versions of traumatic experience; trauma, voyeurism and sexual violence; and the clash between private histories and public representations.

Organization

The collection is divided into five parts, respectively, on the "Archive" of trauma, on "Wartime" and "Postwar" experiences, then on "Recollection" and "Representation". Each part addresses a theme that has emerged in recent thinking on historical trauma studies; any of these headings might be the basis for more sustained investigations.

"Archive", Part I, explores some of the recent thinking on alternative sources, but also on why and how this research area might be reconfigured. Both of the authors here consequently look at important ways in which historical trauma studies can be enriched and expanded to create a fuller cultural history of trauma. Sophie Delaporte's essay, "Making Trauma Visible", by one of the leading French scholars of war trauma in the twentieth century, puts forward an alternative history of diagnosis and treatment. By contextualizing its history anew—initial conceptualization, competing schools of interpretation and treatment—Delaporte challenges fundamental assumptions about the nature of trauma and the way it is understood in both past and present. In particular, she notes the tendency, built into the Anglo-American tradition from its beginnings, to abandon psychoanalytic explanations in favour of more pragmatic and environmental interpretations. In place of this approach, Delaporte calls for historians to give new emphasis to the psychic experience of individuals, to the ways in which they respond to the encounter with death, which she argues is the source of trauma. In a detailed case study, Delaporte refines this down to a "visualizing" of trauma through an analysis of one remarkable piece of evidence from the First World War, the "Amiot Object", a painting maquette made by a French soldier following his experiences on the Western Front in 1915. The implications of this analysis are not only in the artwork itself and the conclusions Delaporte draws from it, but also in the detailed engagement with an object made in the aftermath of traumatic experience, in this case very directly interpreting that experience. Such objects are rare, but the idea of reading visual evidence—sketches, photographs, home movies—as a way to reach the "unspeakable" experience of trauma and its aftermath ("traumatography") is timely and evocative.[10] Two other themes emerge from Delaporte's essay, which echo through the studies that follow: first, the limitations of what is clinically defined as trauma, and the way in which such definitions mismatch the social reality of those who experience traumatic aftershocks; second, and related to this, the continuing "invisibility" of the traumatized as historical subjects, or rather the very selective description of legitimate or "acceptable" trauma in any particular time and place.

Susan Derwin's exploration of "moral injury" poses another critique of PTSD as a diagnostic category. She stresses that in the recent experience of traumatized individuals survivor guilt, injury through the transgression of moral boundaries, and a sense of betrayal by leaders are often present, but beyond any clinical remit. In the setting of this collection, Derwin's observation that the moral uncertainties of modern, non-conventional warfare (how to identify the enemy, how to safeguard the innocent) is especially pertinent, though it would be wrong to assume greater moral certainty in the past. The question of return and the morally ambiguous situation of the ex-combatant are also highlighted. Here, it is the reluctance of peacetime society to accept the violence it sanctions during wartime which causes damage: when killing becomes taboo, the killer is a reminder of acts which in retrospect come to be seen as all the more shameful. Derwin's case study parallels Delaporte's attempt to explore different trauma archives. The problem of addressing moral injury to the perpetrator is, if anything, harder to consider, making imaginative interpretations in fiction or film one of the few sources available. Through a reading of Toni Morrison's *Home* (2011), Derwin raises critical questions about how the experiences of peace and war are inseparable, how those who are violated may themselves become violators, and how injury is done to those who are required to commit acts of violence on behalf of the state and its citizens. This raises a wider question about the ways in which the experience of traumatized perpetrators should be further explored in other historical situations, and the rationale for any such investigation.

"Wartime", Part II, returns to two apparently familiar areas, but in so doing, challenges existing understandings of traumatic experience. What becomes immediately apparent in these essays by Lisa Pine and Hazel Croft are the ways in which material, ideological, and political circumstances frame concepts of mental health and illness. To put it another way, how the perceived presence or absence of trauma depends on surrounding vested interests in the immediate aftermath of traumatic events, but also at greater distance among various interest groups. Local conditions alter drastically the conception, expression and articulation of trauma both inside and outside the clinic. Consequently, some groups are granted recognition, while for others it is denied. Lisa Pine's work on "Testimonies of Trauma: Surviving Auschwitz-Birkenau" addresses this question directly. Pine stresses the gendered nature of traumatic experience, and the superimposition of gender, patriotic, and other ideological values onto its interpretation. Using survivor testimonies from the Auschwitz-Birkenau death camp, the study explores aspects of women's dehumanization, the ways in which they sought to maintain connections with their former lives and identities, and aspects of camp life—non-compassionate responses, or the giving of sexual favours, for example—which have often been passed over. This is one of the first historical studies to outline a possible future gendered history of trauma, and it is an especially welcome example for its investigation of the nuanced ways in which both women and men experienced gender identity as an enabling resource towards their psychological survival.

Hazel Croft's study of "Civilian Neuroses in Second World War Britain" illustrates a different aspect of the ways in which trauma has historically been erased or downplayed for ideological reasons - what we might call the "myth of resilience": the tendency to emphasize ideals of heroic self-sacrifice, of inherent "national" courage, of a "no neurosis" society. Croft details the emergence of this idea in the recollection of Britain's Home Front during the Second World War, but it is hardly a unique instance, and tends to recur wherever political advantage, national self-respect or prestige are in play. As Allan Young noted in his keynote speech at the Copenhagen AfterShock conference in May 2013, "resilience" became a prominent theme in public discourse after the US terrorist attacks in 2001.[11] In Britain's case, the difficulties of managing "shell shock" for propaganda and military advantages during the Great War led to a later "no shell shock" policy for combatants, and a parallel "no neurosis" policy for non-combatants. Croft points out that these policies, political decisions as much as clinical judgements, resulted from anxiety about psychological damage due to large-scale civilian bombardment campaigns. A reluctance to acknowledge such conditions is not, though, the same as their absence. Croft's investigation into the medical encounters between doctor and patient during the Second World War begins to reveal, then, how medics served as the frontline police for such conditions. While this non-conceptualization of trauma had all too obvious financial and practical advantages to the state, the reality of trauma could only be de-emphasized, not eliminated. Hence, medics tended to suggest the best cure was tea and rest, while patients turned to stronger sedatives such as alcohol. The standby treatments from the trenches of the Western Front were still very much used by civilians during the Second World War. By the Second World War though, soldiers' traumatic conditions sometimes obtained social prestige, which might be parlayed into heroic status or victim compensation. Civilian trauma, by contrast, was much less likely to accrue benefits. Rather, anxiety, depression and "hysteria" suffered the same under-funding, overcrowding and social stigma as was attached to those who actually entered "mental hospitals".

"Postwar", Part III, addresses the immediate conditions of return and re-stabilization following the cessation of World War Two hostilities. Soldiers returning to civilian society and home societies adapting to the new conditions of peace, exist in a system of mutual reciprocity: each perceives, shapes and responds in light of the other. The exact nature of postwar material circumstances, medical insights and morale is critical to the ways in which each understands the other, and the extent to which "bad events" are transformed into traumatic responses. Here too there is the likelihood that traumatic conditions among both soldiers and civilians will go unacknowledged, be disguised or otherwise be rendered more or less invisible. Robert Dale's essay "'No longer normal': Traumatized Red Army Veterans in Postwar Leningrad" provides a parallel to the case of women as trauma victims in the death camps by exploring a similar ideological erasure among Russian veterans of the Second World War. Yet, the elusive nature of traumatic responses, and the very different conditions in which its presence might be acknowledged or retarded, makes any such parallels less than straightforward. It turns out not to be the case that war-traumatized soldiers were entirely unacknowledged in late Stalinist society, but their conditions were nevertheless not as much acknowledged or treated clinically as managed socially. Traumatized ex-servicemen were re-acclimatized or failed to reintegrate within the postwar context of family and community life. The development of medical ideas in 1920s and 1930s Russia was organic and materialist in ways that were not very different, for example, from those of the inter-war German medical establishment. The consequences of traumatic wartime experience were, therefore, much more likely to be expressed in alcoholism, criminal and anti-social behaviour. Political ideology may partly account for the failure of medicine or state institutions, but it appears too that there was a genuine cultural difficulty in conceptualizing and naming trauma both by professionals and within communities of wider social interest: in families, in the courts. Since medical definitions of traumatic aftereffect were so narrow, their range and extent could never be fully acknowledged or measured, only glimpsed at a distance. One important implication of Dale's essay is that unexamined ideological assumptions dating back to the Cold War have stymied our historical understanding of trauma as it existed in eastern central Europe, when the subject is considered at all, which is rarely.

The ways in which trauma can be manipulated—stressed, repressed, reworked—for social and political ends come to the fore in a different way in Mikkel Dack's essay on the Fragebogen, denazification, and trauma in

Post-WWII Germany. Dack's argument is that the denazification survey undertaken by the Allies at the end of the war implicitly invited Germans to identify themselves as victims, and thereby to dissociate themselves from difficult or uncomfortable past identifications and events. Against this is the need to understand historically the human, social and psychological destruction not just of individuals, but of an entire defeated nation, and, again, the difficulty—both archival and moral—of exploring the experience of perceived perpetrator trauma. In Dack's view, the long-lasting effect of this victim identification was a collective failure to process suffering and loss. Deceit and denunciation seemingly sanctioned by the state bureaucracy made it all the more difficult to reframe individual life stories or to reconnect communal bonds. Compared to Russia, the advantages to claiming the status of a traumatized victim in postwar Germany were significantly greater. Yet while there was the opportunity to articulate a "useable" past, the implications of that use were not fully thought through, nor perhaps could they be under the circumstances of a defeated, troubled nation struggling with loss and attempting to survive the difficulties of day-to-day living. It is no surprise that many were convicted of falsifying the facts of their former lives. All of this raises important questions about the complex psychological, social and political reasons why traumatic pasts might be falsified or exaggerated, about the kinds of traumatic experience which are socially acceptable, and about the historical conditions which might lead to a particular instance of trauma commodification or vilification.

"Recollection", Part IV, considers the retroactive interpretation of traumatic experience within public discourse, and extends the theme of ideological manipulation or reworking for explicitly nation-state political purposes. The role of ideology is highlighted by Sandra Kessler in her essay on remembering the Korean War. "Public and Private: Negotiating Memories of the Korean War" explores a less well-known setting for traumatic experience, and in so doing her essay calls into question many of the current western assumptions about the nature of trauma. With particular stress on memory making in South Korea, and with a particular interest in cross-cultural communication, Kessler's essay highlights the rarity of discussion, not least across generations, and the ways in which public, politically charged readings of the war can be internalized. This study reveals, then, how traumatic response may be changed by the very different cultural context of the Korean War, and in particular what it meant for South Korean participants. The most intense period of memory suppression, it turns out, was during the military dictatorship of 1961–1987. During this time, "wrong" memories were viewed as politically subversive counter-narratives; bereaved families were actively silenced.

Kessler's account describes too the subsequent era of liberalization in the 1990s and the Truth and Reconciliation Commission in 2005, yet the social dynamics of remembering are not only about political ideologies. The setting for active recollection—individual, familial, professional—is also essential to any understanding of how traumatic memory functions in South Korea today. To examine these processes, Kessler gives a detailed analysis of the War Memorial of Korea, with its symbolic embodiment of state ideology. She also reports on two discussions with Korean War veterans, with as much interest in how they remember as in the content of their accounts. This is a study of the interrelationship between private and public memory, of the ways in which political conditions can confuse and destabilize personal understandings of the past. It is also a study that reveals the extent to which trauma requires cross-cultural "translation", of how clinical categorization and cultural norms differ, and cannot be understood as commensurate.

Maria Kobielska's account of the Katyń Massacre in Contemporary Polish Culture "Endless Aftershock" addresses public and private memory from another perspective. This chapter is a case study on the public repression and release of traumatic memory. Kobielska describes some of the ways in which the traumatic memory of a community, those whose relatives were murdered in 1940, is partially erased, only to find its way back into public consciousness, reactivated by political changes and later events. This raises the question of how and in what ways traumatic memory functions under politically repressive regimes such as those in eastern central Europe during the Cold War. In Kobielska's account, the repression of events within public discourse led eventually to a powerful counter-narrative which emerged around anniversary events in the early twenty-first century. The new prominence of Katyń in Poland's memory landscape has developed from a variety of factors, some relatively recent political developments, but also well-established national traditions: the imposition and subsequent demolition of the communist state in postwar Poland, the older political and religious martyrological mythologies, and the Smolensk air crash of 2010. The methodology of this essay is also worth dwelling on for a moment. First, this analysis moves away from the idea of trauma defined in relation to a generation that directly experiences it, and towards the examination of a more dispersed realm of public discourse.

Second, like Susan Derwin, Maria Kobielska makes a close reading of cultural artefacts. Not an "internal" analysis of the text within itself, but a social reading of how particular items—a state-sponsored commemoration campaign, a feature film, a poem published in the wake of 1989—express an evolving, re-interpretive use of the past. This broader form of cultural analysis is familiar in relation to some well-known, major events such as the First World War, but remains underused for the examination of many other moments less familiar in the western memory "canon". Here again, by considering the differences between particular kinds of memory formation, by exploring the ways in which it is directed according to localized cultural scripts, it becomes possible to give a more fully historicized account of traumatic recollection which also has implications for individual rememberers.

"Representation", Part V, gives further insight into trauma historically defined and erased according to gender, manipulated for metaphorical and ideological advantage, but equally the ways in which film can reimagine traumatic memory for witness and healing. Marzana Sokołowska-Paryż's essay on "War Rape: Trauma and the Ethics of Representation" addresses the question of what place rape has in the representation of war, and how this expresses wider attitudes towards the traumatic experiences of women. While it is apparent that scholarly interest is extensive and varied, it is equally clear that rape is especially difficult to describe as an event in itself rather than as an expression of some other aspect of wartime experience. More often than not, films which feature war rape view it through the eyes of the perpetrator, stress dominant and submissive gender roles, and are comments on character or situation. Film therefore provides as ideal medium through which to consider the cultural position of rape in wartime. Through a series of case studies, the author analyzes filmic representations of rape as metaphor and their failed expression of traumatic experience. The author's analysis is especially intriguing for its breadth of references, which nevertheless shows a common set of themes across films from Germany, Poland, Croatia, Russia and the USA. Such an analysis indicates too that cinema has an important place in the visual analysis of historical trauma, and that cultural historians of film might well extend and refine the kinds of analysis initiated by Anton Kaes in *Shell Shock Cinema*, and by Sokołowska-Paryż.[12]

Peter Leese takes this filmic analysis in a different direction by reading the work of two post-World War Two directors as "ego documents" in the archive of traumatic experience. Film is read here as a compulsive re-iteration of personal traumatic memory through which individuals remake successive versions of "bad events". The forms of these events can be directly historical, metaphorical, dialogical or even allegorical. The implication here is that present circumstances direct each successive interpretation of the past, that negotiations to constitute meaning from an irreducible traumatic memory may succeed, but that such memories are just as likely to remain stubbornly meaningless. Jonas Mekas and Robert Vas are also significant, as mentioned at the beginning of this introduction, because their experiences and recollections are beyond the boundary of what would normally be identified as traumatic. Nevertheless, both men were caught up with the events of their early years and with their agonizing moments of departure. Such a reading has much in common with cultural, media and social studies interpretations of film, but equally stresses the historian's craft by examining the process and procedures of change across time. Finally, this examination suggests that traumatic memory is less a question of binary opposites than a scale of responses, only some of which have financial, clinical or political implications.

New Directions in Historical Trauma Studies

For the "Coda" to the collection, we invited Joanna Bourke, a leading researcher in the field, to provide a commentary on some of the critical issues raised by *Traumatic Memories*, and on possible future directions for historical trauma studies. Bourke stresses themes that are now emerging more fully in current research: the history of emotions as a framework, the language and cultural "reach" of trauma as a concept, and its particular historical origins and trajectory. Critical difficulties of language, method and ethics are also raised by *Traumatic Memories*, not least the problematic ambivalence of trauma scholars towards perpetrators of violence. The question then arises as to how legitimate it might be to view perpetrators of violence as victims of trauma. To name two among the many other critical issues which demand further investigation: to what extent is "trauma" a colonizing concept that imposes a western set of expectations and behaviours inappropriately and unproductively? How might it help in understanding the cultural construction of trauma to consider it as a kind of "performance", which can be carried off successfully or fail with disastrous personal consequences, and which depends on the particular expectations of any given context and audience?

Finally, thinking of the emerging themes that run through this collection, and which might be further developed by researchers, the editors suggest the following. First, historically changing definitions of trauma: there is an implicit challenge in several of these studies (Croft, Pine, Dack) to the current PTSD definition of trauma as well as to the conditions in which it might exist, or be partially erased, and to its "gender neutral" interpretation. Second, sources for the study of trauma: the use of alternative written and other non-written materials of *historical* analysis, for example, fiction and poetry, art objects and films, oral history and survivor testimony, museums and memorials (Delaporte, Derwin, Sokołowska-Paryż's). Third, trauma and agency: to what extent, and in what ways, do the traumatized have control over their own circumstances? In what ways is trauma made or unmade by those who experience it (Pine, Kobielska, Leese)? Fourth, trauma and return: the varied circumstances and meanings of homecoming, how personal and communal responses change the experience, and forgetting as an aid or hindrance to postwar social development (Dale, Dack, Kessler). Fifth, trauma as ideology: the bureaucratic procedures, political interests, and social processes which act upon trauma to manipulate its meaning through the suppression or promotion of particular symptoms; the wider context of state, communal values, and, for example, the Cold War as they shape medical discourse and popular culture (Pine, Croft, Sokołowska-Paryż). Sixth, trauma and memory: the interconnectedness of family, communal, state social dynamics of recollection within a particular society; late memory and its transmission across generations (Croft, Kessler, Leese).

This collected volume is intended to be a companion to *Psychological Trauma and the Legacies of the First World War*, which also emerged out of a conference at the University of Copenhagen in May 2013. Both of these volumes contend that the traumatic impact of the world wars was more complex than the particular, limited symptoms identified by military-medical establishments. Historians can reconstruct subjective traumas by using more diverse sources produced by wider groups beyond medical and political authorities that have been the epicenter of recent scholarship, including family archives, documents from film and photography, and memoirs of soldiers and civilians. In this context, both combat and non-combatant wartime experience can be seen as an initial encounter with trauma. War equally unleashed waves of violence that eventually resulted in socio-economic marginalization, and sometimes in abuse at the hands of medics; soldiers, civilians and physicians could all be affected by wartime brutalization and its after effects. Wartime psychological trauma was thus not confined to the battlefield: combat was the epicenter of a chain reaction of traumatic experiences that require historians to broaden their approach, to locate "hidden" psychological wounds, and to confront the continuing, long-term effects of war.

Notes

1. On Mekas and Vas, see Chap. 12 in this collection. Also Maureen Turim, "Reminiscences, Subjectivities and Truths", in: James, D.E. (ed.) *To Free Cinema. Jonas Mekas & the New York Underground.* (Princeton, NJ: Princeton University Press, 1992), 193–212; Robert Vas and Alan Rosenthal (1980) "*My Homeland* and *Nine Days in '26*", in: Alan Rosenthal, *The Documentary Conscience. A Casebook of Film Making* (Berkeley, Los Angeles and London: University of California Press, 1980), 261–75.

   On the changing nature of definitions and diagnostic labels related to traumatic experience, see, for example, Edgar Jones and Simon Wessely, "War Syndromes: The Impact of Culture on Medically Unexplained Symptoms", *Medical History* 49 (2005), 55–78; and Tracey Loughran, "Shell Shock, Trauma, and the First World War: The Making of a Diagnosis and Its Histories", *Journal of the History of Medicine and Allied Sciences*, 67 (1) January 2012, 94–119.
2. Among the most important attempts to open out and explore the meanings of trauma in relation to history are Dominick LaCapra, *Writing History, Writing Trauma* (Baltimore, Md: Johns Hopkins University, 2001); Cathy Caruth, ed., *Trauma: Explorations in Memory* (Baltimore, Md: Johns Hopkins University, 1995); Cathy Caruth, *Unclaimed Experience: Trauma, Narrative and History* (Baltimore, Md: Johns Hopkins University, 1996); *Trauma: Explorations in Memory* (Baltimore, Md: Johns Hopkins University, 1995).
3. The introductory essays to these collections show how quickly thinking on historical trauma studies is now developing. Mark S. Micale, Paul Lerner, "Trauma, Psychiatry, and History: A Conceptual and Historiographical Introduction" in: Mark S. Micale, Paul Lerner, eds, *Traumatic Pasts. History, Psychiatry, and Trauma in the Modern Age, 1870–1930* (Cambridge: Cambridge University Press, 2001), 1–28; Richard Bessel and Dirk Schumann, "Introduction: Violence,

Normality and the Construction of Postwar Europe", 1–13, but also Alice Förster and Birgit Beck, "Post-Traumatic Stress Disorder and World War Two: Can a Psychiatric Concept Help Us Understand Postwar Society?" 15–35, both in Richard Bessell and Dirk Schumann, eds., *Life After Death. Approaches to a Cultural and Social History of Europe During the 1940s and 1950s* (Cambridge: Cambridge University Press and the German Historical Institute, Washington, DC, 2003); Jolande Withuis, "Introduction: The Politics of War Trauma", in J. Withuis and A. Mooij, eds., *The Politics of War Trauma: The Aftermath of World War II in Eleven European Countries* (Amsterdam: Askant, 2010), 1–11.

4. On the First World War, for example, Peter Leese, *Shell Shock: Traumatic Neurosis and the British Soldiers of the First World War* (Basingstoke: Palgrave Macmillan, 2014); Fiona Reid, *Broken Men: Shell Shock, Treatment and Recovery in Britain, 1914–1930* (London: Bloomsbury, 2011) and Gregory M. Thomas, *Treating the Trauma of the Great War: Soldiers, Civilians, and Psychiatry in France, 1914–1940* (Baton Rouge: Louisiana State University Press, 2009); Michael Roper in *The Secret Battle: Emotional Survival in the Great War* (Manchester: Manchester University Press, 2009); Jason Crouthamel, *The Great War and German Memory: Society, Politics and Psychological Trauma, 1914–1945* (Liverpool: Liverpool University Press, 2009) Peter Barham's *Forgotten Lunatics of the Great War* (New Haven: Yale University Press, 2007).
5. One suggestive theoretical model put forward in recent years is Part 1 of Graham Dawson's *Making peace with the past? Memory, trauma and the Irish Troubles* (Manchester: Manchester University Press, 2007). See also, for example, Ruth Leys, *Trauma: A Genealogy* (Chicago: University of Chicago Press, 2000). The basis for a broader framework is beginning to take shape though, in attempts to historicize memory or diagnostic categories. For example, T.G. Ashplant, Graham Dawson and Michael Roper, "The politics of war memory and commemoration: contexts, structures and dynamics" in: T.G. Ashplant, Graham Dawson and Michael Roper, eds., *The Politics of Memory: Commemorating War* (New Brunswick and London: Transaction, 2009), 3–85; or Edgar Jones and Simon Wessely, "War Syndromes: The Impact of Culture on Medically Unexplained Symptoms", *Medical History* 49 (2005), 55–78.

6. Ben Shephard, *A War of Nerves: Soldiers and Psychiatrists in the Twentieth Century* (London: Jonathan Cape, 2000); Edgar Jones and Simon Wessely, *Shell Shock to PTSD: Military Psychiatry from 1900 to the Gulf War* (Abingdon: Psychology Press, 2006).
7. Nigel Hunt, *Memory, War and Trauma* (Cambridge: Cambridge University Press, 2010); Allan Young, *The Harmony of Illusions* (Princeton: Princeton University Press, 1997); Roger Luckhurst, *The Trauma Question* (Routledge: New York, 2008); E. Ann Caplan, *Trauma Culture. The Politics of Terror and Loss in Media and Literature* (London: Rutgers University Press, 2005).
8. Among these are Jenny Edkins' *Trauma and the Memory of Politics* (Cambridge: Cambridge University Press, 2010); Kirby Farrell's *Post-Traumatic Culture: Injury and Interpretation in the Nineties* (London: Johns Hopkins University Press, 1998); and Ron Eyerman, Jeffrey C. Alexander, and Elizabeth Butler Breese, eds., *Narrating Trauma: on the impact of collective suffering* (Boulder, Col., Praeger, 2011).
9. See especially Judith Herman, *Trauma and Recovery: From Domestic Abuse to Political Terror* (New York: Basic Books, 1992).
10. Ludmilla Jordanova, *The Look of the Past. Visual and Material Evidence in Historical Practice* (Cambridge: Cambridge University Press, 2012); Gillian Rose, *Visual Methodologies: An Introduction to Researching with Visual Materials* (London: Sage, 2011).
11. Allan Young, "Resilience and the Traumatic Neuroses of War following 9/11" Keynote presentation at the Copenhagen conference, "AfterShock: Post-traumatic cultures since the Great War" 23 May 2013. See also Allan Young, 'Resilience for All by the Year 20-' in: D. Cantor and E. Ramsden, eds., *Stress, Shock and Adaptation in the Twentieth Century* (Rochester: Rochester University Press, 2014) 73–95.
12. Anton Kaes, *Shell Shock Cinema. Weimar Culture and the Wounds of War* (Princeton NJ: Princeton University Press, 2009).

PART I

Archive

CHAPTER 2

Making Trauma Visible

Sophie Delaporte

The question of psychic trauma first arose in the late nineteenth and early twentieth century in the exchanges between Freud and Breuer. Thus, it was during these prewar years that the initial framework for understanding trauma was outlined. In a text published in 1895, *Studies on Hysteria*, Freud wrote: "Psychical trauma—or more precisely the memory of the trauma—acts like a foreign body." He also highlighted the suffering endured by the patient when confronting reminiscences: "The traumatic memory does not wear away", adding: "It must be abreacted." The theory of abreaction came a little later, in 1905, in the text entitled *Psychical (Or Mental) Treatment*, the mental treatment advocated by Freud being that of a "treatment (whether of mental or physical disorders)[…] that uses words, the essential tool of mental treatment". Freud goes on to evoke the "magical power" of words in this respect. His analytical technique as well as his concept of trauma thus gradually came to be defined in the course of these writings, nourished by the discussions he maintained with his main disciples: Ferenczi, Abraham and Jung.

From this point of view, the question of psychic trauma would appear to be inextricably linked to the birth of "psycho-analysis", and on the eve of the Great War a rough outline of Freud's clinical theory and his

S. Delaporte (✉)
University of Picardie Jules Verne, Amiens, France

P. Leese, J. Crouthamel (eds.), *Traumatic Memories of the Second World War and After*, DOI 10.1007/978-3-319-33470-7_2

definition of trauma would already seem to be in place. While "Freudian" thinking had reached the USA, the UK, Germany and France, the number of converts remained fairly low. The one element missing from the construction of this thinking on trauma was supplied by the Great War, which transformed the relationship to death due to the very high number of casualties and to the violence of their deaths (let us recall that death in war now almost exclusively meant violent death). Added to the great number of dead were the huge numbers of psychically wounded and the diversity and spectacular nature of their psychic suffering in its various expressions, particularly through the inscription of traumatic experience in the body. The number of traumatic experiences observed and the variety of their forms were a factor in heightening the awareness of medical staff in their examination of the sources of the trauma as well as in their responses to it.

The various studies on the subject produced by historians highlight the great variety of terms used in the medical discourse to qualify the trauma: mental shock, shell shock, "commotion", psychoneurosis, *Kriegsneurose* (war neurosis) and so on. But the words used to describe the observed phenomena, the causes identified to explain them and the methods used to treat the men suffering from mental and/or nervous disorders attest to the medical staff's powerlessness to grasp the mechanisms of psychic trauma and to conceive of it as a clinical entity. The descriptions essentially point to organic causes and predispositions as triggers for war trauma.

Care practices emphasized brutality as a means of flushing out simulators. Rather than a simple denial of psychic suffering, this approach must be seen as a failure to understand the symptoms being observed. But the war helped change the conditions of care for the psychically wounded: doctors insisted on the need to provide care rapidly by having medical facilities set up near the battlefield, as early as February 1915 in the French case, so as to avoid creating a rupture between the injured soldier and the primary group, or of separating him from the "battle atmosphere". The organization of these conditions was elevated into a set of principles by the American psychiatrist Thomas Salmon, now a reference for all contemporary scholars of the psyche.

As Freud stated in 1920: "The question [of psychic trauma] was not closed." He had already written in August 1919: "I have now chosen as nourishment the theme of death." The fundamental step in the construction and articulation of thinking on the question of psychic trauma occurred after the war, with the text written between March and April 1919 and published in 1920, *Beyond the Pleasure Principle*, not long after his *Reflections on War and Death*, which appeared in 1915. In *Beyond the Pleasure Principle*, Freud describes the psychic apparatus and the infraction caused by the direct experience of death. This text therefore completed his thinking on trauma by identifying the decisive element in psychic trauma: death. It describes the terror caused by being confronted with death and its breach of the psychic membrane where it poses as a foreign body in the psyche, obsessively and recurrently presenting itself to the patient in the form of reminiscences.

Beyond the Pleasure Principle provided Freud with the arguments he needed to affirm his clinical conception of trauma. The paradox here is that Freud theorized psychic trauma without ever treating psychically wounded soldiers. While he had an intimate relationship with the war, as his sons were on the battlefield, his relations with the psychically injured were indirect: they were based on the experiences and analyses of Ferenczi, Simmel or Abraham, his main disciples, who were all involved in the war (Figs. 2.1, 2.2, 2.3, and 2.4).

Distinguishing between the impact of stress and trauma on the psyche does not come from Freud, although he described it in so many words. In

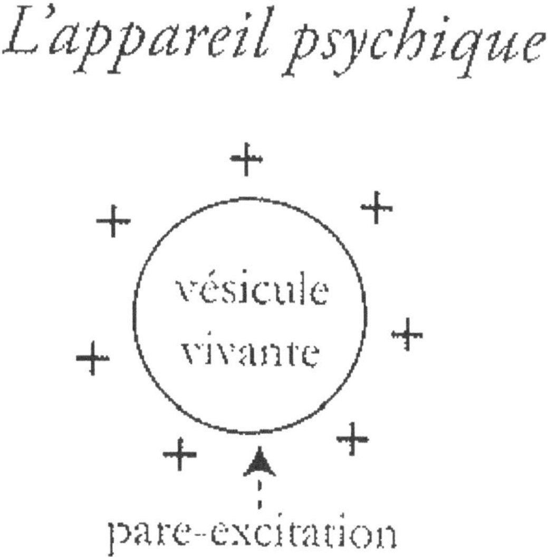

Fig. 2.1. The psychic apparatus. *Source:* Adapted from *Stress et Trauma* 2009; (9) 4: 201–204

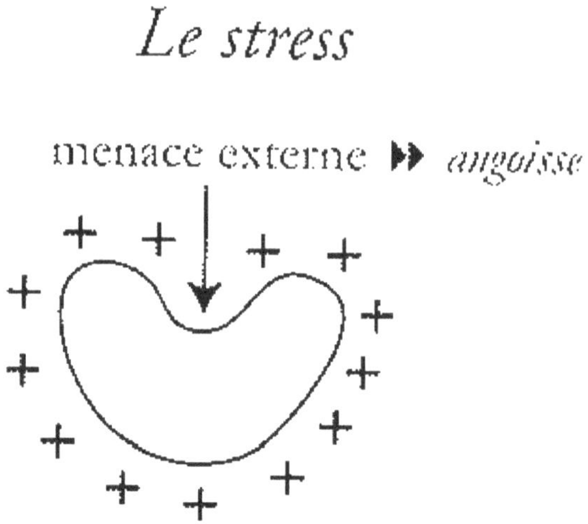

Fig. 2.2. Stress. *Source:* Adapted from *Stress et Trauma* 2009; (9) 4: 201–204

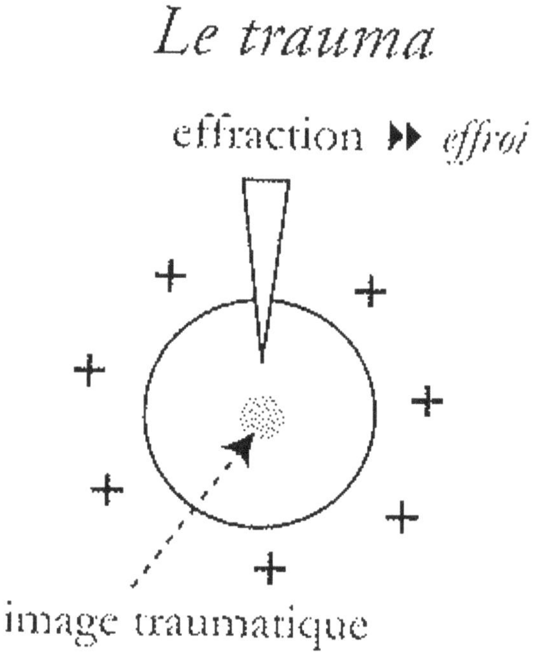

Fig. 2.3. Trauma. *Source:* Adapted from *Stress et Trauma* 2009; (9) 4: 201–204

Fig. 2.4. Post-traumatic stress. *Source:* Adapted from *Stress et Trauma* 2009; (9) 4: 201–204

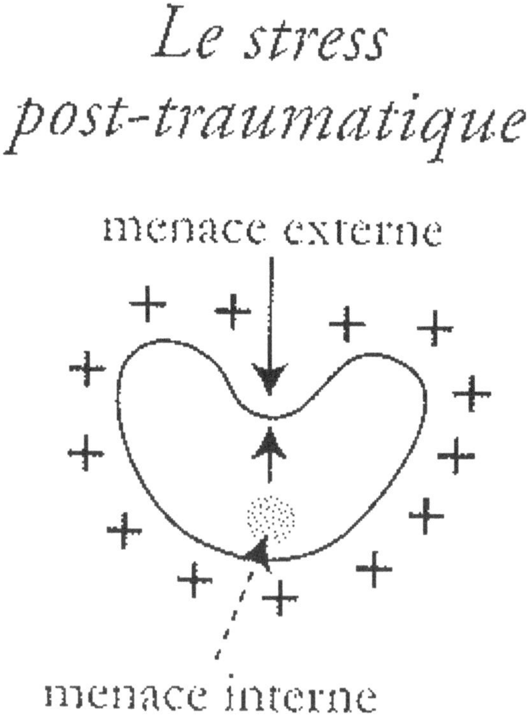

fact, these diagrams are taken from a journal founded in 2000 by French and French-speaking psychiatrists, *La revue francophone du stress et du trauma*. Almost all the contributors are military psychiatrists—François Lebigot, Guy Briole, Louis Crocq, Bernard Lafont, Dominique Vallet and so on—and belong to the new school of Val-de-Grâce, founded in the early 1990s. In France, the question of psychic trauma occupies a small number of psychiatrists (again, almost exclusively military psychiatrists), who have the triple qualification of psychiatrist, psychologist and psychoanalyst. The journal publishes the results of their clinical experience of the trauma induced by war and peacetime attacks (notably those perpetrated in Paris in 1986) and presents their thinking on psychic trauma.

These psychiatrists propose a "conception" that wishes to be "innovative" but is primarily a reappropriation of Freud's theory, to which they adhere very closely. This adherence is reflected in the vocabulary of their discourse but also in their clinical principles. Creating a journal provided an outlet for their theories. This school of thought was born out of opposition to the conceptions advocated in the 1980s in the English-speaking world, in particular the inclusion in the third edition of the *Diagnostic and Statistical Manual of Mental Disorders* (DSM-III) of the "post-traumatic stress disorder" (PTSD) diagnosis favoring the "stressing" dimension of trauma (as reflected in the term "post-traumatic cultures").[1]

From 1914 onwards, behind the diagnosis of "mental shock" and "shell shock" used by doctors to label mental and nervous disorders, one comes across terms such as "strain", "exhaustion" and "anxiety" in the common medical language. From the following year, the word "stress" appears, cited by the physician William Osler, who, in June 1915, stated: "An explanation is to be found [for nervous disorders] in the extraordinary stress and strain of trench fighting."[2] The term "stress" was widely taken up by doctors until the end of the war as one of the causes of "shell shock". For example, in a paper published in the leading medical journal *The Lancet* in 1916, the psychiatrist Elliot G. Smith presented shell shock as "the culmination of months of mental strain" and "emotional stress".[3]

While doctors emphasized exposure to exploding shells in their analysis of "shell shock", they also identified other primary sources. Indeed, there were many for whom the etiology of nervous and mental disorders could be traced to a combination of factors conducive to both physical and emotional exhaustion, factors related to the permanent state of strain to which the combatants were subjected. As one author noted: "These phenomena are particularly likely to occur under the effects of the shock of an explosion and prolonged exposure to states of nervous strain and physical exhaustion, all superimposed."[4] Another pointed out that "the mental symptoms may come from shell shock or be the result of the prolonged nervous strain imposed by the conditions of war".[5] Doctors were therefore highlighting the accumulation of physical and mental fatigue ("The primary causes are physical fatigue and mental strain"), going so far as to speak of a "nervous breakdown".[6] Shell shock was therefore understood to be caused by a combination of factors that exhausted physical energy and made soldiers emotionally vulnerable.

From this period onwards, English-speaking authors emphasized the various factors that weaken combatants' nervous resistance, even evoking a "breakdown point". The term "stress" again features extensively in the language used in English-speaking commentaries during World War II. Indeed, in the course of the war, the use of "stress" became increasingly prevalent in descriptions of mental disorders, appearing in a variety of designations: "combat stress", "battle stress", "prolonged stress", "emotional stress", "physical stress", "acute combat stress", "stress of battle" and so on.

In *Men under Stress*,[7] published on January 1, 1945, Roy Grinker and John P. Spiegel describe many stress-related patient cases, for the most part Air Force crew members or pilots. This work was a milestone in the study of war-induced "psychoneurosis" for the fundamental importance it attributed to "stress" in the onset of neuroses. Indeed, henceforth "stress" stood out as the main factor in determining psychic trauma. The authors describe the psychological mechanisms subjecting the "normal" individual to situations of stress, and, more particularly, to the stress imposed during wartime. They thereby reaffirm that any given individual placed under "sufficient stress may show failure of adaptation", reaching the famous "breakdown point", an argument they insist on in several places in the text, referring to "Everyman's struggle to master his own environment" or "Everyman's everyday failures or neurotic compromises with reality". The combatant's environment is what determines the breaking point to which stress leads. The key idea therefore remains "stress".

The process started in the middle of the Great War gathered momentum during World War II and during the second half of the twentieth century with various contributions, in particular the study by Hans Selye published in 1956, *The Stress of Life*, which adopted the findings of Grinker and Spiegel that established stress as a doctrine before it became a diagnosis with "post-traumatic stress disorder". Indeed, the DSM-III PTSD diagnosis should perhaps only be viewed as the outcome of a reflection on psychic trauma that started during World War I and was not completed until the Vietnam War.

I will insist here on French and French-speaking descriptions of psychic trauma to highlight the split that occurred with those of the English-speaking world. Indeed, the original split appears to have widened into a huge gap that is particularly difficult for the historian to understand.

Are there different ways of thinking psychic trauma, of defining it, of understanding its mechanisms? Is there a right and a wrong way of thinking through trauma? What is meant by "aftershock" and "post-traumatic": simply after the trauma? Should we focus on the care given in the immediacy of the traumatic event, during and after the war? Does "aftershock" necessarily mean "after war"? And what are the correct equivalents of these terms in French? These questions also invite historians to consider how they should approach the subject: archival research, identification of the issues and analysis. The historical approach proposed here intends to be a reappropriation of the object: psychic trauma. In the French case in particular, psychiatrists for a long time acted as the historians of their discipline, which only serves to highlight the reticence of historians to deal with the subject. In this chapter, I wish to undertake a history of psychic trauma that goes beyond temporal limits, those of wartime and peacetime, so as to properly emphasize the porosity that exists between these two times. One cannot overlook the impact of war experience over time, and this has been the case since the Great War to the present. I will therefore examine the concepts of "aftershock" and "post-traumatic" in terms of the visibility and invisibility of archival tools, while considering how these sources have been questioned by historians in their analysis of how psychic trauma has been theorized and treated.

Aftershock

After the Great War, the demobilization of medical staff and psychically injured patients largely deprived historians of any insight into psychic trauma due to the lack of archival sources. In this context, the studies of the American physician Thomas Salmon have become essential reading. Shortly after the signing of the Armistice, while working under the auspices of the National Committee for Mental Hygiene in New York, Salmon undertook an interesting study of psychically injured patients he had observed during the war at Base Hospital 117, in La Fauche, France.[8]

In fact, this was to be the first statistical study providing "follow-up" and visibility of the psychic patients who returned to the USA after the war. It was an "epidemiological" study, based on a small number of people already treated for mental/nervous disorders, gathering feedback on their posttreatment situations. A second survey on the same population was conducted a little later again, in 1924–1925.[9]

This experiment would appear to be the first of its kind and without equivalent in the other countries involved in the war. While these studies chart the condition of veterans suffering from war-induced psychic injury/neurosis in the short and medium term after the war, other categories of veterans—the able or physically disabled—fall outside of this type of survey. This omission underlines the non-inclusion of disorders that manifested themselves after the end of the Great War.

The purpose of these studies was to define the conditions in which a small group of combatants diagnosed as "war neurotics" had returned to civilian life and the ways in which they were or were not rehabilitated. To this end, a questionnaire was designed and a letter was personally addressed to each "shell-shocked veteran" in order to determine how these men had re-adapted to civilian life, especially their ability to work and to reintegrate socially. Out of the 2590 veterans contacted, 758 responded. Although we will not go into the details of the results here, it is worth noting that Salmon's classification identified the following categories: normal, neurotic, fatigued, disabled and psychotic.

For Thomas Salmon, the most important factor in the reintegration of veterans into civil society was the efforts made by government agencies.[10] These agencies strove to help veterans socially, by finding them employment or vocational training, but they also provided them with housing, care and, most importantly, financial assistance through pensions. Thus, in the rehabilitation process, acquiring or returning to a job emerged as an essential step because it opened the door to easier reintegration with the rest of the civilian community. The other key element in this process was highlighted by the study on veterans of the two world wars published by Willard Walter Waller in 1944 entitled *The Veteran Comes Back*, and more precisely the contribution of one of his chapters, "The Veteran Must Adjust To Family Living." Waller stressed the importance of emotional and family ties in returning to civilian life, a process that often required the veteran to "readjust", which in fact meant lowering the violence thresholds acquired on the battlefield.

In the American case, the tools devised during the Great War to monitor and help veterans readjust to civilian life were taken up and developed for the second global conflict of the early twentieth century. Such efforts to assist veterans during and after World War II were made primarily in English-speaking countries, especially in the USA, which had an estimated half a million veterans with neuropsychological disorders.[11] Many follow-up studies are available in which the rehabilitation efforts undertaken are highlighted, particularly regarding the establishment of hospital and social structures for veterans, programs favoring admission into schools or re-enrollment and the allocation of financial assistance.[12]

Here again, the efforts undertaken to assist the "readjustment" to civilian life support Salmon's idea concerning the importance of employment as a means of fitting back into society. However, the place assigned to delayed trauma in this range of measures appears nonexistent, with practically all the surveys conducted on populations of "war-neurotic" veterans. In fact, it was not until 1965, with the study by H. Archibald and T. Tuddenham,[13] 20 years after the end of World War II, that attention focused on the occurrence of aftereffects. In this study, the authors drew a comparison between "neurotic" and "non-neurotic" patients. They emphasized the persistence of common symptoms in these two groups: high anxiety, loss of attention and concentration, sleep disturbance, recurring nightmares and various somatizations, a set of symptoms that characterize psychic trauma.

Specialists of the psyche then began to include a very large new group in their studies, that of nontraumatized veterans, who had been neglected until the Vietnam War.

In the British case, there had been no follow-up in the form of surveys in the interwar period. The bulk of the efforts went to allocating pensions, which in its own way was a form of recognition. The medical establishment gradually followed the American practice of conducting surveys among veterans.

In the French case, the psychically injured veterans still in hospital after the Armistice were demobilized and transferred to psychiatric facilities, that is to say asylums. The option of internment had been chosen to the exclusion of financial compensation or pensions. At the same time, psychically injured veterans were left out of organizations founded to represent valid or maimed veterans, which often acted as substitutes for the state, especially in finding employment for disabled veterans. Moreover, most of the organizations' discourse focused on improving veterans' rights, in particular with regard to pensions and jobs; in some cases, their demands concerned "rest homes" (*maisons de repos)*, types of shelters for veterans who were rejected or marginalized in postwar French society.

Overall, the discourse employed by the organizations was very assertive. They also largely took over the role of representing the views of former veterans, whether able or disabled, during the war, but especially after the war, in a way preventing veterans from speaking for themselves, including about their suffering, as in the case of amputees.

Subsequently, in the second half of the twentieth century, there was little change in France in the approach to mental trauma, in terms of both the recognition and the consideration of delayed trauma. The words used to describe disorders closely followed the language used during the Great War and the care methods were modeled on US and British practices, as shown in one of the few French contributions on this subject for World

War II (Sutter).[14] In total, there were very few publications and there are very few archives to speak of either.

In Indochina, psychic trauma was treated as a social disease in the same way as alcoholism and tuberculosis. Doctors recorded almost 35,000 cases of neuropsychiatric ailments, of which 20,000 involved hospitalizations and 5000 repatriations to France.[15] However, in light of the high frequency of observed cases, they pointed to predisposing factors: debility (including reference to "mental defectives" and "unstable" personalities), regretting that such cases had not been filtered out before departure, and alcoholism, which sometimes was also present before enlistment. But they did not tie alcohol use to confrontation with "traumatic" events, despite alcohol being at the time the only treatment available to soldiers to try to tame "the beast within".

One finds the same discourse and attitude in the Algerian War. There seems to have been no care provided to the men of the French Expeditionary Corps in Indochina during and even after the war upon their return to France, despite some enduring particularly harsh experiences, notably those held captive in Viet Minh camps. Certainly, no follow-up study on their condition has ever been conducted. One of the most revealing examples of this "abandonment" was described by Louis Crocq at a symposium at the Val-de-Grâce in 2009–10 and included in his latest publication in 2012, *16 leçons sur le trauma*",[16] where it is discussed in the tenth lesson on "Trauma and sleep" (I have collated both accounts here). The case concerns a former legionnaire who fought in Indochina from 1950 to 1954 and participated in the Battle of Dien Bien Phu, during which he experienced an "explosion-induced concussion": he was sent flying by an exploding shell and remained unconscious for a few moments. After the battle, he was taken prisoner, so, in addition to his battle experience he endured captivity, hunger, thirst, torture (physical and psychological) and exhausting marches. One night, during one of these walks, he collapsed and was left for dead by the roadside. Taken in and fed by Vietnamese peasants, he preferred to give himself up to be with his comrades rather than escape.

His captors, a little surprised to see him again, assigned him to a small team of prisoners in charge of burying their comrades who died in the camps. Every morning, when they came to bury new bodies, they discovered that the rats had dug up the corpses buried the day before, and had begun to devour them. This experience marked him deeply and left him with feelings of guilt.

After his demobilization, he was confronted with reminiscences that occurred primarily at night in the form of sleepwalking nightmares, which became particularly frequent after he retired from the army in the early 1980s. Several times a week, he would rise from his bed in the middle of the night, go downstairs and outside into his garden, where he picked up a shovel. After making holes larger than 40-cm deep, he went back to his room and in the morning, his wife informed him that he had got up in the night again to dig holes in the garden. It was not until 50 years after his experience at Dien Bien Phu that he decided to consult a psychiatrist, at his wife's insistence. For all the intervening years, he had been haunted by those terrible images and dug holes in the garden! For all those years, he received no help to process his reminiscences and overcome the guilt attached to his trauma.

No provision of care, no recognition and therefore no pensions. Let us note that here it is the patient who goes to the doctor, not the other way round. This situation has persisted right up to today, resulting in an attitude verging on negation. Let us consider this statement by Maurice Bazot, the former head of psychiatry at the Val-de-Grâce: "When a patient comes to see me in order to be examined and for us to grant him a pension, I say to him, 'And what can you do for yourself?'"[17] Thus, French psychiatrists played their part in the French state's failure to provide care to veterans suffering from trauma as well as its nonrecognition of their suffering. Recognizing veterans' trauma means recognizing their right to a pension and therefore has financial consequences.

Making Trauma Invisible

The experience of the Vietnam War appears to have played a crucial role in understanding the impact of traumatic experience over time, with many studies stressing the influence this event had on how doctors took the delayed onset of trauma into account. I will not dwell on it further here; we are all familiar with the way it shaped thinking on psychic trauma.

The DSM-III immediately sparked strong resistance among French psychiatrists. First, because there was already a French classification, drafted by researchers at the *Institut national de la santé et de la recherche médicale* (INSERM) and published in 1968, which recognized "neuroses and neurotic states". Second, because more generally in Europe, classifications are based on the notion of disease and therefore on the elaboration of psychopathological theories that support nosology. Above all, the nosological framework of "neuroses"—a Freudian concept—is nullified in the DSM-III and replaced by disorders classified on a descriptive basis. In the English-speaking world, in its acute form, the state of post-traumatic stress is considered as lasting longer than one day and up to four weeks, whereas in the French-speaking world, it is understood as not exceeding one hour. However, no distinction is made here between stress and trauma, and the use of the term "traumatic stress" in the English literature is indicative of the confusion that exists between the two concepts. The view in the French-speaking world was that stress disappears or else signs of a durable traumatic neurosis in its latent or "meditation" phase begin to appear, accompanied by the first flashbacks (post-immediate phase).

Consequently, French doctors categorically refuse to use the word stress to define these symptoms. In their analysis, stress is defined as "the immediate, biological, physiological and psychological reaction to an alert, the individual's mobilization and defense against aggression or threat". As such, it remains a short-lived response, the stress disappearing along with the "stressor". The DSM preferred to abandon the concept of traumatic neurosis in favor of PTSD; however, in the PTSD diagnosis, the use of the word stress poses a problem. For this reason, French clinicians prefer the term "deferred psycho-traumatic syndrome".

The conceptions developed in the DSM-III became established as the international standards used by the World Health Organization (WHO) and the International Classification of Diseases (ICDs) in 1992. The ratification of the PTSD diagnosis thus affirmed the hegemony of American thinking on trauma. Let us recall here the example of the recent operations in Iraq (Operation Iraqi Freedom) and Afghanistan (Operation Enduring Freedom). While exact figures exist for the number of fatalities and injuries, the number of "psychically injured" appears more difficult to quantify.

The medical discourse is predominantly based on epidemiological surveys. For the historian, these surveys are easy to use: the essential information is found in the summary while the rest of the survey is generally confined to statistical methods. Indeed, given their statistical nature, these studies make no allowance for the individual experiences endured by psychically injured veterans. In almost all cases, they insist on the precocity and intensity of the occurrence of psychiatric disorders, in particular upon returning home; they also provide a record of the moment of the trauma's occurrence and the number of traumas that occurred. While the percentage of medical evacuations for psychic trauma seems very low, the figures are clearly much higher for deferred disorders diagnosed upon the veterans' return home.

As pointed out by Sandor Ferenczi: "Psychoanalysis has taught us that it is not so much the statistical analysis of a large number of cases but the comprehensive investigation of individual cases that may lead to progress in the theory of neuroses."[18]

More surprisingly, in the American (and British) medical discourse, we find a new category of trauma called "Mild Trauma Brain Injury", designated by the term MTBI and applied by English-speaking psychiatrists in their clinical approach to "shell shock", one symptom of which is minor concussion.[19] MTBI is involved in approximately 20 % of such injuries. However, doctors try to distinguish these mild concussions from states of post-traumatic stress. Indeed, concussions tend to fade quickly with rest. The blasts of the shells produce lesions that could explain the psychic trauma—the proof is provided by medical imaging!

Even more than the ineffectiveness of the methods used, what is particularly striking here is their powerlessness to prevent and curb the occurrence of psychic trauma, as well as to attenuate its manifestations (self-inflicted violence). The other aspect that emerges from this set of studies—which attest to a particularly dense medical discourse—is the attention devoted to war experiences. However, sequences relating encounters with death, so crucial in the Freudian conception of trauma, are almost entirely absent from these accounts. When it is mentioned, death is part of a much wider array of "stressful" factors. When I questioned François Lebigot, one of the leading French specialists in war-induced psychic trauma, about the omission of the factor of death in the English-speaking research, he replied: "It is because they haven't read Freud."[20]

One of the consequences of this "rejection" of Freud in the English-speaking world is evident in the types of responses to veterans' psychological suffering, which primarily seek to treat the symptoms including sleeping pills for insomnia, antidepressants for a state of depression, thus masking the core of the problem and refusing "intellectual" therapies, to borrow the idea put forward by Rivers in *Instinct and the Unconscious* (1920).[21]

As the medical discourse does not always give insight into the patients' views, it is important for the historian to draw on other types of sources. The purpose here in using these sources is not to proceed in the manner of a clinician, for that would be overstepping the bounds of the historian's function, rather it is to more closely examine the viewpoint of the survivors of traumatic events however they may seek to express it.

Indeed, while the suffering endured by the vast majority of survivors is shrouded in silence, we have access to a number of written, oral and pictorial testimonies that have been overlooked by the medical world. It is important for the historian to use these sources, to understand them as acts of representation and to analyze their content in terms of encounters with death. This is the approach we shall emphasize in the following section.

Making Trauma Visible

The historian's ability to see the trauma endured by the psychically wounded is largely dependent on the work of specialists of the psyche. Until the end of the two world wars, the latter, as we have seen, emphasized the rehabilitation of "shell-shocked" veterans at the expense of undiagnosed, "concussed" veterans who also suffered as a result of their war experience.

Many of them kept this suffering quiet, out of modesty or due to an inability to express or articulate it, or simply because there was no one to listen. In fact, very few were able to represent their psychic trauma, in the sense given by Freud, namely their encounters with death. Their suffering thus does not seem to have received any support or any consideration for the delayed occurrence of trauma. Consequently, it also escaped the attention of historians, who have almost exclusively relied on the medical sources for their analyses. The historian is apparently at a loss when faced with the silence of the medical establishment regarding this population of the interwar and postwar periods. But silence does not equate with an absence of pain related to the experience of death.

To overcome the almost total lack of medical sources, the historian must therefore look beyond the medical discourse, especially since this discourse was increasingly founded, or in some cases exclusively founded, on epidemiological surveys. To grasp the viewpoint of the psychically injured person, it is necessary to reinterpret veterans' representations of the experience of war upon their return. In adopting this approach, the aim is not to propose a psychiatric evaluation, much less a therapeutic analysis, but to understand how they lived with this foreign body in their minds and above all what the content of this foreign body was. Can the historian identify or recognize trauma? Without trying to replace the specialist of the psyche, the historian can proceed by focusing more closely on the representation of the psyche's relationship with death, in other words, on traumatography, whatever the modes of expression used: writing, painting, handicraft, the spoken word, cinema and so on. The core idea is to render the suffering linked to the psychic trauma visible beyond a medical discourse and to closely study the sequences in which the witness expresses his relationship with death. It is an invitation to examine all accounts afresh, to understand the history of psychic trauma, the impact of the encounters with death, what words are used to express the closeness to death, the death of one's loved family and friends, one's own death and that of the anonymous other. Analyzing this encounter with death is also part of the historian's job.

Let us turn our attention to an object here (Fig. 2.5). It is in fact an object that was held in storage at the Historical Museum of the Great War in Péronne, France, which describes a "traumatic experience". We can safely state that it was made after the war, imagined or manufactured following the war experience. It is certainly clear that it does not belong to the "trench crafts" category. Upon closer examination therefore, this three-dimensional "painting maquette" represents the narrow plot of the battlefield in Champagne on which, on October 27, 1915, the Germans launched an attack using chemical weapons. The representation of the event is not solely based on the object in its materiality. It is also based—as is the case for most pictorial representations—on a representation in writing, which is inscribed in the object itself and its header, thus orienting the viewer's interpretation, as if the three-dimensional image alone could not give sufficient meaning to the event.

"Memory of my 21st birthday. On way back from the Sabot woods on October 27, 1915, the 13th Dragoon regiment relieved the old infantrymen stationed at La Ferme des Marquises in Champagne at 4 am. We were waiting on orders. As the wind was from the north, the squaddies were eager to leave. So we took the full brunt of the attack. The whole first line was gassed. As the wind changed from north to south the second line was spared. The Krauts weren't able to come out of their trenches. At least our artillery gave them a good pounding. While the second line came up to take position on the first line those of us still alive were taken back to the first-aid station located in a deep shelter, left to lie on the ground until night fell and then evacuated in darkness to Mourmelon-le-Petit through the fields, on the back of baggage train carts. We were bumped around so much on the potholed roads so that the most badly injured comrades

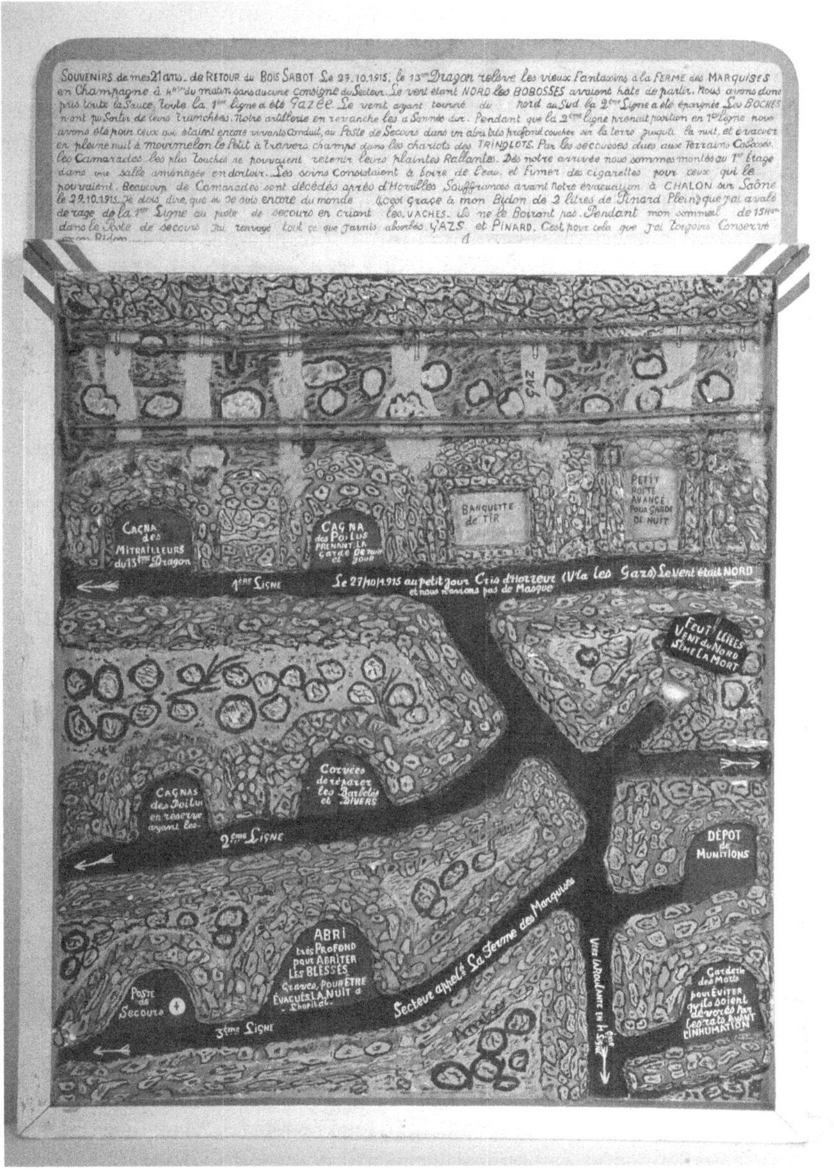

Fig. 2.5 The Amiot object

couldn't help groaning with pain. As soon as we arrived, we were taken up to the second floor to a room laid out as a dormitory. The only treatment available was to drink water and to smoke cigarettes for those that could. A lot of comrades died after horrible suffering before our evacuation to Chalon-sur-Saône on October 29, 1915. I have to say that if I am still alive, "I have my full 2-litre can of wine to thank". I drank it in a rage between the front line and the first-aid station shouting the bastards, they won't drink it while I'm asleep. At 3 pm at the first-aid station I spewed everything I had absorbed, gas and wine. That's why I've held on to that can ever since. Amiot."

TEXT ON THE PAINTING (left to right, by line)

Machine gunners' dugout, 13th Dragoon regiment	Dugout for *poilus* on guard during night and day	Firing bank	Small advanced post for night sentry
1st line: on October 27 1915, in the early hours, screams of horror (the gas arrives) The wind was from the north and we had no masks.			
			The wind from the north brings death
Dugout for *poilus* in reserve with–2nd line	Barbed wire repair work and other tasks		
First-aid station	Very deep shelter to hold the badly wounded to be evacuated at night to the hospital.		
Sector known as La Ferme des Marquises			
			Ammunition depot
		Toward the field kitchen on the 4th line.	Storage area for corpses to avoid them being eaten by rats before being buried.

Amiot, the witness to the event, has depicted a section of the battlefield in Champagne located at a place called La Ferme des Marquises, where the Germans launched a chemical weapons attack on October 27, 1915.

Based on the journey he made from the front during his medical evacuation, Amiot represented the organization of the sector that was the scene of the traumatic event. He relates, through the means of the modeled object, what he saw of the event and what he heard. This sensory perception of the event is typical of a trauma, here that of an encounter with death caused by asphyxiating gases.

The witness was struck above all by the "spectacular" nature of death by gas, despite the relatively low mortality rate. Here, I refer to the example given by the psychiatrist Thomas Salmon in his postwar report on psychic trauma: "One morning a large number of soldiers were returned to the field hospital diagnosed as gas casualties. The influx continued for about eight days, and the number of patients reached about five hundred. The divisional gas officer failed to find any clinical evidence of gas inhalation or burning [...] Physical and neurological examination was practically negative, and the mental findings were inconclusive. Most of the patients had the fixed conviction that they had been gassed and would usually describe all the details with convincing earnestness and generally with some dramatic quality of expression. [...] It was obvious on examination that they were not really gassed. Further, it was inconceivable that they should be malingerers."[22]

But on closer inspection, one can see that Amiot has only depicted a portion of the Champagne battlefield. This object made by one of the survivors of the attack—a gas victim, like many of his comrades in the front line—in fact represents a pulmonary tree with thick black veins and alveoli, the same black as the asphyxiated soldiers' oxygen-deprived blood.

The alveoli filled with lymph and black blood, this liquid flooding the alveolar sacs until the entire lung cavity was submerged. Pulmonary edema resembles a "sponge when taken out of water". This is what causes the gas victim to die by asphyxiation.[23]

The victims literally drowned in their own body fluid. But Amiot could not have depicted the alveoli without having seen them, nor could he have depicted a part of a drowned/congested lung without also seeing one firsthand.

It is likely that the witness had to endure serious sequelae as a result of the attack on October 27, 1915, perhaps to the point of having a lung partly or fully removed. Or, more simply, perhaps he saw a large diagram of a lung in a medical office, or had it pointed out to him by the doctor who treated him after the war.

The representation may have another explanation: Amiot left the part of his body injured by the gas released on October 27, perhaps also the day of his twenty-first birthday, behind on the battlefield. Thus, the object is primarily the representation of the gas attack, that is to say the moment of infraction, through the confrontation with death, others' death in "horrible suffering" and his own too. Furthermore, it is a representation of the aggression against his lungs and the serious aftereffects he endured as a result. The object is at once a representation of mental distress and of an attack on his body.

The Amiot object[24] also raises the question of the psychological impact of chemical weapons and the treatment or lack of treatment thereof by doctors during and especially after the war. It is a question that is mainly palpable through the English-speaking medical discourse. The writings of French doctors, whose primary interest was in the visible, anatomical effects of gas, are almost entirely devoid of reference to psychological sequelae.

The English-speaking literature on the subject assimilates it with the issue of shell shock, even if the studies do take note of the specific body movements observed in gas victims, described in particular by Harold Hulbert.[25] However, the medical discourse does not recognize any psychic "specificity" with regard to the victims of chemical weapons. Terms such as "gas syndrome", "gas hysteria" or "gas neurosis" occur, but these are used in reference to a diagnosis of shell shock, namely the inscription of the relationship with death in the body through somatization (tics or unconscious hand movements such as raising the hand to the throat or putting a mask on), signs of anxiety and suffocation (gasping for air), paresthesia, attacks of delirium or stupor, signs of convulsions, for example. These symptoms may also be associated with nightmares and the reliving of past experiences. The only sequelae accepted by the American and British doctors essentially emphasize—as is the case with French doctors—respiratory, cardiac and pulmonary complications, but not trauma.

Above all, as notably illustrated by a recent study based on veterans' records by Edgar Jones,[26] the doctor's reports note symptoms such as shortness of breath, chest pain, wheezing, heart palpitations and chronic bronchitis without organic lesions. In 1929, Thomas Salmon wrote in *Neuropsychiatry*, one of the volumes published in the *Medical Department of the USA in World War*[27] series, that there were as many cases of gas neurosis as there were of exposure to gas (US records list some 70,000 soldiers exposed to chemical weapons and admitted for treatment).

What the studies based on this type of analysis show is, first, the uniqueness of each of the soldiers' experiences, and second, that a common thread emerges, the crux of the soldiers' experience being based on their encounter with death, whether consisting of one or several encounters. There are no rules and there is not always a hierarchy set by the witnesses with regard to their encounter with the death of the other, or the intimate encounter with their own. A considerable sensory dimension is associated with their relationship with death, which is related in visual, tactile, olfactory and acoustic terms and sometimes in terms of taste.

It would seem almost impossible to claim that the act of representation enables the survivor to definitively put the traumatic event at a distance. All the more so in the Amiot case given that there is no record of the patient beyond the object he produced. Nevertheless, one may consider that representing the event or events that have assaulted the psyche is a way for the person who experienced them to assert some form of ownership and distancing, which in itself is significant.

Conclusion

It is not for the historian to take sides with one or the other camp, but to assess the facts and to emphasize the rigidity of the stances taken by both, as broadly described here, in relation to the thinking and treatment of psychic trauma, whether in the immediacy of the event or at a later stage. The challenge for the historian is therefore to go beyond the medical discourse that for a long time concealed the suffering endured by veterans, particularly in the first half of the twentieth century, in order to make this highly particular trauma visible.

While the concept of "stress" first emerged in 1915, with English and American doctors emphasizing the impact of the soldier's environment in their diagnoses of "shell shock" and subsequently "war neuroses", it became more prominent during World War II, to the point of being identified as the main factor in pushing soldiers to "breaking point". Paradoxically, the medical discourse in the English-speaking world disregards Freud's theory regarding death as the factor fragmenting the psyche but adheres to the therapies advocated by Freud, particularly abreaction.

The principal arguments of Roy Grinker and John Spiegel's *Men Under Stress* were largely taken up by neurophysiologist Hans Selye in the mid-1950s, contributing to the dissemination of the stress doctrine until it was definitively defined as a diagnosis in 1980 under "post-traumatic stress disorder". Its adoption by the international classification attests to the hegemony of American thinking on trauma. French psychiatrists tried to resist this hegemony, preferring to insist on the basis of Freudian thought and emphasizing death as the only element that causes an infraction in the psyche. These two ways of thinking draw on rather disparate therapeutic approaches: one (American and English) promoting drug-based responses; the other (French) essentially advocating verbal therapy. What strikes the historian today are the difficulties that both approaches experience in their efforts to relieve the victims' suffering.

Notes

1. American Psychiatric Association, *The Diagnostic and Statistical Manual of Mental Disorders,* 3rd edition (Washington DC: American Psychiatric Association, 1980).
2. William Osler, "Functional nervous disorders", *Journal of American Medical Association,* June 12, 1915, 64, 2001–2002.
3. G. Elliot Smith "Shock and the soldier", *Lancet,* 1916, 813–817 and 853–857.
4. Charles S. Myers, "Contributions to the study of shell shock; being an account of certain disorders of cutaneous sensibility", *Journal of the Royal Army Medical Corps,* 1916, June, 782–97.
5. Craig Maurice, "The more common neuroses: psychoneuroses occurring in men exposed to shell-shocked and strain of war" (Philadelphia: Blakiston, 1917), 300–11.
6. Arthur F. Hurst, "Functional nervous disorders" in: *Medical Diseases of the War* (London: Arnold, 1917), 1–40.
7. Roy R. Grinker and John P. Spiegel, *Men under Stress. On the war neuroses of Air Force crews and their psychiatric treatment* (Philadelphia: Blakiston, 1945), 484.
8. When the USA entered the war, Salmon set up a hospital at La Fauche in France. See: T.W. Salmon, "Care and treatment of mental diseases and war neuroses 'shell shock' in British Army" (New York: National Committee of Mental Hygiene, 1917) 102; "War neuroses 'shell shock'", *Military Surgeon,* 41, Dec. 1917, 674–93; *Psychiatric lessons from the war* (Reprinted from transactions of the American Neurological association, Forty-Fifty Annual Meeting, Atlantic City, 1919).

9. Norman Fenton, "A Post-was Study of a Typical Group of War Neurosis Cases in 1919–1920 and 1924–1925", in: T.W. Salmon, *The Medical Department of the USA in World War I, Section II: In the American Expeditionary Forces, vol. X, Neuropsychiatry* (Washington: Government Printing Office, 1929) 444–74.
10. In 1923, the American Congress created a Veterans Bureau, placed under the general authority of the President of the USA. The Bureau federated two US agencies responsible for the care and rehabilitation of disabled ex-service men: the "war-risk insurance bureau" and the "United States Public Health Service and the Federal Board for Vocational education, established, respectively, in 1914 and 1917.
11. Nolan D.C Lewis and Bernice Engle, eds., *Wartime Psychiatry. A Compendium of the International Literature*, Section X "Problems of demobilization and Rehabilitation", (New York: Oxford University Press, 1954), 599. Lewis and Nolan noted "In the Middle of 1947, nearly half a million patients (475, 397) from WWII of all patients in veterans' hospitals were neuropsychiatric" (952).
12. See: Norman Q. Brill, "Report, Committee on Veterans", *Am. J. of Psychiatry* 105, 1949, 934–35; Daniel Blain, John H Baird, "The neuropsychiatric program of veterans administration", *Am. J. of Psychiatry*, 103, 1947, 463–65.
13. H. Archibald and T. Tuddenham, "Persistent stress reaction after combat: a 20 year follow-up", *Arch. Gen. Psych.*, 1965, 12, 475–81.
14. J. Sutter, H. Stern, R. Susini, "Psychonévroses de guerre. Etude d'une centaine de cas personnels", *Annales médico-psychologiques*, 1947, 496–525; J. Sutter, H. Stern, R. Susini, "Evolution des psychoses de guerre", *Annales médico-psychologiques*, 1947, 249–270; J. Sutter, "Suites lointaines des émotions de guerre", *Evol. Psych.*, 1950, Jan.–March, 1, 101–6.
15. *Le service de santé en Indochine* (Edité et imprimé à Saïgon: Bibliothèque du Val-de-Grâce, 1955). Chapitre LIV, "Maladies sociales, A6 Alcoolisme, B-Affections neuropsychiatriques C-Tuberculose", 828–854.
16. Louis Crocq, *16 leçons sur le trauma*, 10e leçon, « Trauma et sommeil » (Paris: Odile Jacob, 2012), 161–166.
17. Maurice Bazot, statement made during a meeting of the "Guerre et Médecine" Association, 2003.
18. In: "Deux types de névrose de guerre", article published following a lecture given at the scientific conference of doctors of the Maria-

Valéria military hospital, *Psychanalyse II*, Œuvres complètes, 1913–1919 (Paris: Payot), 238.
19. Y. Bhattacharjee, "Shell shock revisited: solving the puzzle of blast trauma", *Science*, 2008, 319, 406–408; CW Hoge, CA Castro, SC Messer, "Combat duty in Iraq and Afghanistan, mental health problems, and barriers to care", *N Engl J Med*, 2004, Jul. 1, 351, 1, 13–22; CW Hoge, A Terhakopian, CA Castro, SC Messer, "Association of post-traumatic stress disorder with somatic symptoms, health care visits, and absenteeism among Iraq, War Veterans", *Am J Psychiatry*, 2007, 164, 150–3.
20. Entretien avec François Lebigot, psychiatre aux armées, juillet 2010.
21. William H. Rivers, *L'instinct et l'inconscient, Contribution à une théorie biologique des psychonévroses* (Paris : L'Harmattan, 1999) 313.
22. Thomas W. Salmon, *Psychiatric lessons from the war*, June 16–18, 1919.
23. Istin Héderer, *L'arme chimique et ses blessures. Etude générale sur les gaz de guerre* (Paris: Baillère, 1935) 285.
24. "L'objet Amiot", Historial de la Grande Guerre, Péronne, Somme.
25. Harold Hulbert, "Gas neurosis syndrome", *Am J of Psychiatry*, 1920, 77, 213–6.
26. Edgar Jones and Simon Wessely, *From shell shock to PTSD, Military Psychiatry from 1900 to the Gulf War* (Hove and New York: Psychology Press, 2005) 320.
27. Thomas W. Salmon, op. cit.

CHAPTER 3

Moral Injury: Two Perspectives

Susan Derwin

There is a growing awareness that the diagnosis and treatment of post-traumatic stress disorder (PTSD) in military service members has not been an effective means of dealing with the psychological trauma of war. Mental health professionals who treat soldiers returning from Iraq and Afghanistan have perceived a disparity between soldiers' psychological responses to combat and the officially identified cause of PTSD), which is fear. William Nash, who in 2004 served in Iraq as a combat psychiatrist, notes that after the Battle of Fallujah, not fear, but "survivor's guilt, moral injury, [and] feeling betrayed by leaders" were the predominant reactions among soldiers.[1]

The mental health profession is working to find ways to address this newest iteration of these invisible wounds of war, which are being referred to as "moral injury." In what follows, I will discuss a current therapeutic approach to moral injury, focusing on its conceptualization and recommended treatment, which I will then compare to the representation of moral injury in Toni Morrison's 2012 novel *Home*. In its consideration not only of a therapeutic, but also of a literary perspective, the following discussion of moral injury is indebted to the age-old recognition that literary representations of war and its aftermath, including those written by

S. Derwin (✉)
University of California, Santa Barbara, CA, USA

P. Leese, J. Crouthamel (eds.), *Traumatic Memories of the Second World War and After*, DOI 10.1007/978-3-319-33470-7_3

civilians, can offer singular insight into the situations of returning soldiers seeking to reintegrate into their communities. For while modern industrialized society entrusts the psychological care of soldiers to the mental health profession, as David J. Morris reminds in his study *The Evil Hours: A Biography of Post-Traumatic Stress Disorder*, this has not always been the case: "For most of human history, interpreting trauma has been the preserve of artists, poets, and shamans. The ways in which a nation deals with trauma are as revealing as its politics and language [...]." In the classical world, the ancients in the wake of trauma might look for answers in epic poetry, such as *The Iliad* or *The Odyssey*. Today, we turn to the most current edition of the *Diagnostic and Statistical Manual of Mental Disorders*. This fact alone is worthy of further exploration: most of us no longer turn to poetry, our families or the clergy for solace post horror.[2] As a literary and pragmatic response to the recent wars in Iraq and Afghanistan, *Home* can be read as advocating a relocation, or better, a *return*, to the community as the locus of the warrior's post-combat psychological, spiritual and moral healing.

Moral injury is rapidly gaining currency as the designation for a constellation of feelings about "perpetrating, failing to prevent, bearing witness to, or learning about acts that transgress deeply held moral beliefs and expectations."[3] Unlike the diagnosis of PTSD, moral injury is intended to identify the distinctly ethical suffering borne of perpetrating, or witnessing the perpetration of, violence against others. Journalist Nan Levinson has described moral injury "as the result of taking part in or witnessing something of consequence that you find wrong, something which violates your deeply held beliefs about yourself and your role in the world. For a moment, at least, you become what you never wanted to be. While the symptoms and causes may overlap with PTSD, moral injury arises from what you did or failed to do, rather than from what was done to you. It's a sickness of the heart more than the head."[4]

Like Levinson, Rita Nakashima Brock and Gabriella Lettini, co-directors of the Soul Repair Center at Brite Divinity School, formulate moral injury as an inner conflict that results from a disharmony between the self's moral beliefs and actions not in keeping with those beliefs. They write, "Moral Injury disrupts [the] relationship with [the] self when [the] inner moral core is doubted,"[5] when "you feel like you violated some deep part of yourself."[6]

Moral injury has been cited to account for the high suicide rate among veterans—on average 22 per day.[7] Between 2009 and 2011, there was a

44 percent increase in the number of male veterans younger than 30 who committed suicide and an 11 percent increase in suicide among female veterans.[8] According to data released by the military in January 2013, the previous year saw the highest number ever of active duty personnel committing suicide, almost one a day, a statistic that puts suicide ahead of combat as the cause of death among active duty soldiers.[9]

The departments of Veterans Affairs and Defense have backed a 4-year study of moral injury in Marines.[10] The researchers conducting the study believe that the recent wars have had a greater potential than conventional wars for producing ethical damage, and they cite factors such as fighting against an unmarked enemy, civilian threats and improvised explosive devices, all of which produce "greater uncertainty, greater danger for non-combat troops, and generally greater risk of harm among non-combatants."[11] The multiple deployments of troops have also been identified as a contributing factor.[12]

Even with this new acknowledgement that troops are particularly vulnerable to ethical trauma, neither the Veterans Administration nor the American Psychiatric Association considers moral injury an official diagnosis. The 2013 *Diagnostic and Statistical Manual of Mental Disorders* recognizes guilt and shame as symptoms of PTSD but persists in identifying fear as its cause.[13] Nash notes that the military is resistant to acknowledging the reality of moral injury, because "just using the term is somehow pejorative [...] They think we're saying they're immoral. But the exact opposite is true. It's because soldiers have such high standards that they're vulnerable to moral injury."[14]

Moral injury is an experience of the self as an agent of harm. Those with moral injury feel responsible for harm they have done to others and morally compromised because of their roles as perpetrators: in harming others they have also caused damage to themselves.[15] The uniqueness of moral injury may be that the self experiences itself as subject and object of victimization, as if trapped inside a closed loop of psychological wounding. That moral injury can result from witnessing the harm done to others and feeling compromised for failing to have taken action to prevent it makes its psychological self-enclosure all the more salient.

The description of the work researchers are doing suggests that their approach to healing is predicated on validating the morally injured soldier's feelings of guilt. Brett Litz, a lead researcher on the study, writes, "In the case of morally injurious events, [soldiers'] judgments and beliefs about the transgressions may be quite appropriate and accurate."[16] These beliefs and judgments are reassuring. Litz notes, because "inherent in our working definition of moral injury is the supposition that anguish, guilt, and shame are signs of an intact conscience and self- and other expectations about goodness, humanity and justice. In other words, injury is only possible if acts of transgression produce dissonance (conflict), and dissonance is only possible if the service member has an intact moral belief system."[17] Litz's characterization reflects the assumption that it is the therapist's role to affirm the service member's moral self-judgment, a point I will return to later.

Describing their therapeutic approach, Litz writes: "We want to promote—to a degree—a confession-like experience. We do this in a highly evocative, highly emotionally charged way. We want it to be very real and very powerful: In this charged moment, a Marine begins a conversation with their most compassionate, forgiving loved one—someone who will listen to all the horrible details of their injury and still remind the Marine that they can have goodness in their life [...] That they deserve it, but that they have some work to do. And it's the work to do which we're just setting in motion."[18] The morally injured service member is encouraged to take responsibility for the past by "making amends [...] drawing a line between past and present and in some way changing one's approach to how he or she behaves and acts so that one moves towards the positive, towards better living."[19] Such an approach to rehabilitation is designed to echo the voice of conscience of the service member and guide him or her to examine wartimes experience within an ethical framework that affirms belief in civic virtues. The therapy encourages behavioral changes through reflection that also reinforces the morally injured person's sense of personal agency as he or she strives toward "better living," and hence leaves behind prior, morally deficient behaviors.

This therapy has much in common with religious approaches to sin, and as such it bears comparison with the early Christian church's rehabilitation of soldiers. Morris notes that during the Middle Ages, "the post-traumatic condition, such as it was, was treated as a question of theology and, secondarily, as a matter of tending to the moral needs of warriors returning to their communities after war [...] leaders in the early Christian church assumed that warriors returning from battle would be racked by feelings of guilt and shame over their role in breaking the 'Truce of God,' and they paid an unusual amount of attention to their plight, providing them with what could generously be described as a sort of religious medicine."[20] Warriors were assigned rituals of repentance and reconciliation as a means of "ensuring that the potential sins associated with warfare were properly understood and accounted for and that a sort of balance could be maintained between the politics of the time and the need to please God."[21] Morris's account suggests that the concern of Church authorities for the spiritual well-being of soldiers constituted an acknowledgement of the irreconcilable tension between the demands of warfare, on the one hand, and Christian morality, on the other. In this regard, the Church's involvement in the healing of soldiers' spiritual wounds reflected both an understanding of those wounds as an inherent liability of war and a recognition that the process of reintegrating soldiers into the community was a societal responsibility.

Whereas the Medieval Christian Church recognized that the soldier's spiritual injuries were born of the competing demands made by allegiance to God and service to feudal lords, the spiritual injuries of today's service members are seen as a private consequence of war, a view that is consistent with the split that currently exists between the US military and the rest of the society. As Mark Thompson writes, "The past decade of war by volunteer soldiers, sailors, airmen and Marines has acted like a centrifuge, separating the nation's military from its citizens [...] Over the past generation, the world's lone superpower has created—and grown accustomed to—a permanent military caste, increasingly disconnected from U.S. society, waging decade-long wars in its name, no longer representative of or drawn from the citizenry as a whole. Think of the U.S. military as the Other 1 %—some 2.4 million troops have fought in and around Afghanistan and Iraq since 9/11, exactly 1 % of the 240 million Americans over 18. The U.S. Constitution calls on the people to provide for the common defense. But there is very little that is common about the way we defend ourselves in the twenty-first century."[22] In the absence of a collective societal investment in the military, the warrior's moral injury has come to be understood as an existential liability of having voluntarily served, one that does not implicate the larger society. In this regard, the confessional exercise of the experimental therapeutic approach could be seen as symptomatic of the divide between military and civilian culture, insofar as it bespeaks a receptivity to certain emotional effects of combat—guilt, shame, self-loathing—and a disinclination to recognize other feelings for which a confessional approach may be inadequate. Guilt and shame are responses that civilians can accept, and even feel reassured by, insofar as they indicate that the warrior has an intact conscience and hence will not be a societal danger. But sympathetic attunement to warriors' remorseful emotions may also discourage warriors from sharing more volatile emotional responses to having served that cannot be assimilated to a civilian frame of reference.

In his memoir *What It Is Like To Go To War*, Vietnam veteran Karl Marlantes writes that warriors hold dual memberships in worlds whose codes of conduct are antithetical to one another; they inhabit two worlds, "the world where they are acting in the role of God [i.e. where they have the power to deprive others of life] and the world where they are acting in an ordinary societal role."[23] Warriors kill because they are ***authorized*** by society to "take life away from others."[24] In Marlantes' words, "Killing is what warriors do for society. Yet when they return home, society doesn't generally acknowledge that the act it asked them to do created a deep split in their psyches, or a psychological and spiritual weight most of them will stumble beneath the rest of their lives."[25] In gradually allowing himself to examine his feelings about his service in Vietnam, Marlantes discovered that the guilt and self-blame he felt about decisions he made and actions he took as a 23-year-old Army lieutenant were in fact defenses against other emotions that were more difficult for him to acknowledge—rage, helplessness and grief.[26] In light of Marlantes' self-discovery, we might ask what effect a therapy has that seeks to strengthen the warrior's voice of self-judgment, and even encourages that voice to dominate, and also ask whether such an approach does not send a message to warriors that they will be accepted back into the community on the condition that their perspective on their military experience affirms civilian expectations and frames of reference. As Marlantes reminds, "War is the antithesis of the most fundamental rule of moral conduct we've been taught—do unto others as you would have others do unto you. When called upon to fight, we violate many codes of civilized behavior"(48). It is perhaps because of these violations that there is little support in the community for warriors as they "learn how to integrate the experience of killing, to put the pieces of their psyche back together again" and why, "for the most part, they have been left to do this on their own."[27]

Psychoanalyst Martha Bragin has addressed the difficulty civilians have in admitting veterans back into society, noting that too often they are perceived as "unwelcome reminders of the violence that the whole society pays for and of which [...] all people are capable [...] but which they wish to forget.[28] The waging of the recent wars in Iraq and Afghanistan by a "volunteer" army has made it easier for civilians to disavow the violent propensities of individuals and of society more broadly.[29] Jonathan Shay has also noted the widespread resistance among civilians to recognizing the universal human capacity for violence that Bragin calls attention to and that manifests in ambivalence toward soldier. Shay writes that when civilians are terrified and enraged by an "enemy attack," we value the soldier's fighting qualities.[30] "In fear of the enemy, nothing is too much or too good for the 'great hearted spirit' (*thumos*) of our fighting men,"[31] but "when the enemy no longer scares us, and the soldiers come home as veterans [...] we see their needs as greedy, demanding, uncultivated."[32]

Psychoanalyst Tom Helscher believes that in face of this societal ambivalence toward veterans, moral injury may serve a self-preservative purpose.[33] Through self-condemnation, the logic goes, the veteran takes the badness of the world upon him or herself. Believing that he or she is "bad" enables a veteran to preserve belief in the goodness of the world. Such loss of faith in one's own rectitude, though painful, nonetheless protects against an even more devastating loss of faith in the community, whose acceptance the veteran may perceive as conditional, because predicated on preconceived ideas about what "acceptable" responses to war are. Many veterans of the recent wars have observed how little interest there is in nonconventional accounts of soldiers' experiences and how, instead, a "stubborn and misleading narrative [...] persists in the minds of many Americans: Every veteran is either a hero or damaged."[34] On a similar note, Iraq veteran Roy Scranton has criticized "the continuous media appetite for war as narratives of derring-do and of heroism, [...] and [...] an appetite for war where soldiers are just pawns in various political polemics. It's all for people who often, to the soldier, seem like they have no genuine interest in what it's really like, they just want to be entertained or have their opinions validated."[35] Helscher's view suggests that experiencing moral injury, while devastating, nonetheless helps maintain the connection to the civilian world in face of its resistance to recognizing the totality of the warrior's emotional responses to wartime violence. Painful as moral injury is, the alternative may be even more intolerable for the warrior: admitting to feelings other than those associated with contrition, and thereby risking rejection by the community.

The foregoing discussion has endeavored to present, and raise questions about the therapeutic understanding of moral injury as an individual and private consequence of war, and to argue instead for a conception that takes into account the social component of the injury. The absence of such a social component in the therapeutic discourse raises the possibility that the discourse itself may be more a symptom of the military-civilian divide than an objective narrative about the psychic wounds of war. Indeed, it is crucial to bear in mind that moral injury *is* a narrative about the warrior's psychic and spiritual burdens, and as such, that it lends itself to comparison with other narrative accounts of war trauma, such as Morrison's novel.

In distinction to the individualistic and moralizing narrative characteristics of the recent clinical approach to moral injury, *Home* brackets the question of individual guilt and expiation in favor of a collective, social understanding of wartime violence and the reparative work that needs to be undertaken in its aftermath. In exposing the unrecognized societal tributaries that feed into the warrior's post-war feelings of guilt, *Home* offers an understanding of moral injury as a societal wound. In so doing, it demonstrates the broad relevance of what novelists know first-hand: that the creation of narrative is a social and socializing activity. As we will see, the literal journey of Morrison's protagonist from a mental ward back into the community is simultaneously a journey from silence into narrative in which the community plays a crucial role—as a receiver/container of the soldier's traumatic experiences and co-constructor of its meanings. As itself such a narrative, the novel is also an exemplary social space for the holding and containment of the trauma of war.

In *Home*, an African-American veteran of the Korean War, named Frank Money, is suffering from moral injury, because he has killed innocent Korean civilians; one of those killings is especially traumatic. Frank relates his memories of the events surrounding this killing to an unidentified narrator, who includes Frank's words verbatim in the text. In one respect, the novel's dialogical structure is reminiscent of the relationship between the mental health professionals treating moral injury and the soldiers undergoing treatment. But the similarities between the medical and novelistic approaches stop here, for in addition to Frank's story, the narrator of *Home* also provides the histories of the significant people in Frank's life, thereby indicating the importance of societal context and the veteran's pre-combat history in coming to terms with moral injury. And whereas the therapeutic discourse of moral injury understands guilt as an indicator of a soldier's ethical soundness, in the novel, Frank's post-war feelings of guilt serve as a point of departure for an exploration of their connection to the societal traumas that predate Frank's military service.

When the novel opens, Frank has returned from Korea and is confined in a mental ward, having lost the two close childhood friends who had enlisted along with him, and now suffering from PTSD. As Frank thinks about how his friends were killed on the battlefield, he is reminded of his sense of helplessness and of his desire for revenge, both of which drove him to commit the acts that caused his moral injury. He recalls, “And all of that killing you did afterward? Women running, dragging children along. And that old one-legged man on a crutch hobbling at the edge of the road so as not to slow down the other, swifter ones? You blew a hole in his head because you believed it would make up for the frosted urine on Mike’s pants and avenge the lips calling mama. Did it? Did it work? And the girl. What did she ever do to deserve what happened to her? All unasked questions multiplying like mold in the shadows of the photographs he saw.”[36] The mention of the girl is a reference to a particular killing whose memory is the greatest source of Frank’s guilt and shame. It took place at a time when Frank was guarding the hills above the village where his army unit would dump its trash. On the particular day of the incident, Frank hears a crackling in the bamboo. First thinking it is a tiger, since enemy soldiers never traveled singly, and then a dog, Frank is surprised to see the hand of a young girl emerge from beneath the bamboo, patting the ground in search of scraps to eat. Frank does not disturb the girl, who returns almost daily to scavenge. The first time Frank relates this incident to the narrator, he recalls how his relief guard approached the girl as she was reaching for a rotting orange. Frank states that upon seeing the guard, the girl stands up and “in what looks like a hurried, even automatic gesture she says something in Korean. Sounds like `Yum-yum.’ She smiles, reaches for the soldier’s crotch, touches it. It surprises him” (95). As Frank is looking into the girl’s face, the other guard “blows her away” (95). “Only the girl’s hand remains in the trash, clutching its treasure, a spotted rotting orange” (95). Frank supplies an interpretation for the guard’s actions: “Thinking back on it now, I think the guard felt more than disgust. I think he felt tempted and that is what he had to kill” (96).

Towards the end of the novel, Frank narrates the same scene again, this time with a crucial alteration. He states, “I have to tell the whole truth. I lied to you and I lied to me. I hid it from you because I hid it from me. [...] I shot the Korean girl in her face. I am the one she touched. I am the one who saw her smile. I am the one she said ‘Yum-yum’” to. I am the one she aroused. A child. A wee little girl. I didn’t think. I didn’t have to. Better she should die. How could I let her live after she took me down to a place I didn’t know was in me? How could I like myself, even *be* myself if I surrendered to that place where I unzip my fly and let her taste me right then and there? And again the next day and the next as long as she came scavenging. What type of man is that? And what type of man thinks he can ever in life pay the price of that orange" (134). Frank's motive for killing the girl suggests that he was attempting to hold on to an image of himself that was threatened by the desire he felt for her: "How could I like myself, even *be* myself if I surrendered to that place," he states (134). To his mind, letting the girl live would have meant surrendering to a bad temptation. According to Frank's logic then, killing the object that tempts him is actually a way of ***upholding*** the moral order of the world, insofar as it prevents Frank's evil impulse from injecting its toxicity into the world. And because violence is the quotidian norm of war, and given that Frank is enraged by the loss of his closest friends, killing the girl is an expedient way for Frank to make his own badness disappear, after first projecting it onto the girl. But once Frank is back from Korea and immersed in civilian culture, his prior attempt to preserve the goodness of the world now feels like a morally injurious act that dogs him with guilt. His "self-loathing disguised as somebody else's fault" leads him to seek outlets to relieve his self-condemnation: he picks fights, curses strangers and schoolchildren, and urinates on the sidewalk (15). And he also targets himself, banging his head against walls, "weeping before trees—apologizing for acts he had never committed" (15).[37]

Neither condoning nor condemning Frank's actions, the narrator offers a perspective on Frank's pre-war life that brings into view connections between the badness Frank perceives within himself and the social determinations of this perception. The social origins of Frank's bad internal objects—his evil desire—is saliently represented in the first scene of the novel, which takes place in Lotus, a small town in segregationist Georgia, where Frank and his family settled after being chased from their home in Texas. In Lotus, Frank's parents spend their days laboring in the fields and their nights working other menial jobs, leaving Frank and his younger sister, Cee, to the care of unsympathetic and angry relatives who neglect and abuse them. In the novel's opening scene, Frank recalls an event that occurred on a day when he and Cee had wandered into a fenced field on the outskirts of town. There, they behold two male horses, rising on their hind legs, fighting one another to determine who would have first rights over the mares. As they are leaving the field, the children hear the voices of approaching men. Hiding themselves in the tall grass, they witness the men dumping the body of a black man into a shallow grave. Cee begins to tremble when she sees "that black foot with its creamy pink and mid-streaked sole being wacked into the grave (4). Confronted with this graphic exercise of racial violence, under whose threat the children perpetually live, Frank does his best to protect his sister. He recalls, "She trembled when we hid from the shovels. I covered her face, her eyes, hoping she hadn't seen the foot poking out of the grave [...] As a brother four years older, I thought I could handle it" (4). The scene concludes with Frank's comment to the narrator: "Since you're set on telling my story, whatever you think and whatever you write down, know this: I really forgot about the burial. I only remembered the horses. They were so beautiful. So brutal. And they stood like men"(5). The horses represent to Frank an image of compelling strength and action: upright like men, they fight one another as equals, in contrast to the relationship of inequality between the white murderers and their black victim, who, the novel later discloses, had been captured and forced by his captors to battle his own son in a "men-treated-like-dog" fight to death (138). The horses thus provide an idealized image for Frank of his own role as the fierce protector of his sister. In contrast to her passivity, which is registered in her "sad waiting eyes," Frank can identify with the active fearlessness of the horses, which in turn enables him to repress his more threatening identification with the dead black victim (103).

The black man's burial is the repressed primal scene of violence that haunts Frank's later encounter with the Korean girl. When he first observes the girl rummaging for food, Frank associates to his own past: "I have eaten trash in jail, Korea, hospitals, at table, and from certain garbage cans. Nothing, however, compares to the leftovers at food pantries [...] I remember standing in line at Church of the Redeemer waiting for a tin plate of dry, hard cheese already showing green, pickled pigs' feet—its vinegar soaking stale biscuits" (40). The sight of the girl's reaching for a rotting orange triggers Frank's memory of his own scavenging. He recalls: "[We] used to steal peaches off the ground under Miss Robinson's tree, sneaking, crawling, being as quiet as we could so she wouldn't see us and grab a belt" (94). If, in Frank's mind, the girl is a version of his earlier self, when she comes too close to him, she triggers a defensiveness that interrupts his identification with her and instead aligns him with the threatened Mrs. Robinson, who did not tolerate children in her garden. From this point on, the girl ceases to exist as a distinct other in Frank's eyes, and the assumptions he makes about her own neglect cannot be disentangled from the abandonment he experienced as a child. He states, "Every civilian I ever met in that country would (and did) die to defend their children. Parents threw themselves in front of their kids without a pause. Still, I knew there were a few corrupt ones who were not content with the usual girls for sale and took to marketing children" (95–96).

The significance of the desire the girl triggers in Frank is overdetermined. It can be read as a sign of Frank's wish to "approach" the very vulnerability that had to be split off from his inviolable "protector" self.[38] By the same token, insofar as that vulnerability stood to undermine Frank's ability to protect his sister, it remained a threat. In killing the girl, Frank thus destroys that vulnerable, split-off part of himself. Killing her can also be seen as a displaced enactment of Frank's rage against the social environment's failure to have provided him the necessary protections, since, like the girl, he too had been a child lacking "parents who threw themselves in front of their kids without a pause" (95). Finally, as a symbolic attempt to destroy the evil within himself, the killing can also be understood as Frank's attempt to uphold the order of the world that had abandoned him, notwithstanding the fact that in the eyes of that world, as embodied, for example, by Mrs. Robinson, he, like the girl, held little value.

Frank's experience of loss in Korea also reduplicates his prior societal abandonment. Discussing the fatal wounding of the childhood friends with whom he had enlisted, he recalls, "I dragged Mike to shelter and fought off the birds but he died anyway. I held on to him, talked to him for an hour but he died anyway. I staunched the blood finally oozing from the place Stuff's arm should have been. I found it some twenty feet away and gave it to him in case they could sew it back on. He died anyway" (103). The following internal dialogue reflects the link between the rage Frank expresses through civilian killings, and his sense of helplessness: "Why didn't you hurry? If you had gotten there sooner you could have helped him. You could have pulled him behind the hill the way you did Mike. And all of that killing you did afterward? Women running, dragging children along. And that old one-legged man on a crutch hobbling at the edge of the road so as not to slow down other, swifter ones? You blew a hole in his head because you believed it would make up for the frosted urine on Mike's pants and avenge the lips calling mama. Did it? Did it work? And the girl? What did she ever do to deserve what happened to her?" (21–22).

By including Frank's backstory, the text establishes a framework through which to grasp the connection between Frank's moral injury and the societal persecution and neglect to which he was subjected as a child. Frank's transgressions come into focus not as the acts of an autonomous self that has betrayed its core values, but as events in which the prior failures of the social environment continue to exact their price. The rage that motivates his killing of the girl attests to his inability to accept that he could not have prevented his friends' deaths. His helplessness is unbearable, and so he projects it onto the girl and destroys it, in an act that symbolically replicates his prior childhood experiences of psychic annihilation.

Upon returning from Korea, Frank receives a letter alerting him to his sister's precarious situation. The letter acts as a summons for him to resume his earlier role as her protector. Impelled by the thought that "maybe his life had been preserved for Cee, which was only fair since she had been his original caring-for, a selflessness without gain or emotional profit," Frank breaks out of the mental ward and makes his way to Atlanta, where Cee is being held captive by her white employer, a physician who conducted life-threatening experimental procedures on her reproductive organs (34–35). As Frank travels to Georgia, the train he is on stops on the tracks for a necessary repair. While waiting for the trip to resume, Frank takes a walk, and he stumbles onto a scene of two women fighting one another as a man stands by watching. When the man aggressively approaches Frank, he counter-attacks, pushing the man to the ground and beating him. "Unable to stop and unwilling to, Frank kept going even though the big man was unconscious," until the women pull at Frank, screaming at him to stop (101). Afterwards on the train, "Frank wondered at the excitement, the wild joy the fight had given him. It was unlike the rage that had accompanied the killing in Korea. Those sprees were fierce but mindless, anonymous. This violence was personal in its delight. Good, he thought. He might need that thrill to claim his sister" (102). The scene suggests that Frank does not feel the weight of civil society's prohibition against killing, and as such, it recalls his feelings while watching the fighting horses with Cee: "guarding her, finding a way through tall grass and out of that place, not being afraid of anything—snakes or wild old men. I wonder if succeeding at that was the buried seed of all the rest. In my little-boy heart I felt heroic and I knew that if they found us or touched her I would kill" (104). Now with only himself to rely on to save his sister, he is prepared to kill if need be.

It is only after rescuing Cee, who is feverish with infection, that Frank, frantic to save her, has no other recourse than to enlist the help of the community. He brings Cee to the home of Ethel Fordham, a woman who lives in the neighborhood where he grew up. Ethel, along with the other women in the neighborhood, takes charge of Cee, admonishing Frank to stay away from his sister, because "his maleness would worsen her condition" (119). This marks a shift in Frank's relation to his community. He experiences a "feeling of safety and good will,"a feeling that, he writes, is "exaggerated, but savoring it was real." (118). Frank's feeling of well-being, however qualified, gives him a sense, for the first time, of the social environment as a supportive, rather than neglectful, presence, and it enables Frank to accept the limits of his ability to protect his sister without plunging into the rage that had accompanied feelings of powerlessness in Korea.

Before Frank returned with Cee to Lotus, she had been a vulnerable "someone" for him to protect, not a person whose otherness Frank could recognize. Frank tells the narrator, "She was a shadow for most of my life, a presence marking its own absence" (103). But as she heals, Cee becomes a presence, now changed by Ethel's nurture and counsel: "'Look to yourself. You free. Nothing and nobody is obliged to save you but you. Seed your own land [...] Somewhere inside you is that free person I'm talking about. Locate her and let her do some good in the world'" (126). Determined to become "the person who would never again need rescue," Cee accepts the reality of her loss—the doctor's experiments have left her unable to bear children (129). When she tells Frank about the reason for her grief, Frank tries to offer his customary words of comfort, which Cee refuses: "'I can be miserable if I want to. You don't need to try and make it go away. It shouldn't go away. It's just as sad as it ought to be and I'm not going to hide from what's true just because it hurts'" (131).

While Cee was convalescing, the women of the neighborhood taught her to quilt. They "took over the sickroom and started sorting pieces [...] while they stitched together the palette they had agreed upon," practicing a skill that their mothers had taught them (141). Once recovered, Cee, who now "could know the truth, accept it, and keep on quilting," becomes a model for Frank (132). When she tells Frank about the unborn baby whose presence she senses, Frank thinks of the unmourned losses of his own life, coming to the realization, "Maybe that little girl wasn't waiting around to be born to her. Maybe it was already dead, waiting for me to step up and say how" (133). The text of *Home* is the "how" that Frank offers in concert with the narrator. Unlike individual confessional stories, such as the ones that current clinical approaches to moral injury are eliciting from soldiers, Frank's story is a communal one, constructed like the quilts of the Lotus women: as a patchwork of individual stories placed in constellation with one another, so as to reveal a pattern of racial discrimination that implicates the social world in the acts that engendered Frank's moral injury.

At the conclusion of the novel, Frank and Cee return to the unmarked grave of the nameless black man, so that Frank can exhume the buried bones, enshroud them in Cee's quilt and give them a proper burial. After carrying "the gentleman"(143) — a descriptor that emphasizes the humanizing effect of Frank's actions — to a stream on the outskirts of Lotus, Frank digs a narrow grave beneath a sweet bay tree "split down the middle, beheaded, undead—spreading its arms, one to the right, one to the left" (144). Frank and Cee slide the shroud-turned-coffin into the vertical grave, and on the tree trunk Frank nails a wooden marker bearing the epitaph "Here Stands A Man" (145). Having rescued the dead man from oblivion, Frank asserts his newfound sense of agency by laying the dead man's bones to rest, an indication that Frank has gotten past the rage born of helplessness. He has done so by creating a space of meaning where the death of the black man, which was denied a place within the symbolic order, can now be inscribed into it. The anthropomorphic description of the tree underscores its iconic status as an emblem of Frank himself—split between the military and civilian worlds, a survivor of traumatic loss (beheaded), but still receptive (open-armed) to the future. After finishing his task, Frank relates,

> I stood there a long while, staring at that tree.
> It looked so strong
> So beautiful.
> Hurt right down the middle
> But alive and well (147).

Like the tree, which is permanently split but still able to thrive, Frank may now be able to thrive, not because the "psychological and spiritual weight" that comes with killing can ever be lifted, but because it can now be shared by the community.[39] Just as the man buried beneath the tree has been encased in Cee's quilt, itself a symbol of the community's role as witness to his death, so too have Frank's war secrets been folded into and disclosed through a narrative that enables the public to become a custodian of those stories.

In *The Evil Hours* David Morris writes, "In the wake of overwhelming events, after the fateful moment has passed, the mind is often consumed by questions of cosmic responsibility and the dimensions of one's role in the world. For the veteran, in particular, these sorts of questions carry a special weight because, as a device of the state, the fateful responsibilities of soldiering were never intended to be borne alone [...] Soldiers are ultimately vessels and vassals of the state, and they do not go to war of their own accord, so why shouldn't the state or the community help relieve them of their guilt when they return home?[40] *Home* offers an approach to moral injury that resonates with Morris's call for the community's engagement in the process of healing. The novel constructs a communal narrative that does not judge Frank but that instead considers his moral injury within a framework of social violence and thereby "takes the problem out of the hands of the mental health profession and the military and attempts to place it where it belongs—in society, in the community, and in the family [...] It transforms 'patients' back into citizens and 'diagnoses' into dialogue."[41] The account Frank and the narrator co-construct represents healing as an experience of the social environment's supportive capacities, demonstrated through the integration of Frank's war trauma it into the larger "quilt" of a literary text, an integration that serves to distribute the burden of Frank's wartime guilt between himself and the community. Now that this has happened, Frank stands a chance of finding his way home.

Notes

1. Tony Dokoupil, "A New Theory of PTSD and Veterans: Moral Injury," *Newsweek*, December 3, 2012, http://www.newsweek.com/new-theory-ptsd-and-veterans-moral-injury-63539.
2. David J. Morris, *The Evil Hours: A Biography of Post-Traumatic Stress Disorder* (New York: Eamon Dolan/Houghton Mifflin Harcourt, 2015) 2–3.
3. Doloupil, "A New Theory."
4. Nan Levinson, "Mad-Bad-Sad: What's Really Happened to America's Soldiers," *Huffington Post*, June 28, 2012, www.huffingtonpost.com/nan-levinson/mad-bad-sad-whats-really-_b_1633856.html.
5. Rita Nakashima Brock and Herman Keizer, Jr., "Helping Veterans Suffering Moral Injury After War" (PDF), accessed December 10, 2013, http://network.crcna.org/sites/network.crcna.org/files/Slides_HelpingVeteransSufferingMoralInjuryAfterWar.pdf. The Soul Repair Center is dedicated to furthering research on moral injury and educating the public about how to support returning service members who suffer from moral injury; see http://brite.edu/academics/programs/soul-repair/.

6. "'Soul Repair' examines how military vets suffer from moral injury." *Take Two.* WNPR, Southern California Public Radio, Pasadena, California, KPCC, December 12, 2013.
7. Janet Kemp, RN Ph.D. and Robert Bossarte, Ph.D., "Suicide Data Report," Department of Veterans Affairs Mental Health Services Suicide Prevention Program, 2012, http://www.va.gov/opa/docs/Suicide-Data-Report-2012-final.pdf.
8. Leo Shane III, "Report: Suicide rate spikes among young veterans," *Stars and Stripes*, January 9, 2014, http://www.stripes.com/report-suicide-rate-spikes-among-young-veterans-1.261283.
9. Timothy Williams, "Suicides Outpacing War Deaths for Troops," *New York Times*, June 8, 2012, http://www.nytimes.com/2012/06/09/us/suicides-eclipse-war-deaths-for-us-troops.html?r=0.
10. Dokoupil, "A New Theory of PTSD."
11. Brett T. Litz et al., "Moral Injury and Moral Repair in War Veterans: A Preliminary Model and Intervention Strategy," *Clinical Psychological Review* 29 (December 2009) 695–706.
12. David Wood, "The Grunts: Damned If They Kill; Damned If They Don't," *Huffington Post*, March 18, 2014, http://projects.huffingtonpost.com/moral-injury/the-grunts.
13. Dokoupil, "A New Theory of PTSD."
14. Dokoupil, "A New Theory of PTSD."
15. In this regard, the affective experience of moral injury represents an altogether different psychological response to killing than that of soldiers who have undergone brutalization and barbarization. For a discussion of these conditions in relation to the psychological states of German soldiers, see: Georg L. Mosse, *Fallen Soldiers: Reshaping the Memory of the World Wars* (New York: Oxford University Press, 1990); and Omer Bartov, *The Eastern Front, 1941–45, German Troops and the Barbarisation of Warfare* (Basingstoke: Palgrave Macmillan, second edition, 2001).
16. Litz et al., "Moral Injury," 702.
17. Litz et al., "Moral Injury," 701.
18. Martha Beginger, 'Moral Injury': Gaining Traction, But Still Controversial," *On Point,* WNPR, Boston, WBUR, June 25, 2013, http://www.wbur.org/2013/06/25/moral-injury-research.
19. Litz et al., "Moral Injury," 704.
20. Morris, 77.

21. Morris, 77–78.
22. Mark Thompson, "The Other 1 %," *Time Magazine*, November 21, 2011, http://www.time.com/time/magazine/article/0,9171,2099152,00.html.
23. Karl Marlantes, *What It Is Like To Go To War* (New York: Grove Press, 2011) 26.
24. Marlantes, *What It Is Like*, 26.
25. Marlantes, "*What It Is Like,*" 26.
26. For a discussion of the way writing enabled Marlantes to discover buried emotion, see Susan Derwin, "The Warrior's Subjectivity," *MLN*, Volume 129, Number 3, April 2014 (German Issue), 504–13.
27. Marlantes, *What it is Like*, 26.
28. Bragin.
29. Thompson.
30. Jonathan Shay, *Odysseus in America: Combat Trauma and the trials of Homecoming* (New York: Scribner, 2002) 13.
31. Shay, *Odysseus*, 13.
32. Shay, *Odysseus*, 13.
33. Thomas P. Helscher, Ph.D., FIPI, "Moral Injury: Environment, Culture and Mind," presentation, UC Interdisciplinary Psychoanalytic Consortium, Lake Arrowhead, May, 2013.
34. Gen. James Jones and Dan Goldenberg, "Put Veterans To Work," *Los Angeles Times*, Opinion/Op-Ed, November 11, 2013, http://www.latimes.com/opinion/op-ed/la-oe-jones-employ-veterans-20131111-story.html#axzz2kMCYJGVO
35. NPR Books, Interview: Roy Scranton, "In 'Fire And Forget,' Vets Turned Writers Tell Their War Stories," Terry Gross, host, November 11, 2013, http://www.npr.org/2013/11/11/244520706/in-fire-and-forget-vets-turned-writers-tell-their-war-stories.
36. Toni Morrison, *Home* (New York: Alfred A. Knopf, 2012) 22–23; subsequent references will be included in the body of the text.
37. Helscher proposes a connection between bad internal objects and moral injury in relation to Morrison's novel, drawing upon Ronald Fairbairn's concept of "moral defense" as presented in W.R.D. Fairbairn, "The Repression and the Return of Bad Objects (with Special Reference to the 'War Neuroses')," *Psychoanalytic Studies of the Personality* (Routledge: London and New York, 1990) 59–81.
38. That is why Frank's erotic ties are predicated on his attraction to indicators of vulnerability. About women, he states, "I like the small

breakable things inside each one. Whatever their personalities, smarts, or looks, something soft lay inside each. Like a bird's breastbone, shaped and chosen to wish on. A little V, thinner than bone and lightly hinged, that I could break with a forefinger if I wanted to, but never did. Want to, I mean. Knowing it was there, hidden from me, was enough" (68–69). When he meets Lilly, "He could not take his eyes away from the backs of her knees. As she stretched, her dress of a soft cottony flowered fabric rose up, exposing that seldom noticed, ooo-so-vulnerable flesh. And for a reason he still did not understand, he began to cry. Love, plain, simple, and so fast it shattered him" (22).

39. Karl Marlantes, *What It Is Like*, 26.
40. Morris, 80–81.
41. Tyler Boudreau, "The Morally Injured," *The Massachusetts Review*, Autumn/Winter 20ll, Vol. 52, Issue 2/3, 746–54.

PART II

Wartime

CHAPTER 4

Testimonies of Trauma: Surviving Auschwitz-Birkenau

Lisa Pine

Introduction

The emerging field of trauma studies from the 1990s onwards has engendered a variety of important new research in this area of scholarship. The Second World War and the Holocaust provide the context for a crucial moment in the social and cultural history of trauma. This chapter considers the historical implications of the traumatized body, mind and emotions at a particular time and place within this context, analysing the psychological trauma of the impact of the Holocaust upon its victims at Auschwitz-Birkenau. The research for this chapter is based on the testimonies of male and female survivors of Auschwitz-Birkenau. This type of witness testimony to trauma forms a significant part of our understanding of the Holocaust as a whole. This chapter analyses how male and female survivors have remembered their experiences and how they have written their narratives about Auschwitz-Birkenau. These testimonies of trauma detail events in the death camp most associated with the horrors of the Holocaust and the atrocities carried out by the Nazi regime during the Second World War.

This chapter examines some of the distinctions faced by victims of the Nazi regime in regard to their gender, as men's and women's testimonies

L. Pine (✉)
London South Bank University, London, UK

P. Leese, J. Crouthamel (eds.), *Traumatic Memories of the Second World War and After*, DOI 10.1007/978-3-319-33470-7_4

have many aspects in common, but also some significant differences. The distinctions in their memories are of much interest because they illustrate subjectivities of trauma. Furthermore, the experiences faced by survivors of Auschwitz had a great impact on their own subsequent lives and on how they chose to relate their narratives and histories. This is especially noteworthy in terms of the development of the historiography—whose traumatic experiences gain attention and why, and whose have been ignored? Women's Holocaust histories and narratives have not been examined until comparatively recently. No longer are women's voices unheard and there is now substantial literature on women's writing and the Holocaust.[1]

This is an area of research that is constantly growing. The diversity of experiences faced by Holocaust victims requires greater scrutiny. Furthermore, particular aspects of experience that have been difficult or taboo subjects have also been neglected in the historical writing. However, such angles are important to our knowledge of the Holocaust as a whole because they give us a breadth of comprehension and a greater insight into the diversity of victims' experiences.

This chapter begins with a discussion of survivor testimonies as historical sources. It then analyses the writings of both male and female Auschwitz survivors, illustrating the specific experiences they faced as men and women and examining the coping and survival strategies they adopted. It explores both men's and women's experiences and behavior that challenged gendered expectations. A gendered approach has now become a mainstream part of the history of the Holocaust.[2] Yehuda Bauer has suggested that "the problems facing women as women and men as men have a special poignancy in an extreme situation such as the Holocaust".[3] Dalia Ofer and Lenore Weitzman emphasize that rather than distracting us from the Nazi brutality against all Jews, a gendered approach enhances our understanding of it "by locating it in the specificity of individual experiences".[4] It expands our knowledge base and provides a greater and more differentiated understanding of the experiences of victims. Pascale Bos has examined the place of gender in the study of Holocaust victims and survivors.[5] She calls for a more critical approach to the evidence of gender distinctions in Holocaust narratives, emphasizing the discursive construction of the experience, memory and representation of the past. Indeed, Bos argues that "precisely in acknowledging (and highlighting) the elements of choice and subversive power in the creation of (gendered) personal narratives we can conceive of survivors' agency in compelling new ways".[6] Hence, she underlines the need for and movement towards a significant change in our understanding of what narrative truth means and how it is used in historical analysis. The lens of gender enables readers to consider what is distinctive between the ways in which women and men have selected and constructed their narratives. As Bos rightly argues: "Men and women experience, remember, and recount events differently", because of their socialization.[7] The particularity and diversity of individual experiences makes it impossible to universalize Holocaust experiences, whether these are female or male ones.

Survivor Testimonies as Historical Sources

Holocaust survivor testimonies—both written and oral—are essential historical sources, which provide a unique insight into the unfolding of events precisely because they are reflections of personal and individual experiences.[8] Langer's work on the oral testimony of survivors illuminates the forms and functions of memory in the reliving of traumatic events and experiences by Holocaust survivors. He argues that oral narratives allow an unshielded truth to appear.[9] Representations of memories and experiences in written and published memoirs and testimonies are also powerful and significant as historical sources. As Benzion Dinur has stated: "from every point of view, memoirs and reminiscences of persons who witnessed and experienced the European catastrophe, watched it develop… are of major importance".[10] They offer fruitful opportunities for analysis of the diversity of traumatic experiences during the Holocaust with wide-reaching implications for our understanding of this historical event. Paul Bartrop underlines the crucial role of testimonial accounts in forming our understanding of what life was like in the Nazi camps.[11] The richness of the narratives in written testimonies allows readers to gain a greater understanding of the Holocaust. Each writer has a different story to narrate, even in the description of intrinsically similar events, because it is the way in which the writers have comprehended and related their experiences that comprises the true core of their work. However, it is important to take into account that such written accounts yield "a represented rather than an unmediated reality" and to comprehend the constructed nature of evidence itself in written testimony.[12] Holocaust survivor narratives have been written in a variety of circumstances—some soon after the event, some after the passing of several decades, some with the help of a ghostwriter. Whilst this does not make them less legitimate or valuable as historical sources, there may be problems such as the accuracy and reliability of recall, of which historians must be aware. Moreover, on the whole, the people writing down their narratives were not practiced authors and survivor testimonies are not always elegant or polished. Furthermore, as they were written for publication, a sifting process took place in the mind of the writer and/or the editor. This means that some memories were omitted and others retained or even enhanced. The writing, as Waxman notes "comes from the careful representation of experience, or the perceived 'appropriateness' of experiences for publication".[13] This means that traumatic events have been rendered invisible because they were too hard or distasteful to write down. Difficult aspects of traumatic experiences can be erased from the historical narrative, as survivors' reconstructions of their experiences may "smooth corners" in their stories, particularly of events or episodes that they find painful or hard to confront. As Waxman notes: "published accounts not only relate witnesses' experiences, but also tell us something about collective understandings of the Holocaust".[14]

Nevertheless, published survivor accounts are certainly "subjectively true".[15] Their authors chronicle events they witnessed themselves. As Bartrop states, they "do no attempt to make magic, nor do they attempt to imagine the unimaginable. They simply try to tell the stories from their own individual perspectives".[16] It is their intention to tell the "truth" as they comprehend it, as clearly as possible in order to convey the essence of their experience to their readers. This chapter uses published testimonies as its main source base. Whilst there may be some qualitative distinctions between published and unpublished accounts, these are not of a nature to make a difference to understanding the gendering of narratives. For example, archival testimonies of the responses of German Jews to Nazi persecution during the 1930s yield very similar gendered perspectives to those sources used here, in terms of men's and women's experiences and how they were remembered and described.[17] Do these narratives tell or intend to tell the full or the only story? The answer is no. Holocaust survivors may have different reasons for writing down their narratives, but none of them claim to tell the full or the only story of the Holocaust. The historian must keep this in mind and not have unrealistic expectations about the nature of these sources. In Holocaust testimony, "the writer's personal experience is representative and used to provide a perspective on the common plight", not to give full histories of camps or even necessarily to relate major incidents that occurred.[18] Not one of them can tell the whole story on its own and nor do they intend to do so. Survivor testimonies are intimate accounts of personal experiences, which the writers wish to convey to their readers. The process of testifying then is "not merely to narrate, but to commit oneself, and to commit narrative, to others".[19] In so doing, for many survivors, the process of writing their narratives was also a means of resurrecting their identities, which had been so starkly removed from them by the Nazi camp system.

Furthermore, historians may overlook difficult subjects or types of behavior that are not expressed in written memoirs or testimonies, thus excluding them from the historical narrative. Testimonies that homogenize women's experiences and identities can be misleading.[20] The tendency in historical writing has been to define Jewish women as mothers, sisters and nurturers, "with a very particular notion of what constitutes female behavior".[21] Sara Horowitz challenges the type of interpretation that "erases the actual experiences of women and, to an extent, domesticates the events of the Holocaust".[22] Anna Hardmann cites examples of women fighting for their own existence at the expense of others.[23] Zoe Waxman has also argued that assumptions that women only had motherly and care-giving roles "obscure the diversity of women's Holocaust experiences".[24] She further argues that the valorizing of sacrifice also means that the struggles surrounding temptation are "glossed over". Waxman states that "the collectivization of Holocaust memory has led to a homogenization of Holocaust comprehension that eschews difficult testimony or stories that fall outside accepted narratives".[25] As many people find it difficult to confront the full horrors of the Holocaust, the literature has tended to overlook the desperate actions undertaken by victims in order to survive under the appalling conditions in which they found themselves. But this does not mean that they did not occur. As so much of the existing literature has represented women as nurturers, the intention here is to form a more nuanced picture by looking at different types of action or conduct among women and men than traditionally accepted normative behavior. An analysis of survivor narratives allows for a greater awareness of these distinctions.

Men's Experiences and Behavior at Auschwitz

The terrible privations and circumstances of internment at Auschwitz included thirst and hunger, extremes of temperature, arduous physical labour, overcrowding, inadequate food and foul water, lengthy roll calls, exhaustion, illness, injury and the constant fear of "selection" for the gas chambers. In terms of men's behaviour, gendered expectations were centred on strength and hardness, toughness and determination.[26] Signs of weakness fell short of normative behaviour for men. Viktor Frankl states that "it was necessary … to keep moments of weakness and furtive tears to a minimum".[27] Men did not wish to appear cowardly or weak. As a result of different social constructions of gender, men were less likely to discuss emotions, admit to weakness or the need for another person with whom to share their burden. Lagerwey notes that "male survivors framed their narratives in order and coherence, and often de-emphasized emotions" and that they told of "personal isolation, personal survival at any cost, ruthless competition".[28] It appears that because men had been socialized into being independent and autonomous, that these characteristics were the ones most often portrayed in their narratives. Male and female survivor accounts also represent work as a means of survival very differently. Pride in work and its impact on their identities is much more common in male writings. By contrast, female accounts have tended to be much less specific on work and how it was conducted. This suggests that work was more central to men's experiences in line with contemporaneous gendered norms. Whilst "food talk" amongst women at Auschwitz has been much analysed, Viktor Frankl also recounts men engaging in food talk. He states that the majority of prisoners, when they were working near each other and not closely watched by guards "would immediately start discussing food" asking each other about their favourite dishes. Frankl writes: "Then they would exchange recipes and plan the menu for the day when they would have a reunion—the day in a distant future when they would be liberated and return home".[29]

Male memoirs have tended to underplay bonds and relationships and to emphasize instead examples of individual valour, strength or autonomy. Bruno Bettelheim has explained his view on the subject of survival in the camps as follows: "Survival in the camps—this cannot be stressed enough—depended foremost on luck … While nothing one could do could assure survival, and while chances for it at best were extremely slim, one could increase them through correctly assessing one's situation and taking advantage of opportunities; in short, through acting independently and with courage, decision, and conviction, all of which depended on the measure of autonomy one had managed to retain".[30] Dutch survivor, Loius de Wijze, underlined the need for care of the self in his memoirs as well: "Everyone lives for himself. Our one and all-encompassing credo is: Survive! Between the outer limits of life and death, previous values and norms lose their meaning, and our spiritual baggage gradually erodes. The only norm that counts is 'I'".[31]

It is important to note and add, however, that references to close relationships do appear in male narratives and there are instances of male writing that show men behaving in ways that differed from expected male gender norms. Primo Levi tells of an Italian civilian worker, Lorenzo, who brought Levi "a piece of his bread and the remainder of his ration every day for six months".[32] Without Lorenzo, Levi believes that he would not have survived Auschwitz. He states that this was: "not so much for his material aid, as for his having constantly reminded me by his presence, by his natural and plain manner of being good, that there still existed a just world outside our own, something and someone still pure and whole, not corrupt, not savage … Lorenzo was a man; his humanity was pure and uncontaminated, he was outside this world of negation. Thanks to Lorenzo, I managed not to forget that I myself was a man".[33] He later describes a "tight bond of alliance" with Alberto, another prisoner.[34] Hence, social bonding was significant to male experiences, not only to female ones.

Furthermore, the testimonies of other male survivors underline the importance of the father-son relationship to survival, when fathers and sons had managed to avoid separation and stay together. Henry Wermuth recalls: "The presence of my father was, without a doubt, a major factor in my survival; but it also meant that I did not have, nor was I in need of, any other social contacts".[35] This suggests that the father-son relationship was so powerful, that it completely replaced the necessity for other bonds. On the death march from Auschwitz, Elie Wiesel recalls his momentary desire to fall out of line, to the edge of the road and die: "My father's presence was the only thing that stopped me … He was running at my side, out of breath, at the end of his strength, at his wit's end. I had no right to let myself die. What would he do without me? I was his only support".[36] Wiesel shows here the significance of his relationship with his father and their mutual support.

The death marches have been described in many memoirs and testimonies as driving Holocaust victims to increasingly desperate behavior. Hans Winterfeld recalls the death march from Auschwitz: "Normally, one could talk to the other prisoners, but when food was distributed, they began to look and act like lunatics: their eyes stared rigidly at the ladle or at the arm that distributed the bread. When they received their ration, they constantly watched other prisoners to check that nobody had been given more. It was completely irrelevant what kind of person it was: uneducated and primitive, or educated and intellectually superior. I often wondered how cultivated human beings could behave like animals".[37]

Indeed, Levi comments too on the aim of the Nazi camps to "reduce us to beasts". But, he writes, "we must not become beasts; that even in this place one can survive, and therefore one must want to survive, to tell the story, to bear witness; and that to survive we must force ourselves to save at least the skeleton, the scaffolding, the form of civilization".[38] His desire to survive was thus underpinned by his desire to bear witness. He was determined to defend his strength and dignity for this purpose. As Eva Kolinsky has noted, many other survivors defined their own personal code of behavior in a bid to maintain a sense of their own self-value.[39] In Levi's *Survival in Auschwitz*, for example, Steinlauf insisted on washing, even though washing did not get him clean, because it enabled him to keep his dignity and demonstrated his refusal to become a beast, thus undermining German goals. This type of behavior is also evident in the writings of female survivors. Men's experiences bore both similarities and differences to those of women. Their responses to them were equally complex, nuanced and influenced by normative gendered expectations. The determination to survive and their capacity for survival was based on whatever resources they could use—including supportive relationships, ingrained cultural norms, the attempt to maintain dignity, stealing or procuring food, or sheer luck.

Women's Experiences and Behavior at Auschwitz

Female prisoners at Auschwitz had to deal with a number of problems that affected them specifically as women. Their testimonies highlight the traumas of losing their sense of their physical selves. One significant aspect of this was the SS camp ritual of shaving the inmates on their arrival. Having their heads shaved was a much more traumatic and degrading experience for women than for men. Whilst all prisoners were deeply shamed by this measure, for women this was a blow to their feelings of femininity and to their sexual identity. Livia Bitton-Jackson writes of newly arrived female prisoners having their hair shaved from their heads, under their arms and in the pubic area: "The shaving of hair has a startling effect. The absence of hair transforms individual women into like bodies. Indistinguishable … We become a monolithic mass".[40] Rena Gelissen describes the humiliation of being "naked in front of strangers" and of being shaved by male prisoners: "They shear our heads, arms; even our pubic hair is discarded just as quickly and cruelly as the rest of the hair on our bodies".[41] Another survivor, Isabelle Choko, in her memoir, also relates that, at Auschwitz, "at the precise moment my head was shaved, I ceased to exist as a human being".[42] Rose Meth, born in 1925 into a Hasidic family in Zator, Poland, who was deported to Auschwitz in August 1943, gives a similar account of her arrival: "I can't begin to describe the shock and the humiliation. We were sheltered children. They made us undress completely in front of the Nazi soldiers. We wanted to die. They shaved our heads. They shaved all our hair, everywhere. We were given numbers".[43]

The tattooing of their camp numbers was described by survivor Eva Schloss as "part of the process intended to strip me of my pride and identity. When I was marched away from Auschwitz railway station, I left the girlish Eva Geiringer and her dreams, behind".[44] Olga Lengyel describes the degrading and humiliating treatment of female inmates on their arrival, having to undress and undergo physical examinations, before being allowed to dress in camp clothes. Gelissen mentions the gynaecological examination for new female prisoners as well. These gynaecological examinations were invasive and humiliating for female prisoners. They were painful and traumatic experiences recounted with much horror by female survivors.

The distribution of random and unfitting clothes had a significant impact on women as new camp inmates. Their individuality and their sense of identity were entirely removed by all of these actions. Gelissen recounts her feelings of despair when she noticed her "lovely white boots with their red trim" being worn by an SS woman.[45] Lengyel describes the "bizarre rags that were handed out for underwear" that were "not white or any other colour, but worn out pieces of coarse dusting cloth".[46] In addition, tattered dresses were randomly distributed with no regard to size. In terms of the emotions these circumstances generated, Lengyel states: "In spite of the tragedy of our situation, we could not help but laugh as we saw others so ridiculously outfitted. After a while, it was a struggle to overcome the disgust we felt for our companions, and for ourselves".[47] A similar reaction to their "grey, sack-like dresses" is described by Bitton-Jackson, as she compares herself after her arrival at Auschwitz with inmates who had been there longer: "The strange creatures we saw as we entered the camp, the shaven, grey-cloaked bunch who ran to the barbed wire to stare at us, we are them! We look exactly like them. Same bodies, same dresses, same blank stares. They, too, must have arrived from home recently. They, too, were ripe women and young girls, bewildered and bruised. They too longed for dignity and compassion. And they, too, were transformed into figures of contempt instead".[48]

After the initial shock and horror engendered by their new appearance, some women attempted to ameliorate their outfits. In the space of twenty-four hours, they adjusted their ill-fitting garments to their bodies and sewed up the holes, "using needles made out of wooden splinters and threads pulled out of the one blanket allocated to them".[49] Isabelle Choko describes feeling a need to hide her shaved head and tie up her dress which was much too large: "I ripped a piece from the bottom of my pale pink shirt to tie around my head like a turban and another piece to roll into a belt. My mother helped me since I had no mirror … Other women, too, were trying to 'look human' again".[50]

Menstruation became a significant biological problem that women had to face in Auschwitz-Birkenau. Bitton-Jackson describes a girl in front of her at roll call: "the blood simply flows down her legs".[51] When they menstruated, women and girls had no way of stopping the flow of blood, which was extremely difficult and humiliating. Gelissen recalls her first period at Auschwitz: "I scour the ground for anything that might help me hinder the flow. There is nothing".[52] Over time, in the abnormal circumstances in which they were living, women stopped menstruating. Whilst this removed the problem of humiliation, the cessation of menstruation created other concerns for many women. Some felt a loss of their identity as women, whilst others feared they would never be able to have children. Lengyel attributes the ceasing of menstruation partly to "the constant anguish under which we lived", but she also suggests a "mysterious powder" or "substance" mixed into all the food given to the inmates.[53] Gelissen writes similarly that "most of the girls and women in camp" lost their periods.[54] Female inmates specifically faced these biological and psychological issues relating to menstruation and its cessation.[55]

In addition, some girls and women were subjected to appalling violence, as well as sexual abuse and violations. In her desperation for some string to use as shoelaces, Gisella Perl hoped to exchange her bread ration for a piece of string from a Polish male prisoner: "I stopped beside him, held out my bread and asked him, begged him to give me a piece of string in exchange for it. He looked me over from head to foot, carefully, then grabbed me by the shoulder and hissed in my ear: 'I don't want your bread … You can keep your bread … I will give you a piece of string but first I want you … you … ' For a second I didn't understand what he meant … His hand, filthy with the human excrement he was working in, reached out for my womanhood, rudely, insistently. The next moment I was running, running away from that man, away from the indignity that had been inflicted on me, forgetting about the string, about the shoes, about everything but the sudden realization of how deeply I had sunk".[56] After this shameful experience, she was determined to maintain her dignity in the face of every humiliation, every torture. Women's vulnerability, their fear of rape and their reactions to humiliation is amply evident in the narratives of female survivors. For example, the fear of rape and the theme of humiliation run through the account of Judith Magyar Isaacson, a Hungarian Jew, deported to Auschwitz in 1944.[57] Schloss too writes: "it seems hard to believe that the German SS guards would take a sexual interest in the starving, dirty, ragged women they were ruling over—but some of them did".[58] Hence, whilst rape was not official policy because Nazi racial laws prohibited German sexual relations with Jewish women, there is evidence that at least some German guards and others, including Kapos and other prisoners, raped Jewish women. Women and young girls were subjected to traumatic sexual abuse and violations, often from their very earliest moments at Auschwitz, and whilst this was difficult to narrate, for many it was an unforgettable humiliation.[59]

In Millu's first narrative in *Smoke over Birkenau*, a young inmate, Lili, was the victim of the cruelty of her Kapo, Mia, whose "frustration and impatience" turned to anger if her boyfriend was late or failed to turn up: "A violent shove sent my head slamming against the iron bar".[60] This was commonplace behaviour on the part of the Kapo. Lili's position was invidious and fraught with tension. She was a pretty, young and gracious girl and because of this, she was favoured by the Kapo who gave her good work—sewing. However, Lili was in a very dangerous situation, as Mia's boyfriend liked her. On one occasion, Mia's boyfriend, who had drunk too much, began overtly flirting with Lili and kissing her, "his lips brushing her neck". This proved catastrophic for Lili, as Mia was furious and savagely attacked her, resulting in terrible injuries.[61] She called Lili "a whore" and subsequently ensured that she was selected for the gas chambers.[62]

In another of Millu's narratives, Zina, accused of being "a whore" was violently attacked by an old camp guard: "… raising his club, he began beating Zina furiously on the chest and shoulders. The blows were so fierce that in her frail state she collapsed instantly. He kept on beating her as she lay there on the ground".[63] Bitton-Jackson describes violence from the moment of her arrival at Auschwitz and numerous episodes of random punishments and beatings.[64] Lengyel similarly details the threat of violence from the outset and refers to many occasions on which she and other female inmates were subjected to violence and physical abuse.[65]

Gelissen's writing too mentions many incidences of extreme violence and brutality directed against female prisoners.[66] Apart from such examples of random punishment and brutality, Lengyel further describes "medical" experimentation on female inmates, including experiments in relation to menstruation, subjection to artificial insemination, injection with sex hormones, sterilization and gynaecological experiments.[67] Gelissen's narrative makes reference to such experiments as well.[68] Sterilization experiments on women at Auschwitz took place in Block 10, a place described by Robert Lifton as "quintessential Auschwitz".[69] The notorious Block 10 induced fear and terror in female victims.

At Auschwitz, women tried to adjust and adapt to their changing circumstances. They used resourcefulness, homemaking skills and cleaning in order to establish some modicum of control over themselves and their space. For instance, they tried to clean themselves and to rid themselves of lice. Lengyel recounts how they "passed the single scrubbing brush to one another with a firm determination to resist the dirt and the lice. That was our only way of waging war against the parasites, against our jailers, and against every force that made us victims".[70] Gelissen too writes of how the women engaged in a "ritual cleansing" of lice.[71] Furthermore, there was a need for cooperation in extreme circumstances and self-preservation through mutual help, which has been highlighted, in particular, in many female survivor testimonies. At Auschwitz, women used different strategies to cope with their situation, such as the formation of ersatz families and "camp sister" relationships, the sharing of recipes, cooking methods and memories of Sabbath and Festival meals.

Millu writes of Gustine, a prisoner at Auschwitz from Holland, who talked about her home, "for hours on end", as a coping strategy: "the fire sparkling in the big blue tiled stove and her mother preparing the snacks for tea, the smell of fresh bread, the most comforting smell in the world, and the butter, the ruby-hued currant marmalade, the gaily coloured curtains on the windows. Oh, beloved home, the most cherished place on earth!".[72] Gelissen recalls the Sunday morning picnics with cheese Danish pastries that she used to have with her sister Danka: "Around noon we open Mama's Danishes, still warm from the oven, or maybe the sun kept them warm, and eat them while languishing in the sun … How I miss… eating Mama's homemade sweets".[73] Lengyel talks of reminiscing and reciting poetry as coping strategies, "to escape the frightful present".[74] Furthermore, Gisella Perl recalls: "Later, as we came to know one another better, we invented games and recited poetry to keep our minds off the sordid present". Other evenings, they played "another game, which spread from block to block until every woman in Auschwitz played it enthusiastically. We called the game 'I am a lady' … I am a lady—I said one night—a lady doctor in Hungary. It is morning, a beautiful sunny morning and I feel too lazy to work. I ring for my assistant and tell her to send the patients away, for I am not going to my office today … What should I do with myself? Go shopping? Go to the hairdresser? Meet my friends at the café? Maybe I'll do some shopping. I haven't had a new dress, a new hat in weeks …".[75] The references in this game are clearly gender specific to the women's previous experiences and social construction.

Moreover, kitchen memories reminded women of their former position in their families and communities and reaffirmed their own sense of essential value. Women used conversation as a distraction from their circumstances and talked about their "old" lives. This reminded them of their strengths as nurturers, homemakers and cooks. It allowed them to maintain a sense of identity. Food preparation was part of the ritual of living in family, social and community life, as well as Jewish festivals, and it defined the former status of many women. The sharing of recipes and cooking tips was significant for women psychologically because it indicated a commitment to the future.[76] In addition, they fantasized about the future, a time when the war would be over, as a coping strategy.[77] These types of themes are common in female survivor testimonies and narratives. Furthermore, by describing the food they once cooked to another inmate, "they shared a familiar experience and connected to another person".[78]

Female narratives often describe how inmates shared food with each other. For example, Lili shared a "precious gift" of "some cabbage leaves" with two of her fellow prisoners.[79] Bitton-Jackson recalls smuggling potatoes and how her mother saved hers in order to use them in place of candles on Friday night: "one evening while shoveling snow in the yard, we discover mounds in which potatoes are stored for the winter. We quickly dig them up and, hiding them under our dresses, smuggle enough potatoes into the camp to allow each inmate at least one potato. We wash them in the toilet and eagerly await our bedtime … Noiselessly, with utmost care, so as not to attract the attention of the guard on patrol we bite into the hard, delightful skin of the raw potato. But Mummy saves her potato. 'For Sabbath lights' she says. Friday at sunset Mummy kindles her Sabbath lights in the carved-out potato halves using oil smuggled from the factory and threads from our blankets for wicks".[80] This example illustrates not only the resourcefulness of these women, but also the determination of Bitton-Jackson's mother to try to continue her tradition of lighting candles for the Sabbath. She was caught but not punished on this occasion. Bitton-Jackson goes on to relate how they subsequently saved "potatoes for a Hanukkah celebration with lights". With care and secrecy, they lit "Hannukah oil lamps in carved-out potato halves" and succeeded in kindling the lights for eight nights without being caught.[81] Millu writes of maintaining rituals and the celebration of Hannukah as well.[82] These attempts by women to uphold religious traditions were valuable coping strategies.

Family relationships were of great significance where mothers and daughters, or sisters, could stay together, as illustrated by Gelissen's account. She was fiercely protective of her sister Danka and tried to shield her as much as possible. Rena's promise after all was to protect and look after her sister—indeed, her determination to bring her sister back alive was her *raison d'être* and motivation for survival: "My one great feat in life, my fate, is to survive this thing and return triumphant with my sister to our parents' house … I will succeed because I have no other choice. Failure does not even occur to me. We may die in the interim—death cannot be avoided here—but even that will not dissuade me from my sole purpose in life. Nothing else matters but these four things: be with Danka, be invisible, be alert, be numb".[83] She looked after Danka when she had scabies and procured lotion to treat it for her and cared for her when she became ill with malaria.[84] In Danka, Rena found her "reason and will to live".[85] Gelissen kept up her sister's spirits when she lost the will to go on and swore to her that if Danka was ever selected for the gas chambers that she would accompany her.[86] Ultimately, they both survived. Millu's writing also notes the strength of feeling between sisters in the camp and that most of them loved each other "with an almost morbid attachment".[87]

Moreover, even in ersatz family relationships, such as those of "camp sisters", social bonding, in groups of two or more, helped women to keep up their struggle to survive. Rose Meth describes her ersatz camp sister: "Estusia and I were like sisters. People never knew that we were not really sisters. As soon as all my real sisters were taken away from me and Estusia saw my condition, she helped me a lot morally. She told me I must be strong and survive".[88] Such surrogate families cared for each other and improved women's chances of survival. Lucie Adelsberger describes her camp family in which her "daughters" provided her with clothing and food whenever they could. She states that members of such families often put their own lives at risk and that even for those who did not survive:

"the friendship and love of a camp family eased the horror of their miserable end".[89] This kind of bonding was not exclusive to women, but it appears to have been both much more prevalent among women and to have been expressed and reported more in testimonies written by women, including those of Isabella Leitner and Charlotte Delbo.[90] Female prisoners offered each other support, comfort and solidarity. Women were able to "transform their habits of raising children or their experience of nurturing into the care of the nonbiological family".[91] As isolation and the separation of families was deliberately imposed by the camp system, the creation of new "families" helped inmates by giving them a system of mutual support and a source of material and psychological strength in place of their real families.[92]

There has been a taboo in treating women who behaved differently from perceived gender norms and expectations, largely reflecting a reluctance to deal with a painful or difficult subject.[93] Yet, examples of such behavior in female narratives do exist. Fanya Gottesfeld Heller states in her memoirs that: "The unrelenting fear of death and gnawing pain of hunger led to acts of desperation among many who survived; some stole, others lied and schemed. Still others took comfort in intimate relationships that might be considered illicit or misguided in ordinary times. It was not all pure and righteous, but it happened".[94] Gendered norms about expected types of female conduct such as social bonding and nurturing were contradicted by examples of spiteful and hateful behavior. Millu describes how physical hardship and deprivation produced competitive, self-interested behavior—women who were "ready to pummel and trample over the others in order to get in first and grab a good place".[95] Bitton-Jackson describes an episode when a bed collapsed onto her very weak mother. The other inmates did not care or help as they were awaiting the distribution of food—"they laugh at my alarm … Not one of them pays attention to my frantic pleas".[96] Millu describes the "morbid curiosity" of the women at Birkenau at the selections for the gas chambers. They craned their necks to see "like spectators at a sports match".[97] Such behaviour was at variance with gendered norms about women's conduct.

Millu describes the transformative and destructive effect of Birkenau on the identity and behavior of its prisoners over time. The inmates taunted and abused each other. She writes: "I recoiled in shame from their weary eyes gleaming with malice and their pinched mouths spewing out vulgarities, sick at the sight of what our misery had made of us … Soon I would be a true daughter of the *Lager* [camp] … I would be no different from the old-timers".[98] Lengyel too states that "it seemed as though the Germans constantly sought to pit us against each other, to make us competitive, spiteful and hateful" and notes how even "the most peaceful souls were occasionally seized with a desire to strangle their neighbours" in the overcrowded conditions in the bunks, through exasperation at their circumstances.[99]

Sexuality and sexual conduct could become significant at times in the camp. It is hard to piece together these aspects of camp life for two main reasons. Firstly, they were taboo subjects, which have only recently been discussed in the historical literature.[100] Secondly, it is difficult for survivors to narrate sexual trauma.[101] However, the subjects of lesbianism, the granting of sexual favours and life in the camp brothel all deserve attention. Lesbianism was a taboo form of behavior and references to it are uncommon in survivor narratives. Vera Laska has noted the lack of available documentation on lesbians: "Women's memoirs say little on the subject, either because they considered the subject indelicate or because they chose to remain in the closet. The women who were lesbians when they entered the camps or became so afterward are hidden behind a double veil of hypocrisy and silence".[102] However, there is some mention of lesbianism. Lengyel distinguishes between "three categories" of lesbians: the first group, who were "lesbians by instinct"; the second group, who "because of the abnormal conditions, suffered changes in their sexual viewpoint" and often "yielded under the pressure of necessity"; and the third group, who "discovered their lesbian predilections through an association with corruption". She goes on to describe lesbian "orgies".[103] In Millu's book, there is a reference to a "most evil Kapo" with a "black triangle" on her shirt, portrayed as "fat and sturdy".[104] There is an implicit connection drawn between her appearance, lesbianism and "evil" character. There is reference to another lesbian Kapo, the "Kapo of the dressmakers renowned for her lesbian predilections".[105] The "heavy, resounding footsteps" of the "formidable" Frau Gotti could be heard every morning as "she came to wake her lover with a long kiss as well as a little snack". The suggestion here is not only of lesbian stereotyping, but also of the exchange of sexual favours for food. Furthermore, our understanding of lesbianism is made more difficult because lesbian relationships were hard to identify and distinguish from the numerous close friendships that women formed at Auschwitz and other camps.[106]

Survivor narratives refer to the granting of sexual favours by some girls and women in exchange for food, other items or "camp luxuries".

This was commonplace and formed a significant aspect of what women found to be so humiliating and degrading about the camp experience. Lengyel describes an episode when Tadek, a carpenter who came to mend the bunks, was friendly and attentive to her. She describes him as handsome, tall and smiling. He gave her food, but then made it clear that he expected sexual favours in return.[107] Some women adopted the survival strategy of flirting, bantering or acting coy with men and performing sexual favours, as a way of gaining extra food or luxuries. The impact of the *Puffkommando* (brothel) on different women was significant. There was a marked distinction of attitude between those women inside the brothel and those outside. On one level, there was the moral stance of rejection of a woman for prostituting herself, yet at the same time, there was some jealousy and resentment about the "luxuries" that life in the brothel afforded. References to these are fewer and harder to hard, but they do exist and demonstrate behavior that deviated from perceived attitudes and conceptions about the appropriate conduct of women. Indeed, in the historiography of both women's experiences of the Third Reich and the concentration camps in general, brothels have been mentioned only comparatively recently as these fields have developed to encompass them.[108] Annette Timm has noted that whilst some women were forced into service as prostitutes in the concentration camps, others "chose this option as a way to prolong their lives".[109] Some women welcomed the chance to work in the camp brothel as conditions were better and they had a temporary reprieve from the possibility of being selected for the gas chambers.[110]

Pregnancies had to be concealed at Auschwitz, because all pregnant women were sent immediately to the gas chamber. Pregnant women hid their condition for as long as possible, for "the camp was no maternity ward".[111] Despite the attempts of German officers to trick women into revealing their pregnancies, Lengyel writes: "Incredible as it may seem, some succeeded in concealing their conditions to the last moment, and the deliveries took place secretly in the barracks".[112] At the infirmary at Auschwitz, as soon as a baby was born, both mother and infant were sent to the gas chambers. In order to save the lives of the mothers, Lengyel describes how newborn infants were killed: "And so, the Germans succeeded in making murderers of us … The only meager consolation is that by these murders we saved the mothers".[113]

Gisella Perl, a Jewish doctor from Hungary, who was interned in Auschwitz, also recounts killing newborn children in order "to save the life of the mother".[114] "It was up to me to save the life of the mothers, if there was no other way, than by destroying the life of their unborn children". She recalls that the procedure took place: "In the dark, always hurried, in the midst of filth and dirt. After the child had been delivered, I quickly bandaged the mother's abdomen and sent her back to work". She states that: "I delivered women pregnant in the eighth, seventh, sixth, fifth month, always in a hurry, always with my five fingers, in the dark, under terrible conditions". She concludes: "No one will ever know what it meant to me to destroy these babies. After years and years of medical practice, childbirth was still to me the most beautiful, the greatest miracle of nature. I loved those newborn babies not as a doctor but as a mother and it was again and again my own child whom I killed to save the life of a woman ... and if I had not done it, both mother and child would have been cruelly murdered".[115]

Conclusion

Gender provides a useful tool for interpreting the experiences and behavior of Holocaust victims. Gender is a characteristic of all human experience. Both masculinity and femininity have been socially constructed and shaped by historical circumstances and expectations. Moving away from universal interpretations, both women's experiences as specifically female and men's experiences are significant to our understanding. The field of Holocaust studies that was gender neutral until the 1980s now includes a substantial literature on gender. Furthermore, a comparatively recent, yet substantial output of memoirs and testimonies by female Holocaust survivors, has ensured that women's voices are no longer unheard. This allows us to consider the impact of trauma on women as well as on men. As Kremer notes, female writings have shown that "representation of history through the lens of male hegemony is incomplete".[116] These developments in the historiography have meant that scholars are now in a much better position to comprehend the diversity and complexity of the experiences of Holocaust victims. In the end, both male and female survivors state that luck played a large part in their survival. For example, Eva Schloss, with a similar view on this to Bruno Bettelheim, writes "a large part of my survival was down to pure luck".[117]

Men's and women's traumatic experiences of the Holocaust were not identical, but as Myrna Goldenberg has suggested, they were "different horrors" within the "same hell".[118] Their testimonies illustrate the complexities of their emotional responses to trauma and how they have remembered and written about it. The experiences and memories of their trauma were subjective and distinctive, in certain respects, along gendered lines. During their imprisonment at Auschwitz, women had to opt for agency and make choices in a variety of ways that were distinctive from those made by men. Yet, Frankl notes that for men too, the "choice of action" existed, even in the face of the terrible privations they faced at Auschwitz.[119] In the end, all Jews were equally destined for death, but there were differences on the road to that destination for men and women. The use of survivor memoirs and testimonies enables us to understand the subjectivities of the traumatic experiences faced by prisoners at Auschwitz. The lens of gender was significant both in the experiencing of these events and in the reporting or narrating of them. An analysis of male and female testimonies of trauma adds an important angle to our knowledge and understanding of this dark chapter in human history. It also suggests a way forward in the scholarship of trauma more generally—the development of a history of trauma along gendered lines—especially in circumstances of other wars and genocides, as well as how and why memories and representations of trauma change over time.

Notes

1. This literature includes: M. Heinemann, *Gender and Destiny: Women Writers and the Holocaust* (London: Greenwood Press, 1986); R. Linden, *Making Stories, Making Selves: Feminist Reflections on the Holocaust* (Columbus: Ohio State University Press, 1993); J. Baskin (ed.), *Women of the Word: Jewish Women and Jewish Writing* (Detroit: Wayne State University Press, 1994); E. Fuchs (ed.), *Women and the Holocaust: Narrative and Representation* (Oxford: University of America Press, 1999); S. Lillian Kremer, *Women's Holocaust Writing: Memory and Imagination* (Lincoln: University of Nebraska Press, 1999); S. Horowitz, "Gender, Genocide and Jewish Memory", *Prooftexts: A Journal of Jewish Literary History*, Vol. 20, No. 1 (2000), 158–90; A. Reading, *The Social Inheritance of the Holocaust: Gender, Culture and Memory* (Basingstoke: Palgrave Macmillan, 2002); Z. Waxman, *Writing the Holocaust: Identity, Testimony, Representation* (Oxford: Oxford University Press, 2006).
2. See A. Allen, "The Holocaust and the Modernization of Gender: A Historiographical Essay", *Central European History*, Vol. 30, No. 3 (1997), 349–64. However, Allen's essay mainly addresses women's

roles as perpetrators or bystanders. It does not deal with the subject of Jewish victims.

3. Y. Bauer, *Rethinking the Holocaust* (New Haven: Yale University Press, 2001), 167.
4. L. Weitzman and D. Ofer, "The Role of Gender in the Holocaust", in D. Ofer and L. Weitzman (eds), *Women in the Holocaust* (New Haven: Yale University Press, 1998), 13.
5. P. Bos, "Women and the Holocaust: Analysing Gender Difference", in E. Baer and M. Goldenberg (eds), *Experience and Expression: Women, the Nazis, and the Holocaust* (Detroit: Wayne State University Press, 2003), 23–50.
6. Ibid., 25.
7. Ibid., 33.
8. L. Langer, "Interpreting Survivor Testimony", in B. Lang (ed.), *Writing and the Holocaust* (New York: Holmes and Meier, 1988), 39–40. See also, L. Langer, *Versions of Survival: The Holocaust and the Human Spirit* (Albany: Suny Press, 1982). On oral testimony, see also L. Langer, *Holocaust Testimonies: The Ruin of Memory* (New Haven: Yale University Press, 1991); A. Rubin and H. Greenspan, *Reflections: Auschwitz, Memory, and a Life Recreated* (St. Paul: Paragon House, 2006); J. Matthias (ed.), *Approaching an Auschwitz Survivor: Holocaust Testimony and its Transformation* (Oxford: Oxford University Press, 2009); H. Greenspan, *On Listening to Holocaust Survivors: Beyond Testimony* (Westport: Praeger, 1998), especially 209–11; on survivors and their listeners, see 41–73.
9. Langer, *Holocaust Testimonies.*
10. Cited in J. Young, *Writing and Rewriting the Holocaust: Narrative and the Consequences of Interpretation* (Bloomington and Indianapolis: Indiana University Press, 1990), 29.
11. P. Bartrop, *Surviving the Camps: Unity in Adversity During the Holocaust* (New York and Oxford: University Press of America, 2000).
12. Langer, "Interpreting Survivor Testimony", 33.
13. Waxman, *Writing the Holocaust*, 128.
14. Ibid., 3.
15. Bartrop, *Surviving the Camps*, 47.
16. Ibid.
17. L. Pine, *Nazi Family Policy, 1933–1945* (Oxford and New York: Berg, 1997), 149–75.

18. T. Des Pres, *The Survivor: An Anatomy of Life in the Death Camps* (New York: Oxford University Press, 1976), 38.
19. S. Felman and D. Laub, *Testimony: Crises of Witnessing in Literature, Psychoanalysis, and History* (New York: Routledge, 1992), 204.
20. B. Gurewitsch (ed.), *Mothers, Sisters, Resisters: Oral Histories of Women Who Survived the Holocaust* (Tuscaloosa: University of Alabama Press, 1998).
21. A. Hardmann, "Women and the Holocaust", *Holocaust Educational Trust, Research Papers*, vol. 1, no. 3 (London, 2000), 12.
22. S. Horowitz, "Memory and Testimony of Women Survivors of Nazi Germany", in J. Baskin (ed.), *Women of the Word: Jewish Women and Jewish Writing* (Detroit: Wayne State University Press, 1994), 265.
23. Hardmann, "Women and the Holocaust", 15.
24. Z. Waxman, "Unheard Stories: Reading Women's Holocaust Testimonies", *The Jewish Quarterly*, Vol. 47, No. 177 (2000), 53.
25. Waxman, *Writing the Holocaust*, 186.
26. M. Berger, B. Wallis and S. Watson (eds), *Constructing Masculinity* (New York: Routledge, 1995). On the social construction of masculinity, see also R. Connell, *Masculinities* (Cambridge: Polity Press, 1995).
27. V. Frankl, *Man's Search for Meaning* (London: Simon and Schuster, 2004), 86.
28. M. Lagerwey, *Reading Auschwitz* (London: Sage, 1998), 75.
29. Frankl, *Man's Search for Meaning*, 41.
30. B. Bettelheim, *Surviving the Holocaust* (London: Fontana, 1986), 100–101.
31. L. de Wijze, *Only My Life: A Survivor's Story*, (New York: St. Martin's Press, 1997), 67.
32. P. Levi, *If this is a Man* (London: Abacus Books, 2000), 148.
33. Ibid., 150.
34. Ibid., 168.
35. H. Wermuth, *Breathe Deeply My Son*, (London: Vallentine Mitchell, 1993), 139.
36. E. Wiesel, *Night: with Connections* (London: Holt, Rinehart and Winston, 1988), 92–3.
37. Cited in E. Kolinsky, *After the Holocaust: Jewish Survivors in Germany after 1945* (London: Pimlico, 2004), 27.
38. Levi, *If This is a Man*, 58.
39. Kolinsky, *After the Holocaust*, 14.

40. L. Bitton-Jackson, *I Have Lived a Thousand Years* (London: Simon and Schuster, 1999), 75.
41. R. Gelissen, *Rena's Promise: A Story of Sisters in Auschwitz* (London: Weidenfeld and Nicolson, 1996), 139.
42. I. Choko, in I. Choko, F. Irwin, L. Kahana-Aufleger, M. Kalina and J. Lipski, *Stolen Youth: Five Women's Survival in the Holocaust* (New York and Jerusalem: Yad Vashem, 2005), 42.
43. Cited in C. Rittner and J. Roth (eds), *Different Voices: Women and the Holocaust* (New York: Paragon House, 1993) 136.
44. E. Schloss, *After Auschwitz* (London: Hodder and Stoughton, 2013), 114.
45. Gelissen, *Rena's Promise*, 67.
46. O. Lengyel, *Five Chimneys: The Story of Auschwitz* (Chicago: Academy Chicago Publishers, 1995), 29.
47. Ibid., 30.
48. Bitton-Jackson, *I Have Lived a Thousand Years*, 77.
49. R. Bondy, "Women in Theresienstadt and the Family Camp in Birkenau", in Ofer and Weitzman (eds), *Women in the Holocaust*, 323.
50. Choko, *Stolen Youth*, 48–9.
51. Bitton-Jackson, *I Have Lived a Thousand Years*, 92.
52. Gelissen, *Rena's Promise*, 81.
53. Lengyel, *Five Chimneys*, 98–9.
54. Gelissen, *Rena's Promise*, 139.
55. N. Tec, *Resilience and Courage: Women, Men and the Holocaust* (New Haven and London: Yale University Press, 2003), 168–9.
56. Cited in Rittner and Roth (eds), *Different Voices*, 109.
57. J. Isaacson, *Seed of Sarah* (Chicago: Univerity of Illinois Press, 1991).
58. Schloss, *After Auschwitz*, 127–8.
59. V. Laska, cited in Rittner and Roth (eds), *Different Voices*, 266–7.
60. L. Millu, *Smoke over Birkenau* (Evanston: Northwestern University Press, 1997), 22–3.
61. Ibid., 39–41.
62. Ibid., 47.
63. Ibid., 138.
64. Bitton-Jackson, *I Have Lived a Thousand Years*, 73, 99, 127 and 140.
65. Lengyel, *Five Chimneys*, 26, 108, 131 and 156.

66. Gelissen, *Rena's Promise*, 75, 83, 90–1, 115, 144–5, 166–7 and 172.
67. Lengyel, *Five Chimneys*, 199 and 186–93.
68. Gelissen, *Rena's Promise*, 148 and 183.
69. R. Lifton, *The Nazi Doctors: Medical Killing and the Psychology of Genocide* (London: Macmillan, 1986), 270.
70. Lengyel, *Five Chimneys*, 135.
71. Gelissen, *Rena's Promise*, 80.
72. Millu, *Smoke over Birkenau*, 155.
73. Gelissen, *Rena's Promise*, 225.
74. Lengyel, *Five Chimneys*, 72.
75. Cited in Rittner and Roth (eds), *Different Voices*, 109.
76. M. Goldenberg, "Memoirs of Auschwitz Survivors: The Burden of Gender", in Ofer and Weitzman (eds), *Women in the Holocaust*, 335. See also, C. de Silva (ed.), *In Memory's Kitchen: Recipes from Terezin*, Introduction by Michael Berenbaum (Northvale and London: Rowman and Littlefield, 1996).
77. Goldenberg, "Memoirs of Auschwitz Survivors: The Burden of Gender", 62–3, 122 and 148.
78. M. Goldenberg, "Food Talk: Gendered Responses to Hunger in the Concentration Camps", in Baer and Goldenberg (eds), *Experience and Expression*, 171.
79. Millu, *Smoke over Birkenau*, 29. On sharing food, see also 57.
80. Bitton-Jackson, *I Have Lived a Thousand Years*, 153.
81. Ibid., 154.
82. Millu, *Smoke over Birkenau*, 68–9.
83. Gelissen, *Rena's Promise*, 101.
84. Ibid., 127–8 and 154–62.
85. Ibid., 71. On this, see also 52, 72, 73, 75, 99, and 101.
86. Ibid., 124–5.
87. Millu, *Smoke over Birkenau*, 151.
88. Cited in Rittner and Roth (eds), *Different Voices*, 140.
89. L. Adelsberger, *Auschwitz: A Doctor's Story* (London: Northeastern, 1996), 98–100.
90. I. Leitner, *Fragments of Isabella: A Memoir of Auschwitz* (New York: Dell Publishing Company, 1978), 44 and C. Delbo, *Auschwitz and After* (New York: Yale University Press, 1995), 63, 66 and 103.
91. J. Ringelheim, "Women and the Holocaust: A Reconsideration of Research", *Signs: Journal of Women in Culture and Society*, 10 (1985), 747.

92. Pine, *Nazi Family Policy*, 178.
93. On this, see L. Pine, "Gender and the Family", in D. Stone (ed.), *The Historiography of the Holocaust* (Basingstoke: Palgrave Macmillan, 2004), 371–2. See also, Hardmann, "Women and the Holocaust", 12; Waxman, "Unheard Stories", 53; Waxman, *Writing the Holocaust*, 186.
94. F. Gottesfeld Heller, *Love in a World of Sorrow: A Teenage Girl's Holocaust Memoirs* (New York: Devora Publishing Company, 2005), 10.
95. Millu, *Smoke over Birkenau*, 52.
96. Bitton-Jackson, *I Have Lived a Thousand Years*, 121.
97. Millu, *Smoke over Birkenau*, 46–7.
98. Ibid., 58. See also 65, where Millu uses the metaphor of smoke to describe how the camp transformed prisoners over time.
99. Lengyel, *Five Chimneys*, 36 and 40.
100. See D. Herzog (ed.), *Sexuality and German Fascism* (New York and Oxford: Berghahn, 2005) and D. Herzog, *Sex after Fascism: Memory and Morality in Twentieth Century Germany* (Princeton: Princeton University Press, 2005).
101. N. Shik, "Sexual Abuse of Jewish Women in Auschwitz-Birkenau", in D. Herzog (ed.), *Brutality and Desire: War and Sexuality in Europe's Twentieth Century* (Basingstoke: Palgrave Macmillan, 2009), 221–246.
102. Laska, cited in Rittner and Roth (eds), *Different Voices*, 264.
103. Ibid., 197–9.
104. Millu, *Smoke over Birkenau*, 173.
105. Ibid., 192.
106. Laska, cited in Rittner and Roth (eds), *Different Voices*, 263.
107. Lengyel, *Five Chimneys*, 60–2.
108. On this, see C. Paul, *Zwangsprostitution: Staatlich errichtete Bordelle im Nationalsozialismus* (Berlin: Hentrich, 1995), especially 13–18, 23 and 131; A. Timm, "Sex with a Purpose: Prostitution, Venereal Disease, and Militarised Masculinity in the Third Reich", in D. Herzog (ed.), *Sexuality and German Fascism* (New York and Oxford: Berghahn, 2005), 223–55; R. Sommer, "Camp Brothels: Forced Sex Labour in Nazi Concentration Camps", in Herzog (ed.), *Brutality and Desire*, 221–246.
109. Timm, "Sex with a Purpose", 247.
110. Paul, *Zwangsprostitution*, 134.

111. Lengyel, *Five Chimneys*, 116.
112. Ibid., 115.
113. Ibid., 114.
114. Cited in Rittner and Roth (eds), *Different Voices*, 114.
115. Ibid., 113–4.
116. Kremer, *Women's Holocaust Writing*, 238.
117. Schloss, *After Auschwitz*, 116.
118. M. Goldenberg, "Different Horrors, Same Hell: Women Remembering the Holocaust", in R. Gottlieb (ed.), *Thinking the Unthinkable: Meanings of the Holocaust* (New York: Paulist Press, 1990), 150–66.
119. Frankl, *Man's Search for Meaning*, 74.

CHAPTER 5

Rethinking Civilian Neuroses in the Second World War

Hazel Croft

It might be assumed that 70 years after the end of the Second World War, the issue of wartime neurosis among civilians has been settled. The narrative of civilians' psychological response to the war, set in place by Richard Titmuss' *Problems of Social Policy* published in 1950, has rarely been challenged in the subsequent historiography and memorialization of the war. Titmuss set out the thesis that the war caused few psychiatric breakdowns, and, if anything, civilians were strengthened in their psychological resolve due to wartime camaraderie, full employment, active roles in civil defense and war work.[1] Indeed, during the early years of the war, psychoanalyst Edward Glover bemoaned that psychiatric reports emphasized with "monotonous regularity" how the "incidence of 'bomb neuroses' was 'astonishingly small'".[2] Glover, however, was skeptical as to the veracity of these reports, which he described as being "quite valueless" and subject to "gross error".[3] There was no assessment of the severity of the traumatic experience, no check on patients' psychiatric history, no accurate account of the changes in the population, and "no uniformity of diagnostic approach."[4] Glover even suggested that a pre-war "mass neurosis myth", whereby psychiatrists predicted millions of psychiatric casualties had been transformed into an equally inaccurate "no neurosis" myth.[5]

H. Croft (✉)
Birkbeck College, University of London, London, UK

P. Leese, J. Crouthamel (eds.), *Traumatic Memories of the Second World War and After*, DOI 10.1007/978-3-319-33470-7_5

"The official view developed," he wrote, that "the problem of air-raid shock had solved itself."[6]

This "official" view has often been taken at face value in subsequent histories of the home front. Moreover, the psychiatric response to the war has all too often been treated as a secondary issue or as an adjunct to debates about civilian morale.[7] In 2004, a team of researchers led by historian Edgar Jones undertook a survey of government and medical literature from the war in order to reassess the incidence of civilian neurosis during the Second World War.[8] Although the study provided insights into the impact of government and medical discourses on civilian mental health, it was conducted in light of political concern about civilian reactions to terrorist attacks following 9/11 in New York in 2001 and 7/7 in London in 2005, and thus framed its findings in the context of whether morale held up. As the authors point out, however, morale was always a problematic concept. The plethora of official surveys and reports collected by the Ministry of Information and other government agencies during the first years of the war were infused with propagandistic rhetoric and "institutional bias", and often based on subjective accounts from individuals.[9] Attempts to measure civilian morale were largely concerned with assessing attitudes and behavior, with only speculative references to the collective state of mind of the civilian population.[10] Moreover, morale, however defined, cannot simply be equated with mental health, nor can it be measured and assessed in the same way.

In this chapter, I suggest that stepping outside the framework of morale can shed new light on civilian mental health during the war. Over the last three decades many scholars have begun to challenge what one historian described as the "monochrome picture" of the home front, analyzing how gender, nationality, class and race conditioned and altered civilians' experiences of the war. The work of Sonya Rose, Geoffrey Field and Amy Bell, for example, has attempted to look, in the words of Amy Bell, "beneath the veneer of public descriptions of civilian morale and steadfast national identity" to reveal complexities and nuances in civilians' responses to bombing and to government attempts to police behavior and emotions.[11] Much of the analysis of the psychological effects of the Second World War on civilians has been incorporated in wider studies of everyday life during wartime, [12] or in histories of war trauma spanning the twentieth century.[13] There has also been a substantial historical literature on the psychological effects of the war, particularly evacuation, on children. As sociologist Nikolas Rose has suggested, the war accorded a new "visibility" to the child as an object of psychiatric scrutiny.[14] In this research, however, I have focused attention on the psychiatric judgment and treatment on the adult civilians who have been less visible in the historiography of the psychological effects of the war, but who nevertheless came under the remit of the psychiatric services. My aim is not to claim that in Britain there existed a large number of psychiatric casualties that the authorities covered up, or that historians have simply failed to unearth. Nor do I suggest that civilians were suffering from a neurosis or trauma when neither psychiatrists nor civilians attached a psychiatric label to their emotional states. Rather, I examine how the "no neurosis" narrative was constructed in official government and medical discourse and the ways in which political and medical assumptions shaped and determined psychiatric practice during the war.

I begin by setting out and analyzing the political context in which government ministers, and their psychiatric advisors, decided and limited what disorders were counted as psychiatric casualties caused by the war. I move on to explore psychiatric interventions into the lives of those who had directly experienced bombing raids, focusing on the ways psychiatrists and doctors judged and treated those civilians who sought help at First Aids Posts and GP surgeries. In the final section, I analyze psychiatric practice in the more institutional setting of psychiatric outpatient clinics, drawing on the unpublished reports of the visits to the clinics by two government inspectors. Throughout, I highlight the tensions between official governmental and psychiatric discourses and patients' experiences of the traumas of war. Here it has been useful to consider Raymond Williams' concept of "structures of feeling".[15] The wartime narrative of reliance was not settled at the start of the war, but was constantly in the process of being shaped, reshaped, reiterated and resisted. Williams' concept is useful in developing an understanding of how the dominant wartime "mood" of stoical steadfastness contained within it a range of shifting and contradictory social attitudes, meanings and emotions. For Williams, "structures of feeling" could explain "meanings and values as they are actively lived and felt", and provides insights into the relationship between lived experiences with more formal belief systems.[16] Examining wartime neuroses through this framework thus provides a way in which we can begin to "get at" the multiplicity of responses to traumatic events and the differing ways civilians' articulated and expressed nervous distress during the war.

"Quieten Them Down": The Official View

During the war, whether psychiatric symptoms were attributed to the war was as much a political question as a medical or psychiatric one. In the face of the predictions of mass psychiatric casualties, the government was anxious to avoid not only civilian panic, but also the high financial costs of providing psychiatric treatment and paying out compensation claims. The experience of shell shock in the First World War, and the subsequent high levels of compensation payments for war disabilities, was still fresh in the government's memory. Indeed, the government appointed two former shell shock doctors, the neurologist Gordon Holmes and the psychiatrist Bernard Hart as official advisors. Edward Glover described these appointments as "reverting to the ideologies of the last war but one," and claimed the government had "shut the door on any prospect of systematic research on the psychology of a people at war".[17] Indeed, Holmes was renowned for his uncompromising physicalist views of mental disorder and for his unsympathetic attitude toward neurotic soldiers in the First World War.[18] Holmes and Hart both emphasized that only those civilians who were predisposed to mental disorder would break down in times of war, claiming that the number of psychiatric casualties would be dependent, "not merely on external events and forces, such as the number and size of bombs, but on the preceding mental state of the individuals concerned."[19] Moreover, they urged the government not to pay any compensation to civilians suffering from neurasthenia or other psychiatric diagnoses.[20]

The government set up a plan for what it called "authoritarian" treatment, which aimed to sift and sort patients, so that only those considered to have a long-term, pre-war mental disorder would be sent to already overcrowded mental hospitals. Emotional shock caused by air raids was to be treated as a temporary reaction to bombing, by "front-line" psychiatrists administering tea, sugar, sedatives or barbiturates to patients, and then by sending them home or evacuating them as soon as possible. The government's priorities were made clear in instructions, sent to every medical practitioner in the country, forbidding doctors from using the term "shell shock", in case it garnered too much public sympathy for the victims, and insisting that "reassurance, patriotism and a large dose of bromide should be sufficient."[21] Sir Hubert Bond from the Ministry of Pensions characterized the government's approach: "Do not talk about these things," he insisted. "Get them home at once, in the next hour if possible, and give them some drug—morphia, etc., to quieten them down."[22]

The government's priorities were made clear in its wartime legislation for civilian pension claims. For the first two years of the war, the government enacted a pension policy which meant that no civilian could claim financial compensation unless they had sustained a *physical* injury in a bombing raid. The Personal Injuries (Civilians) Act, passed in 1939, restricted all civilian claims to those who had sustained visible physical injuries which involved "damage to the tissue".[23] The legislation was designed to prevent large numbers of civilians from claiming war injury pensions. As Adair Hore, the permanent secretary at the Ministry of Pensions, explained during its drafting, the purpose of the legislation was "to eliminate the effects of shock, and cut out people who collapse when they hear a shell burst."[24] This sharp distinction between physical and psychological injuries was in some ways a return to First World War debates between commotional or psychological causes of shell shock, and reinforced ideas that physical injuries were more deserving of compensation than emotional and psychological traumas. Indeed, Percy Bolus, the medical director of the Ministry of Pensions, insisted that unless a blast caused bodily damage, such as hemorrhaging or lung collapse, symptoms of shock would only persist in those who had a constitutional weakness.[25] Although the government modified its stance in 1941, conceding that "emotional shock" could be counted as a pension-worthy physical injury even if there was not visible, physical wound, its attitude toward civilian pensions remained very restrictive.[26] Those diagnosed with "emotional shock" could only claim compensation if the shock was considered to be the result of direct exposure to a blast and after they had been admitted to a "neurosis center" in an Emergency Medical Service hospital and subject to psychiatric investigation, treatment and rehabilitation.[27] The Ministry of Pensions insisted that there would be no compensation in cases where "symptoms are induced merely by apprehension and fears occasioned by enemy activity, and which are variously diagnosed as neurasthenia, anxiety neurosis, hysteria, nervous debility, etc".[28]

Although government pension policy was undoubtedly driven by desire to minimize the financial encumbrance on the state, the exclusion of neurosis as grounds for compensation also reflected and reinforced predominant psychiatric theorizations about the causes of neurosis. Bernard Hart, one of the government's chief psychiatric advisors, argued that granting compensation would encourage individuals to "succumb" to neurosis by protecting and rewarding them for the disorder. Embedded in this view was the assumption that psychological illnesses were a form of malingering, whereby the patient attempted, consciously or unconsciously, to use the illness to gain material benefit. As Hart put it, the denial of compensation may "appear superficially to be ruthless and unfair to the individual patients", but it was, he suggested, "salutary to the patient himself, because they may save him from the miseries of a protracted and crippling illness".[29] Similarly, Aubrey Lewis, clinical director of the Maudsley Hospital, wrote to the Ministry of Pensions urging the government not to award compensation because this would only increase the numbers of patients alleging their neurosis was due to bombing. He maintained that the only cases that should qualify as civilian psychiatric casualties were those "in which some form of mental illness in a *previously healthy* person had developed *promptly* under a *near escape* from death or injury by bombing".[30]

Both the Ministry of Pensions and establishment psychiatrists maintained that the "normal" reaction of civilians to air raids was temporary emotional shock and that more protracted and serious neurotic disorders would only develop in those individuals who were viewed as being predisposed to nervous conditions or as having a "faulty" family history. Theories about predisposition were prevalent in psychiatric reports throughout the war. Edinburgh-based psychiatrist Harry Stalker, for example, argued in 1940 that neuroses would only develop in "predisposed persons" whom he judged to have "abnormal" or "grossly abnormal" personalities, which meant they could not adapt to the conditions of war.[31] Yet psychiatrists did not always spell out exactly what they meant when they described patients as being predisposed to nervous disorders—did they mean the patient had previously been diagnosed with a mental illness or did the reference to "predisposition" signify an all-encompassing "abnormal" condition of the whole person, including their social background and personality? In many wartime psychiatric reports, there was an implicit assumption that if a person had previously suffered from a nervous condition, then their wartime disorder could not have been caused by the air raids. It was thus the "abnormality" of the individual, rather than the external traumatic events of the war, which was seen as determining whether nervous states would develop into more protracted mental disorders.

This approach was illustrated in the major government-sponsored survey into neurosis in wartime, conducted by Carlos Blacker, which was published at the end of the war.[32] In the survey, Medical Officers in charge of 216 psychiatric clinics in England and Wales were asked to fill in a questionnaire. In order to determine whether psychological difficulties could definitely be attributed to the war, Blacker asked psychiatrists if their patients:

1. Suffered from a psychiatric condition before 1940. If so, the war was not considered to be the primary factor in the development of neurosis.
2. If they had been the victim of a *direct physical injury*.

This question, the report explained, aimed "at separating persons who are involved in the experience of a direct physical character such as blast or falling masonry from those who were *merely* [my emphasis] exposed to fears or to indirect stresses as are involved in life in shelters or through evacuation".[33]

Moreover, the wording of the questionnaire assumed that air raids would not be the primary cause of neurosis. As Blacker wrote when devising the questions, "The phrase 'associated with air raids' is designedly used in preference to 'caused by air raids' because, in many cases, it is doubtful the air raids are the real cause of the disability".[34] Thus in many ways the construction of the questions, and the assumptions embedded within them, prefigured the survey's main conclusion that air raids had not led to a significant rise in neuroses.

How did these assumptions about the causation of mental disorders shape psychiatric practice during the war? In the following analysis, I suggest that psychiatric practice and diagnosis was determined not only by medical assessment of patients' symptoms, but also by social and economic factors, and the moral and political stance of doctors and psychiatrists. As historian Paul Lerner has emphasized, psychiatric practice can only be understood by considering its "ever-present political and economic dimensions".[35]

Psychiatric First Aid

Civilians, who directly experienced air raids and/or witnessed the death and injury of loved ones and neighbors, and the physical destruction of homes and neighborhoods, could seek respite and help at one of the network of First Aid Posts set up in heavily bombed areas by the government and local authorities. The posts were established in makeshift accommodation, such as requisitioned school buildings, Church halls or rooms in hospitals, and were staffed mainly by A.R.P. wardens and other civil defense workers, along with volunteers from the Red Cross and St. John's Ambulance.[36] Many of the First Aid Posts also had a psychiatrist, usually from a nearby mental hospital, and a psychiatric social worker attached to them. Priority was given to treating those with physical injuries and immediate social needs, such as clothing, temporary accommodation, the salvaging of possessions and financial assistance.[37] One psychiatric social worker working in Southampton described how,

> Everyone is occupied with supplying the material needs of the population, and there is so much uncertainty, anxiety and excitement amongst those who have been rendered homeless that only the more severe forms of psychosis, mental deficiency and epilepsy show themselves.[38]

Despite the priority given to physical treatment, government figures revealed that in 1941, 700 new cases of "emotional shock" were treated every week, amounting to approximately one-fifth of all casualties treated at First Aid Posts.[39] Little is known, however, of what happened either during or after the "psychiatric first aid" administered at the posts. Henry Wilson, a psychiatrist attached to a First Aid Post in London's East End, admitted that, "in the rush of work no adequate notes of follow up of these cases, which ranged from acute emotional disturbance to hysterical paraplegia and stupor, were possible".[40]

One study traced 127 people who had been treated at a First Aid Post after a heavy raid, and who had been sent home after being diagnosed as suffering from "emotional shock". The authors found that 11 percent of these people had subsequently suffered from anxiety, 56 percent from anxiety and depression, 16 percent from depression and 16 percent from anxiety-state hysteria.[41] Of those buried alive for more than one hour during the raid, some 65 percent had suffered from either a temporary neurosis or persistent neurosis, which was serious enough for the individual to have to take extended absence from work.[42] Cases included a married woman in her mid-forties, who had been covered with debris and buried in a gas cupboard for over an hour after her home had been hit. Her son had been injured beside her. She could "scarcely sleep for weeks: and 'one worry after another' had come upon her after this—her son's injury, her husband became ill and her daughter died with TB, arranging a new house, etc.". Remarkably, the woman remained well, apart from spending a few weeks in bed because she felt "run-down".[43]

In contrast to many psychiatric studies conducted during the war, this follow-up study placed great emphasis on the "subjective nature of the experience" of air raids, and on the severity of the traumatic experience.[44] The authors concluded that factors such as abnormal constitution or personality played a part in only a minority of the cases they investigated. Moreover, the authors highlighted how social factors, such as dealing with bombed-out homes, financial strains, long working and traveling hours and a serious upset in the pattern of living, were the major factors for the persistence of neurosis.[45] Similarly, a house-to-house investigation in Bristol, conducted one month after severe bombing raids, found that one-third of the civilians interviewed were suffering from anxiety, depression and various physical illnesses (such as, gastric disorder, bladder dysfunction and menstruation problems), which the investigators attributed to the effects of bombing.[46] Those who were suffering from anxiety or related physical disorders were not being recognized, claimed the authors of the report. There was a time-lag of two to four weeks in the development of such symptoms, which often only manifested after the person had begun organizing repairs, rescuing possessions and contacting relief agencies to obtain financial help.[47] It was impossible, suggested the authors, to calculate how many people never received medical attention or who relied on tonics, alcohol, tobacco or other measures to reduce their anxieties. As the report suggested, those suffering from psychological disorders,

> are often ashamed to report their illness, and do not consult their doctor; this latter class stop working, send for a tonic from the chemist, and may stay at home for some weeks in an apathetic state.[48]

We do not know how many civilians took to their beds, or relied on alcohol, tobacco or tonics to help them get through the war. Some medical and welfare workers at the time were concerned the psychological needs of sections of the population were being overlooked by the authorities, and that psychological problems may remain latent for a period of time. Social workers working for the Mental Health Emergency Committee in Bristol, for example, worried that, "the longer term danger of breakdowns later is ignored, or not understood". Bomb victims could "live for weeks in almost impossible conditions", they noted, and thus "allow illness and nervous symptoms to go untreated and generally plant the seeds of future troubles".[49] As psychoanalyst Edward Glover reported in 1942, countless people suffering from psychological disturbances "filtered back into the general population, where they were dealt with, if at all, by local practitioners having no special psychological training".[50]

It could be very difficult for patients to admit their nervous troubles to their family doctor. Not only was the GP often a friend of the family, the GP surgery itself was still at this time largely a domestic space, situated within the doctor's home, and dominated by personalized relationship between doctor and patient.[51] This domestic set-up could make it harder for patients to admit to what might be seen as a personal failing, especially in the context of the cultivation of an "ideal" stoical citizen, emphasized in press reports and government propaganda. GPs often took on the role of enacting what psychoanalyst John Rickman called "moral reinforcement", rather like a "kindly parent figure" exerting authoritative reassurance over the patient.[52] According to Dr. Geoffrey Evans, writing to the *British Medical Journal (BMJ)*, doctors had a duty to "take pains to determine that our thoughts are those of courage, confidence, faith and hope." Moreover, he argued that doctors must, "sedulously refuse every thought of fear, regret, resentment, and the like, because these thoughts have a weakening effect".[53] Such resolve not to show any "weakening" meant that doctors could often be dismissive of patients' or relatives' subjective feelings about their nervous disorders. As one GP put it, "my people are ashamed to complain of their symptoms".[54] Other doctors, reflecting and reiterating official discourses, suggested the war merely provided patients with an excuse for the existence of a prior mental disorder or weakness. Dr Ellis Sturgo, writing to the *BMJ*, even contended that the war gave neurotics "a superb scapegoat to account for their abnormal personalities".[55]

There was also an important class dimension in the relationship between doctors and patients, whereby for working class patients the doctor was often seen as a figure of authority, and to whom it was hard to admit fears. There was also the very practical matter of cost, which made it impossible for many poorer patients to even consider visiting their doctor about their nervous troubles. As psychoanalyst Melitta Schmideberg observed, many poorer people never visited a doctor due to expense, and others were so "upset or bereaved through bombing it did not even occur that medical help might be desirable."[56] Patients often presented to their doctor with a physical rather than a mental ailment. According to a study on one GP practice in London during 1940 and 1941, half the patients eventually diagnosed with nervous disorders had initially sought advice from the GP about a physical disorder. The study surmised that patients often only felt able to visit their doctor, "when some physical disorder gave them an excuse".[57] This reflected a fear of admitting a mental weakness, especially in the context of the developing "mood" of carrying on amid the material and emotional wreckage of the war. As a doctor from Kent noted in a letter to the *BMJ*, this resulted in a large number of cases being "unrecognised and untreated (unless one describes as treatment an assurance by their private doctor that there is "nothing wrong" with them)".[58]

As noted in the introduction to this chapter, evacuated children were one section of the civilian population which did become a focus of psychiatric concern. As historian Michal Shapira has observed, children occupied a "privileged position" in investigations into the psychological effects of war.[59] In some ways, wartime psychiatric reports underplayed the traumatic effects of bombing on children. Indeed, children were often viewed as being *more* resilient and adaptable than adults in coping with the experience of relentless raids.[60] Thus in many reports of children's psychological reactions, children were assessed in a similar way to adults—with pre-war nervous symptoms being viewed as a more important indicator of a child's mental reactions than the severity of the air raids.[61] A study of 8000 school children in Bristol by psychologist Maureen Dunsdon, for example, found only 300 children suffering from detrimental mental effects of the raids, including psychological symptoms such as trembling and crying, and psychosomatic symptoms such as headaches, anorexia and indigestion.[62] Although psychiatric investigations did not ignore the traumas and fears induced in some children by raids, much of the research focused not on the experience of air raids but on the effects of evacuation, and the psychological traumas children suffered by being removed from their home surroundings. In particular, the separation of the child from the mother was seen as having much greater potential to cause long-term psychological damage than the fears and anxieties of air raids. As historian Mathew Thomson has highlighted, children came to symbolize not the damaging psychological effects of the war per se but deep anxieties about the separation of the child from the home and the mother.[63] Psychoanalysts played a key role in articulating such concerns and in "reifying" the child's psyche as central to the healthy development of future adult civilians, such as in the wartime therapeutic work with disturbed children practiced by Anna Freud and Dorothy Burlington in Hampstead and Donald Winnicott in Oxford.[64]

In contrast to the concern articulated about the mental health of evacuated children, some contemporary observers noted that the psychological needs of many adult civilians experiencing bombardment had been neglected. One Mass Observation report, for example, warned that there was a danger of medics and civil defense workers neglecting the "private feelings" of civilians coping with the aftershock of air raids, leaving people not knowing how to articulate their fears and emotions.[65] The prevalence of such cases prompted Mass Observation founder Tom Harrisson to write to the *BMJ* describing how people could "cave in" after a heavy bombing raid. "In some cases they have simply taken to bed and stayed in bed for weeks at a time", he wrote. These cases were unlikely to have ever come to the attention of a psychiatrist or family doctor because their symptoms did not conform to an official diagnosis of neurosis. "They have not shown marked trembling or hysteria, but an extreme desire to retreat into sleep and into being looked after, as if chronically ill", he suggested.[66] Such examples indicate a multiplicity of psychological reactions to the war, not all of which came under the remit of the psychiatric profession, and to which civilians did not necessarily attach a psychiatric label.

Psychiatric Clinics: In the Shadow of the Mental Hospital

Although the extent and provenance of undiagnosed and untreated nervous problems during the war could only be speculated upon, attendance at psychiatric clinics could provide more tangible evidence of the extent of mental health problems suffered during the war. These clinics, often attached to mental hospitals, were staffed by mental hospital psychiatrists and took referrals from GPs, First Aid Posts and mental hospital psychiatrists. In many ways the clinics traversed the boundaries of psychiatric care, treating both patients considered to have long-term, serious mental disorders and those with more minor and transient psychological problems. Some historians have suggested that many psychiatric clinics stood empty during the war, yet Blacker's official survey found the clinics severely overcrowded, with depleted staff unable to deal with the demand for services.[67]

Despite the importance of these clinics in the psychiatric history of the war, remarkably little has been written of the material conditions or social relationships of these overcrowded and understaffed sites of treatment. To attempt to rectify this, I have drawn on the unpublished reports carried out for Blacker's survey by two inspectors, Catherine Gavin and Isobel Laird, from the Board of Control (the body which oversaw mental institutions before the creation of the NHS) in March and April 1943. Gavin and Laird visited every psychiatric clinic in the Greater London and the North West of England regions respectively, interviewing the psychiatrists, social workers and almoners who staffed them and reporting on the facilities and conditions they encountered.[68] None of this reportage was included in Blacker's final published version, nor has it been the subject of subsequent historical analysis. The value of these reports lies in the detail they provide into the physical conditions of the clinics, and the attitudes and opinions of those who staffed them. Although the reports offer, as Gavin herself said, “nothing more than a bird’s eye picture”, they provide hitherto unexplored accounts of the space and resources of the clinics, and of the relationships between the staff and patients within them.[69]

The inspectors wrote of the clinics as run-down, gloomy, blacked-out and discouraging places for patients. In Barrow, patients waiting for treatment could not fit in the tiny blacked-out waiting room, and queued in a cold corridor with no seats, sharing the space with patients from other clinics. Laird writes, “On certain days the neurotic patients wait among children in various noisy and gory stages of recovery from operations for the removal of tonsils”.[70] In Preston, psychiatric patients were forced to sit or stand, “in a very narrow corridor totally blacked-out, poorly-lit, and ventilated mainly from the large waiting room where about fifty patients with an assortment of skin affections await their clinic”.[71] In the London area, Gavin similarly describes makeshift and inadequate buildings, with crowded waiting rooms, sometimes overflowing into nearby corridors.[72] Gavin and Laird found that patients often faced a lack of privacy, with patients having to reveal details of their nervous complaints to everyone else queuing to see the doctors. At the Warrington clinic, “The dingy waiting hall is filled with fumes from the boilerhouse … [it] is not large, and the hatch at which new patients ask for cards is in one wall. New patients therefore give all the necessary particulars about themselves in full hearing of all waiting patients”.[73] The absence of privacy also sometimes included consultations being carried out in front of other patients or with nurses and relatives moving in and out of makeshift spaces.[74]

Although these conditions were neither unique nor surprising in the context of the scarcity of resources in wartime Britain, the evidence that patients were prepared to queue for hours in cramped halls and cold corridors, and seek services with little privacy, is an indicator of a significant demand for psychiatric help during the war. This is especially the case considering the physical obstacles people had to surmount to reach the clinics, such as traversing bomb-damaged areas. Patients at the clinics also faced the added stigma of the association of the clinics with the large mental hospitals. One-third of all psychiatric clinics in England and Wales were physically attached to the asylum, sharing the same buildings or outbuildings in the grounds of mental hospitals.[75] As many as 150 out of the 216 clinics, including those attached to voluntary and general hospitals, were staffed by psychiatrists and social workers from a nearby mental hospital.[76] As Bernard Hart pointed out, many of the psychiatrists who worked in the clinics tended to view the patients they examined "from the angle of their suitability to be admitted to mental hospitals as voluntary patients".[77] Indeed, Laird estimated that the clinics were "too closely identified in the mind of the population with mental hospitals," and from her observation of patients, she considered that there was a danger of the clinics being regarded "as a recruiting centre for a mental hospital."[78]

Despite the fear of the mental hospital, and the stigma attached to having a mental illness still prevalent in the war period, by the time Gavin and Laird prepared their reports, attendance at the majority of the clinics they visited had exceeded pre-war rates. Although there was a drop in the numbers of new patients attending the clinics in 1940, the numbers of new attendees steadily rose through the next two years.[79] Gavin reported that out of all 44 London clinics she visited, there was only one clinic in central London "where mention was made of any lack of work".[80] Clinics reported fluctuating, but steadily increasing numbers through the course of the war. At the British Hospital for Functional Mental and Nervous Disorders in Camden in North London, for example, patient numbers fell during the Blitz period, even though the clinic was situated in a heavily bombed area. Staff at the clinic believed this was mainly due to the more vulnerable sections of the population being evacuated, the effects of the black-out, which meant evening sessions were canceled, and because they thought the war gave potential patients "something else to think about". At the time of the report, however, patient numbers were steadily rising, mainly due to the relaxation of black-out restrictions and people adapting to living in bombed-out London.[81]

Of course, overcrowded conditions and a steady rise in new patients attending the clinics was not necessarily a measure of a rise in neurosis in the general population due to the war. The numbers attending clinics were affected by multiple factors, such as the numbers of people evacuated from the cities or conscripted into industrial work, and civilians' ability to attend clinics amid bomb damage, transport restrictions and black-out regulations. Blacker suggested the rise in attendances at the clinics was mainly due to increased awareness of the clinics among GPs.[82] Most psychiatrists interviewed in the survey, however, reported that their most prevalent problem was not the numbers referred by GPs, but that psychiatrists were forced to send patients *back* to their GPs due to staff shortages and the lack of inpatient beds. Indeed, some of the psychiatrists interviewed worried about what happened to patients dispatched back home due to lack of facilities. The Central Middlesex County Hospital in West London was staffed by just one psychiatrist who could only attend the clinic on one afternoon per week. The psychiatrist complained that 90 percent of his patients had to be "disposed of at the first interview", and that patients were only returned when they experienced some "social difficulty".[83] As Gavin reported, "The complaint is that such patients are pushed home after a very short time and alleged to have been given no definite treatment".[84] Staff shortages and rising patient numbers resulted in some clinics introducing a rigorous selection of patients. In the London region, half of the 44 clinics held only one half-day session per week at the time of Gavin's visit, and five clinics had suspended their services due to lack of staff and bomb damage.[85] Dr. Grey Clark from West London was one of several psychiatrists interviewed by Gavin who bemoaned that too many patients and too few staff resulted "in a high degree of selection to cope with the pressure of work".[86]

This is not to suggest that all patients at the clinics, and those waiting for treatment, were experiencing nervous problems directly related to the war—indeed, many of the psychiatrists interviewed often denied the influence of air raids in precipitating their patients' nervous disorders. Nevertheless, many of the psychiatrists attributed the onset of neurosis to the wider and longer-term effects of the war, such as the disruption to routine, the dislocations of social life, homelessness, lack of transport and other facilities, the effects of fatigue and loneliness, and grief following the death of loved ones. As psychiatrist Dr. Noel Harris from the Middlesex Hospital psychiatric clinic expressed it, his patients were most upset by the "complete disturbance of normal life".[87] In other words, the effects of the war, and the disturbance to everyday life, were viewed as major contributory factors to the onset of neurosis—even though such disorders were never calculated as being caused by the war.

Conclusion

This re-examination of civilian neurosis has indicated a far more complex picture of the mental health of the civilian population than is often acknowledged in histories of the home front. Official government and medical policy and discourse aimed to contain and to manage psychological problems by strictly defining what mental disorders were "caused by the war" and by attributing wartime nervous conditions to physical and mental disorders which predated the war. In this way, the state sought to deny or minimize the role of the war in causing, or even in exacerbating, civilians' mental disorders. Government and mainstream psychiatric discourse closely reflected and reinforced each other during the war, and theories of predisposition to mental disorder, whether physical or psychical, allowed psychiatrists to explain the development of wartime neuroses without blaming the war itself. This chapter has illustrated, however, that the narrative of "few psychiatric casualties" was not settled at the start of the war, but was always in the process of being redefined, renegotiated and reiterated.

Psychiatrists and other medics were not unanimous in their opinion on the etiology of the mental disorders in the civilians they encountered. Although few psychiatrists believed that air raids were the sole cause of mental illnesses, many feared that nervous problems might manifest after the end of the war, while others highlighted the effects of wider wartime hardships and the "abnormality" of life in wartime for either creating or exacerbating nervous disorders. Moreover, there was always a tension between official discourses which underplayed the effects of the war on civilians' mental ill-health and the lived experiences both of the patients who sought psychiatric help and of the unknown numbers of civilians who experienced nervous traumas but who never visited a doctor or psychiatrist and who remained unaccounted for in the official figures. By viewing the psychiatric story of the war through a new lens, this chapter has aimed to contribute to a deeper understanding of the relationship between war and mental health, and the complex interplay of medical, socio-economic and political factors involved both in psychiatric judgment and diagnosis during the war. Moreover, it has reiterated how conceptualizations of war neurosis and trauma need to be firmly placed in the particular material, ideological and historical circumstances in which they were developed, shaped and articulated.

Notes

1. Richard Titmuss, *Problems of Social Policy*, (London: HMSO, 1950).
2. Edward Glover, "Notes of the Psychological Effects of War Conditions on the Civilian Population III. The Blitz, 1940–41", International *Journal of Psychoanalysis*, Volume 23, (1942), 29.
3. Glover, "Notes of the Psychological Effects of War Conditions on the Civilian Population", 29.

4. Glover, "Notes of the Psychological Effects of War Conditions on the Civilian Population", 29.
5. Glover, "Notes of the Psychological Effects of War Conditions on the Civilian Population", 29, 36.
6. Glover, "Notes of the Psychological Effects of War Conditions on the Civilian Population", 29.
7. More recent examples of the vast literature on civilian morale include Robert Mackay, *Half the Battle: Civilian Morale During the Second World War*, (Manchester: Manchester University Press, 2002); Malcolm Smith, *Britain and 1940: History, Myth and Popular Memory*, (Abingdon: Routledge, 2000); Peter Stansky, *The First Day of the Blitz: September 7, 1940*, (New Haven & London: Yale University Press, 2007).
8. Edgar Jones, Robin Woolven, Bill Durodie and Simon Wessely, "Civilian Morale During the Second World War: Responses to Air-Raids Re-examined", *Social History of Medicine*, Vol. 17, (2004), 463–479; Edgar Jones, Robin Woolven, Bill Durodie and Simon Wessely, "Public Panic and Morale: Second World War Civilian Responses Re-examined in the Light of the Current Anti-Terrorist Campaign", *Journal of Risk Research*, Volume 9, (2006), 57–73.
9. Jones et al, "Civilian Morale During the Second World War: Responses to Air-Raids Re-examined", 469.
10. See, for example, the weekly reports collected from around Britain by the Ministry of Information. The National Archives (TNA), Ministry of Information (INF) 1/292 "Home Intelligence Weekly Reports".
11. Amy Helen Bell, *London Was Ours: Diaries and Memoirs of the London Blitz*, (London: I.B. Tauris, 2011), 80; Geoffrey Field, *Blood, Sweat and Toil: Remaking the British Working Class* (Oxford: Oxford University Press, 2011); Sonya O. Rose, *Which People's War? National Identity and Citizenship in Wartime Britain 1939–1945*, (Oxford: Oxford University Press, 2003). There is a vast literature on the experience of gender during the war. See, for example, Penny Summerfield, *Reconstructing Women's Wartime Lives: Discourse and Subjectivity in Oral Histories of the Second World War*, (Manchester & New York: Manchester University Press, 1998).
12. See, for example, the chapter "The Fear of Fear" in Juliet Gardiner, *The Blitz: the British Under Attack*, (London: Harper Press, 2010), 177–200; Amy Helen Bell, *London Was Ours: Diaries and Memoirs of the London Blitz*, (London: I.B. Tauris, 2011).

13. See Ben Shephard, *A War of Nerves: Soldiers and Psychiatrists, 1914–1994*, (London: Jonathan Cape, 2000).
14. Nikolas Rose, *Governing the Soul: the Shaping of the Private Self*, (London, Free Association Books, 1999, second edition), 162; Recent historical studies about the psychological focus on the child include Michal Shapira, *The War Inside: Psychoanalysis, Total War, and the Making of the Democratic Self in Postwar Britain*, (Cambridge: Cambridge University Press, 2013); Mathew Thomson, *Lost Freedom: the Landscape of the Child and the British Post War Settlement*, (Oxford: Oxford University Press, 2013); Lisa Farley, "'Operation Pied Piper': a Psychoanalytic Narrative of Authority in a Time of War", *Psychoanalysis and History*, Volume 14, (2012), 29–52.
15. Raymond Williams, *Marxism and Literature*, (Oxford: Oxford University Press, 1977), 128–135.
16. Williams, *Marxism and Literature*, 132.
17. Glover, "Notes on the Psychological Effects of War Conditions on the Civilian Population (1)", 133.
18. A.J. Murray, cited in Ian Macdonald, "Gordon Holmes and the Neurological Heritage", *Brain*, Volume 130, (2007), 295.
19. Cited in TNA Ministry of Health (MH) 101/1. " Review of the EMS 1923-May 1940, Sir John Hebb's Report", 70.
20. TNA Ministry of Pensions (PIN) 15/2399 "Conference on Entitlement in Neurasthenia and the Psychoses". Conference of Neurologists and Representatives of the Service Departments, 3 July, 1939.
21. TNA PIN 15/2402 Letter from Adair Hore to William Codling at HMSO; "Neuroses in War Time: Memorandum for the Medical Profession", (London: His Majesty's Stationery Office, 1940); published in *British Medical Journal*, 2, (16 December, 1939), 1199–1201.
22. TNA PIN 15/2399. "Conference of Neurologists and Representatives of the Service Departments: Compensation in Cases of Neurasthenia and Psychosis", 3 July, 1939.
23. TNA PIN 15/2314 "Personal Injuries (Civilians) Scheme. Definition of 'Physical Injury'. Neurasthenia, mental and nervous injury".
24. TNA PIN 15/2399 "Conference on Entitlement in Neurasthenia and the Psychoses". Conference of Neurologists and Representatives of the Service Departments, 3 July, 1939.
25. TNA PIN 15/2946 "Treatment of Neurasthenia". P.R. Bolus, Ministry of Pensions, letter to Dr. L.W. Nicholson, 22 May, 1941.

26. TNA PIN 15/2208 "Neurasthenia. Definition of Nervous Shock in Relation to War Injury". Letter from Adair Hore, Ministry of Pension to G.K.A. Grey, Treasury Chambers, 7 March, 1941; TNA PIN 15/2314 "Personal Injuries (Civilians) Scheme. Definition of 'Physical Injury. Neurasthenia, mental and nervous injury".
27. TNA PIN 15/2314. "Personal Injuries (Civilians) Scheme. Definition of 'Physical Injury'. Neurasthenia, mental and nervous injury". "1235: Cases of Shock", undated.
28. TNA PIN 15/2314. "Personal Injuries (Civilians) Scheme. Definition of 'Physical Injury'. Neurasthenia, mental and nervous injury". "1235: Cases of Shock", undated.
29. TNA PIN 15/2208 "Neurasthenia. Definitions of Nervous Shock in relation to War Injury". Letter from Dr Bernard Hart to Prideaux at the Ministry of Pension, 27 January, 1941.
30. TNA PIN 15/2208 "Neurasthenia. Definitions of Nervous Shock in Relation to War Injury". Letter from Aubrey Lewis, Mill Hill Emergency Hospital, to Dr. E. Prideaux, Medical Division, Ministry of Pensions, Dated 15 January, 1941. Emphasis in the original.
31. Harry Stalker, "Panic States in Civilians", *British Medical Journal*, 1, (1 June, 1940), 889.
32. C.P. Blacker, *Neurosis and the Mental Health Services*, (Oxford: Oxford University Press, 1946).
33. Blacker, *Neurosis and the Mental Health Services*, 165.
34. CMAC Wellcome Library. PP/CPB/D.5/1. "C.P. Blacker. Ministry of Health: Neurosis Survey: Report, analysis sheets, 1942–1944 and 11943 Letters from Ministry of Health". 'Notes on the Questionnaire', 5.
35. Paul Lerner, *Hysterical Men: War, Psychiatry and the Politics of Trauma in Germany, 1890–1930*, (Ithaca & London: Cornell University Press, 2003), 2.
36. TNA Home Office (HO) 199/317 "First Aid Posts"; Mass Observation (MO) file report 271, June 1940.
37. Glover, "Notes on the Psychological Effects of War Conditions of the Civilian Population", 17; Juliet Gardiner, *Wartime Britain 1930–1945*, (London: Headline Books, 2004), 391.
38. TNA Cabinet Office (CAB) 102/719 "Mental Health 1939–1941"—Mental Health Emergency Committee: Summary of Workers' Reports 1.1.41.
39. TNA PIN 15/2208 "Neurasthenia. Definition of Nervous Shock in Relation to War Injury". "Civilian Neurosis. First Aid Posts".

40. Henry Wilson, "Mental Reactions to Air Raids", *British Medical Journal*, 1, (7 March, 1942), 284.
41. Russell Fraser, I.M. Leslie and D. Phelps, "Psychiatric Effects of Severe Personal Experiences During Bombing", *Proceedings of the Royal Society of Medicine*, Volume 36, (January, 1943), 120.
42. Fraser et al, "Psychiatric Effects of Severe Personal Experiences During Bombing", 119–120.
43. Fraser et al, "Psychiatric Effects of Severe Personal Experiences During Bombing", 121.
44. Fraser et al, "Psychiatric Effects of Severe Personal Experiences During Bombing", 122.
45. Fraser et al, "Psychiatric Effects of Severe Personal Experiences During Bombing", 123.
46. TNA CAB 102/719 "Mental Health 1939–1941". Mental Health Emergency Committee: Summary of workers' reports 1.1.41, 7.
47. TNA CAB 102/719 "Mental Health 1939–1941". Mental Health Emergency Committee: Summary of workers' reports 1.1.41, 7.
48. TNA CAB 102/719 "Mental Health 1939–1941". Mental Health Emergency Committee: Summary of workers' reports 1.1.41, 7.
49. TNA CAB 102/719 "Mental Health 1939–1941". Mental Health Emergency Committee. Summary of Workers' Reports 1.1.41, 3–4, 5.
50. Glover, "Notes of the Psychological Effects of War Conditions on the Civilian Population", 17.
51. David Armstrong, *Political Anatomy of the Body: Medical Knowledge in Britain in the Twentieth Century*, (Cambridge: Cambridge University Press, 1983), 21.
52. John Rickman, "The Mental Aspects of A.R.P.", *British Medical Journal*, 2, (26 August, 1939), p. 458.
53. Geoffrey Evans, "Doctor and Patient in War Time", letter, *British Medical Journal*, 2, (7 October, 1939), 742.
54. Cited in Aubrey Lewis, "Incidence of Neurosis in England Under War Conditions", *The Lancet*, 2, (15 August, 1943), 178.
55. Ellis Sturgo, "Psychiatric Casualties in London", letter, *British Medical Journal*, 2, (9 November, 1940), 646.
56. Melitta Schmideberg, "Some Observations on Individual Reactions to Air Raids", *International Journal of Psychoanalysis*, Volume 23, (1942), 171.
57. J. Whitby, "Neurosis in a London General Practice During the Second and Third Years of War", *Proceedings of the Royal Society of Medicine*, Volume 36, (January, 1943), 124.

58. B.H. Kirman, "Psychiatric Casualties," letter, *British Medical Journal*, 2, (30 November, 1940), 761.
59. Shapira, *The War Inside*, 1.
60. Examples of this voluminous literature include, M.I Dunsdon, "A Psychologist's Contribution to Air Raid Problems," *Mental Health*, Vol. 2, (October, 1941), 37–41; Frank Bodman, "Child Psychiatry in War-Time Britain", *Journal of Educational Psychology*, Volume 35 (May, 1944), 293–301; E.M. Creak and B.J. Shorting, "Child Psychiatry", *Journal of Mental Science*, Volume 90, (January, 1944), 265–381; Rosemary Pritchard and Saul Rosenzweig, "The Effects of War Stress upon Childhood and Youth", *Journal of Abnormal and Social Psychology*, Volume 37, (July, 1942), 329–344; Arthur T. Jersild and Margaret F. Meigs, "Children and War", *Psychological Bulletin*, Volume 40, (October, 1943), 541–573.
61. Cyril Burt, "The Billeting of Evacuated Children", *British Journal of Educational Psychology*, Volume 11, (June, 1941), 179.
62. Dunsdon, "A Psychologist's Contribution to Air Raid Problems," 37–41; Frank Bodman, "War Conditions and the Mental Health of the Child", *British Medical Journal*, 2, (4 October, 1941), 486.
63. Thomson, *Lost Freedom*, 16.
64. Shapira, *The War Inside*, 6; Anna Freud and Dorothy Burlingham, *Infants Without Families and Report on the Hampstead Nurseries, 1939–1945*, (London: Hogarth Press, 1974); John Bowlby, "The Influence of Early Environment in the Development of Neurosis and Neurotic Character", *International Journal of Psychoanalysis*, Volume, 21, (1940), 154–178; John Bowlby, *Child Care and the Growth of Love*, (Harmondsworth: Pelican Books, 1953).
65. Mass Observation (MO) File Report 568, "Morale in 1941", 61; See also MO file Report 451, "Reception Areas in Oxford", 17.
66. Tom Harrisson, "Obscure Nervous Effects of Air Raids", letters, *British Medical Journal*, 1 (12 April, 1941), 573–574, (31 May, 1941), 832.
67. See, for example, Rose, *Governing the Soul*, 24; This also suggested by Juliet Gardiner, *The Blitz*, 179.
68. TNA MH 51/663. "Civilian Neurosis Survey". The reports from the clinics are not catalogued in the main file, but are unsorted, in an envelope at the back of the file. There is no record of the reports for the remaining ten regions of England and Wales covered by the survey.
69. TNA MH 51/663 "Civilian Neurosis Survey". C.M. Gavin, 'Confidential Report to Triumvirate on Out Patient Clinics in the London Area', 5.

70. TNA MH 51/663 "Civilian Neurosis Survey". Isobel Laird, "N.W. Region. Report on Fieldwork," 5.
71. TNA MH 51/663 "Civilian Neurosis Survey". Isobel Laird, "N.W. Region. Report on Fieldwork," 7.
72. TNA MH 51/663 "Civilian Neurosis Survey". C.M. Gavin, "Confidential Report to Triumvirate on Out Patient Clinics in the London Area."
73. TNA MH 51/663 "Civilian Neurosis Survey". Isobel Laird. "N.W. Region. Report on Fieldwork", 7.
74. TNA MH 51/663 "Civilian Neurosis Survey". Report from Royal Northern Hospital Neurological Clinic, Holloway Road.
75. Blacker, *Neurosis and the Mental Health Services*, 9.
76. Blacker, *Neurosis and the Mental Health Services*, 57, 69.
77. TNA MH 76/115 "Neurosis: Provision of Psychiatric Treatment. Neurosis Survey". Letter from Bernard Hard to Prof Fraser following the conference on conference on civilian neurosis, undated.
78. TNA MH 51/663 "Civilian Neurosis Survey". Isobel Laird, "N.W. Region. Report on Fieldwork," 11–12.
79. Blacker, *Neurosis and the Mental Health Services*, 146–148.
80. TNA MH 51/663 "Civilian Neurosis Survey". Report from St. Marylebone and Western General Dispensary Psychiatric Clinic.
81. TNA MH 51/663 "Civilian Neurosis Survey". Report from The British Hospital for Functional Mental and Nervous Disorders, Camden Road.
82. Blacker, *Neurosis and the Mental Health Services*, 14.
83. TNA MH 51/663 "Civilian Neurosis Survey". Report from Central Middlesex County Hospital Psychiatric Clinic.
84. TNA MH 51/663 "Civilian Neurosis Survey". Report from St. John's Hospital Psychiatric Clinic, Morden Hill, Lewisham.
85. TNA MH 51/663 "Civilian Neurosis Survey". Catherine Gavin, "Confidential Report to Triumvirate on Out Patient Clinics in the London Area", 1.
86. TNA MH 51/663 "Civilian Neurosis Survey". Report from West End Hospital for Nervous Diseases Outpatient Department.
87. TNA MH 51/663 "Civilian Neurosis Survey". Report from the Middlesex Hospital Psychiatric Clinic, Mortimer Street, London.

PART III

Postwar

CHAPTER 6

"No longer Normal": Traumatized Red Army Veterans in Post-war Leningrad

Robert Dale

On 10 February 1946, Maria Golubeva wrote to her sister in Simferopol describing the difficulties and disappointments of life in post-war Leningrad. Maria was living in one room with five family members. In November 1945, her son Andrei joined them, following his demobilization from the Red Army. His living space had been occupied by other people during the Siege of Leningrad, and he was now attempting to reclaim it through the courts. Andrei was working as an artist in a state institution, although he wasn't receiving a ration card. He had been granted permission to enter university at the start of the next academic year. Andrei's transition to civilian life was anything but smooth. As his mother wrote, "He is after all an invalid and worse still, he is psychologically abnormal."[1]

On 18 September 1952, the Leningrad city court found Vladimir Krymov, a Red Army veteran, guilty of anti-Soviet agitation, a political crime. On 5 August 1952, according to a series of witnesses, Krymov, in a state of intoxication, had created a scandal in a central Leningrad shop, which involved using unprintable language (*netsenzurnaia bran'*), slandering Communist party leaders, expressing anti-Semitic views and spreading rumours of a forthcoming war in front of staff and customers.[2]

R. Dale (✉)
School of History, Classics and Archaeology, Newcastle University, Newcastle upon Tyne, UK

P. Leese, J. Crouthamel (eds.), *Traumatic Memories of the Second World War and After*, DOI 10.1007/978-3-319-33470-7_6

Vladimir was not a dangerous political dissident, but rather an alcoholic ex-serviceman who had failed to readjust to civilian life. In late August 1953, his mother Olga Krymova wrote a letter of appeal to the USSR state prosecutor explaining that her son was mentally ill and needed psychiatric care. She claimed that Vladimir had suffered two traumas (*travmyi*): the first a head injury (*kontuziia golovy*) whilst serving in the Army, the second a nervous breakdown prompted by his wife leaving him for another man. Vladimir, according to his mother "was an abnormal person" and a "typical schizophrenic." She attributed Vladimir's outburst to mental illness, and questioned whether, "Soviet law makes provision to try a psychiatrically ill person for abnormal ravings (*nenormal'nyi bred*)."[3]

These two vignettes, one from the war's immediate aftermath and the other over seven years after the end of fighting, illustrate the difficulties Leningrad's returning soldiers experienced while reintegrating into civilian society, and the responses of Leningraders to the unconventional and disorderly behaviour of traumatized veterans. The war on the Eastern Front between 1941 and 1945 exposed soldiers to years of strain, privation, violence and killing, as well as separation from their families. Many veterans witnessed and participated in deeply traumatic events. In serving the motherland, Red Army soldiers had to be prepared to sacrifice not only life and limb but also their nerves. When Maria Golubeva and Olga Krymova described their sons as no longer normal, they were grasping for a language to describe veterans' traumatic reactions to modern industrialized warfare. According to the official myth, Red Army veterans largely survived the war without crippling mental trauma, and were immune to the aftershocks of war that plagued the capitalist west. In a society where psychological trauma, especially amongst veterans, created ideological difficulties and was frequently repressed, it was difficult to find a suitable vocabulary to discuss war trauma. Veterans, civilians and psychiatrists all found it difficult to frame the psychological and emotional damage of war. These two mothers may have struggled with the medicalized terminology, but "no longer normal" veterans were a social and medical reality in post-war Leningrad.

This chapter argues that Red Army veterans, like ex-servicemen elsewhere, sometimes experienced post-traumatic reactions and mental health difficulties as they readjusted to civilian life. It examines newly discovered archival evidence, alongside published sources, that describes psychological problems and psychiatric symptoms amongst Leningrad's ex-servicemen that in other societies were recognized and treated as trauma. This evidence falls into two main categories: first, the research conducted by Leningrad's psychiatrists, in particular the Bekhterev Institute, a leading psychiatric and neurological research institution with a distinguished history of studying trauma; and second, the traces left across the archival records, such as Maria Golubeva's and Olga Krymova's letters, by traumatized veterans. The influx of approximately 300,000 veterans demobilized in Leningrad between mid-July and the end of 1948 had survived one of the twentieth century's most violent and murderous conflicts, and were returning to a community with its own deeply destabilizing wartime experience. Veterans' prospects must have seemed bleak. However, most veterans proved remarkably resilient in the face of difficult and disquieting experiences, finding their own ways of coping with psychological trauma. Although traumatized soldiers made their presence felt far beyond the consulting room and the psychiatric ward, most were remarkably successful at readjusting to civilian life. Post-war Soviet society, late Stalinist Leningrad in particular, had developed its own unique social, political and clinical understanding of and response to war trauma which shaped veterans' readjustment.

Nowhere was the presence of demobilized veterans more evident than in Leningrad, where they constituted a prominent social constituency. The trickle of returning soldiers that began in July 1945 rapidly became a torrent. In just over two years, 268,376 veterans were demobilized in Leningrad, more than any other Soviet city.[4] A further 53,334 disabled veterans, registered with the city's district social security offices, and tens of thousands of former POWs, partisans and migrants, demobilized through other mechanisms or in other locations, were also resident in the city.[5] Against the backdrop of Leningrad's wartime population collapse, veterans represented between ten and fifteen per cent of the city's population throughout the late Stalinist period. In 1945, the city's population stood at barely a third (927,000) of its 1941 level (2,992,000). By 1947, it had recovered to approximately two-thirds of its pre-war population (1,998,000), but as late as 1953 Leningrad's population was half a million lower than on the eve of war.[6]

Leningrad's veterans were returning to a city whose inhabitants had experienced unimaginable horrors. The Siege of Leningrad (*Blokada*) was a catastrophe for the city and its people. Official figures calculated 632,253 deaths from starvation and associated illnesses, and a further 6747 deaths from bombs and shelling.[7] This was almost certainly an underestimate. Researchers have suggested a death toll between 700,000 and 1 million.[8] Regardless of the precise total, no city in modern history has ever suffered a greater loss of human life. The loss of life was more than ten times that in Hiroshima in August 1945.[9] Yet it was not simply the number of deaths but their manner that was shocking. Besieged Leningraders watched their bodies shrink, their friends and family wither and die, as rations and their nutritional value plummeted. Reserves were exhausted, ersatz foods were developed, pets were eaten, soups were made from wallpaper paste, leather was chewed and frightening reports of cannibalism abounded. In the worst days of the siege, the winter of 1941/1942, death became unremarkable. Corpses were left in apartments, where they fell on the streets or stacked in basements. Blockade survivors (*blokadniki*) were on war's frontlines; the experience left them physically and mentally exhausted.

Trauma and the psychological casualties of modern warfare, both military and civilian, as this volume testifies, are the subject of a rich and expanding historiography. The idea that modern warfare was inherently traumatic and that anybody might have been disturbed by it has entered the western cultural mainstream. Words like "trauma" and "shell shock" have become metaphors for almost any uncomfortable or disquieting experience. This language often obscures the remarkable resilience of individuals and societies in the face of extreme events. "The emphasis on emotional breakdown and psychiatric illness," as Joanna Bourke has argued, "has obscured the fact that most men coped remarkably well with the demands being made upon them in wartime."[10] Assumptions about the universality of war trauma should be guarded against. Different societies respond to trauma in different ways, deploying different diagnoses and terminology to describe the mental breakdown of soldiers and civilians. War trauma has manifested itself in varied and complex ways across time and space. Conditions such as war neuroses, shell shock, combat fatigue and post-traumatic stress disorder were the product of very different historical contexts. As Ben Shephard reminds us, each and every conflict is a unique confluence of social, cultural, economic, political, military and medical factors, which affect how war trauma is diagnosed and treated. Different social attitudes to fear, madness and social obligation all influenced the role of military psychology in treating trauma and even the symptoms observed.[11]

Russia and the Soviet Union had their own history of responding to battlefield trauma, which illustrates these points particularly clearly. Nervous problems on the battlefield had been observed as early as the Russo-Turkish War, but widespread interest in war trauma amongst the psychiatric profession as a whole began during the Russo-Japanese War (1904–1905), a decade earlier than interest in soldiers' nervous and psychological disorders began in Western Europe.[12] Russian physicians and psychiatrists were often uncertain and at odds how to diagnose and explain the unusual symptoms observed during the war. Without standardized diagnoses or even established terminology, medics in different locations often reached different conclusions, sometimes seeking psychological and sometimes physical aetiologies for war neuroses. Some specialists hypothesized that sustained exposure to the concussive impact of explosives caused damage to the brain and nervous system. New terms, *kontuziia* (contusion), *voennaia kontuziia* (military contusion) and *vozdushnaia kontuziia* (air contusion), were coined for these injuries, becoming key vocabulary in the diagnosis of trauma.[13] The First World War brought a worrying surge of psychiatric casualties, for which the Imperial army was unprepared, despite the warnings offered by the Russo-Japanese War. Psychologists and psychiatrists continued to question whether physical, psychological or emotional factors caused war neuroses, and whether wartime psychiatric disorders constituted new illnesses. Medics often sought an explanation for mental trauma in organic physical damage, either injuries or concussions to the brain or nervous system caused by rapid changes in air pressure from shelling. Yet there were also psychiatrists who concluded that war neuroses were the product of psychological trauma.[14] Discussions about war trauma on the pages of learned journals, and sometimes more widely, were disrupted and overshadowed by the Revolutions of 1917 and the Russian Civil War. Trauma, however, never entirely disappeared from scholarly or public view. "Wounded or psychologically traumatized veterans," as Karen Petrone writes, "were ... commonly encountered on the social landscape of the Soviet Union in the 1920s as the living embodiment of war memory and a powerful and daily reminder of the costs of war."[15]

By the start of the Great Patriotic War, Soviet society had endured 25 years of violence. War, revolution, civil war, famine, collectivization and political terror recalibrated attitudes and responses to trauma. These collective experiences, it has been argued, inured Soviet society to privation and suffering.[16] Despite shifting social attitudes and the challenges of squaring Stalinist ideology and psychiatric theory and practice, some researchers continued to study the psychiatric impact of war throughout the interwar years.[17] In 1938, for example, as the threat of war intensified, Viktor Petrovich Osipov, director of Leningrad's Military Medical Academy, began to edit a landmark collection of essays, marking the 140th anniversary of the Academy, studying the psychiatric disorders of previous conflicts, particularly the First World War. It was eventually published in

1941. Amongst the contributions were chapters examining the psychiatric practices of foreign armies between 1914 and 1918, and a survey of wartime psychiatric disorders, such as *kontuziia*, hysteria and traumatic neuroses, based on international and Russian literature.[18] Ospiov's own chapter outlined the basics of identifying psychoses and short descriptions of the psychiatric illness military doctors might encounter during war. The Russian Imperial Army had experienced panic, hysteria, concussion (*kontuziia*) and psychological breakdown. But, Ospiov predicted that in the future the Red Army would be more resilient. He argued that during the Russian Civil War the Red Army experienced significantly lower levels of psychiatric and psychological illness than the tsarist army during the First World War because of higher morale.[19] Soldiers and armies with higher political and class consciousness were better equipped to combat the natural biological, emotional and nervous reactions to war threatening their personalities.[20] V.A. Gorovoi-Shaltan's contribution stressed the importance of social factors in preventing war neuroses, praising the class unity between officers and the ranks, and the role of the party and Komsomol in political education.[21] Osipov suggested that improved economic well-being, higher cultural levels (*kul'turnost'*), lower general infection rates and higher physical indicators amongst youth meant that the nation was more robust.[22] Against a backdrop of shortage, privation and famine, it is hard to read this claim as anything other than a nod to ideological orthodoxy.

By the time these confident predictions were published, an alternative reality was already making itself felt. Despite military psychiatrists' confidence in new Soviet social structures, the Great Patriotic War unleashed a wave of violence, death and destruction. The hyper-masculine world of the Soviet military and the social taboos surrounding mental illness, however, restricted the identification and public expression of war trauma. Soviet soldiers and officers were neither the positive heroes immune to psychological stress familiar from Soviet propaganda, nor the faceless unthinking brutes lacking the emotional and moral makeup of western soldiers, an image peddled during the Cold War. Although it has been suggested that trauma was virtually invisible in the wartime Red Army, psychiatric casualties never entirely disappeared from official history, or from memory.[23] During the war, the pages of psychiatric journals once again filled with studies of the damage done to soldiers' minds. Conferences were organized, research was shared and theoretical debates thrashed out.[24] The multivolume official medical history of the war devoted a volume, published in 1949, to wartime nervous disorders (including neuroses, hysteria and *kontuziia*), a testimony to the efforts of wartime researchers.[25] This was an enormous publishing project, spanning 35 lavishly illustrated volumes with a print run of half a million copies and subsidized prices for doctors and medical students. It was launched and overseen by legislation signed by Stalin, hardly the actions of a state officially denying war trauma.[26]

The gulf between the theory and practice of military medicine, however, was enormous. Amidst the chaos and privations of the frontlines, the treatment of psychiatric casualties bore little resemblance to the textbooks. As Wanke acknowledges, "Soviet military psychiatry struggled to rediscover and implement an organizational structure that that would provide adequate psychiatric care to the military."[27] The best traumatized frontline soldiers could hope for was rest and better rations. The priority was returning soldiers to active duty as quickly as possible. This was often achieved by chemical intervention, a liberal dose of alcohol and sometimes hypnosis. These treatments had the benefit of being quick, easy to administer close to the frontlines and relatively cheap. Anything more advanced was unrealistic, given shortages of medicines, equipment and trained personnel. It seems likely that only a fraction of those suffering from some form of trauma ever received treatment; their symptoms went unrecognized or were ignored.[28] Estimating the number of psychiatric casualties is difficult, particularly as the official history of wartime psychiatric illness gave no absolute figures, just percentages for the distribution of casualties by disorder. One estimate calculates that only 100,000 out of nearly 20 million active service soldiers were recorded as permanent psychiatric casualties.[29] This is almost certainly an underestimate. Wartime and post-war Soviet society tended to treat the war's cost as physical, rather than psychological. "Circumscribed within the limits of a physiological paradigm," as Anna Krylova argues, "the Party press presented the war's legacy as readily remedied by means of reconstructive surgery and high-quality false limbs."[30]

Russia's northern capital had a long track record of studying battlefield trauma. Saint Petersburg had been the centre of psychiatric profession until the 1890s, when Moscow began to compete for this distinction. Following the capital's move back to Moscow in March 1918, the psychiatric profession and funding gravitated towards Moscow. Nevertheless, Leningrad's psychiatrists remained at the cutting edge of Soviet research into wartime nervous disorders. They maintained a strong sense of corporate identity, based upon the institutions where or the professors under whom they had trained, and their own approaches to the discipline.[31] Two institutions were at the centre of this work. First, the Military Medical Academy, which had a distinguished history of studying trauma dating back to the late nineteenth century. It would become the foremost centre of Soviet military psychiatry, at the heart of interwar, wartime and post-war psychiatric research.[32] Although the published research of its psychiatrists, most notably V.P. Ospiov, is available, its archives and patients' medical records remain closed. In contrast, the archives of the Bekhterev Institute, alongside its published output, are relatively accessible. The Institute was established in 1913 by Vladimir Mikhailovich Bekhterev, a pioneer in exploring external causes of mental illness, in order to study psychology, psychiatry and brain anatomy. He had held the prestigious Chair of Psychiatry and Nervous Disorders at the Military Medical Academy from 1893 until 1913, when he resigned in protest over the handling of his evidence at the infamous Beilis Trial.[33] During the Siege, the Bekhterev Institute studied and treated civilians suffering from mental breakdown linked to starvation. Its psychiatrists also worked beyond the institute's walls, regularly treating soldiers in military hospitals. This activity informed future research, leading to a number of important post-war studies of trauma.[34]

Leningrad's veterans were returning to a city and community with greater experience and a better understanding of war trauma than in most other places. The war and blockade made trauma a research priority. Civilian mental breakdowns caused by mass starvation and the front's psychiatric casualties had to be treated and explained. In a paper delivered at a conference organized by the Bekhterev Institute in March 1946, V.N. Miasishchev and E.K. Iakovlenva stressed that the most pressing task for the institute during the Fourth Five Year Plan was to liquidate the nervous-psychiatric effects of the war: "Lately in the seriously shocking conditions of wartime, and in connection with them, the occurrence of psychiatric and other traumas to the nervous system considered as group of illnesses has increased."[35] The blockade extracted a toll on civilian Leningraders' mental health. A number of wartime and post-war studies drew a link between dystrophy (extreme emaciation) and psychiatric breakdown. Severely weakened constitutions were, it was argued, more susceptible to nervous disorders, nightmares, anxiety, depression and emotional instability. The blockade also generated its own specific diagnosis. Amidst the death and starvation, physicians observed an increase in high blood pressure, which was eventually labelled "Leningrad hypertension."[36]

Psychological trauma appears to have been somatized; mental pain turned into physical symptoms, which, with rest and better nutrition, could be overcome. Of course, other researchers from across the Soviet Union studied manifestations of war trauma.[37] Although Leningrad's psychiatrists were not entirely unique, a distinct cluster of researchers centred on the Bekhterev Institute devoted great time and effort to studying locally observed manifestations of trauma. During and after the war they conducted several important studies of traumatic reactions amongst soldiers and ex-servicemen, some of which were published and others survive in archival documents.

In 1944, E.S. Averbukh published a pamphlet entitled *What every doctor needs to know about psychiatric illness and treating psychiatric illnesses in wartime conditions.* It aimed to familiarize civilian and military doctors with the mental disturbances they were likely to encounter, and provide clear guidelines for diagnosing, monitoring and treating psychiatric patients. Averbukh informed doctors that they could expect to encounter patients experiencing memory loss, poor concentration, confused thinking, hallucinations, heightened emotions, paranoia, mania or dementia.[38] During the war and the years that followed, his colleagues dug deeper into these symptoms and their causes. Several psychiatrists studied mental disorders that had started to be diagnosed following concussions, head injuries and other war injuries. There were studies of delayed forms of psychoses, post-traumatic memory loss, vision loss and depressive conditions that developed amongst patients who had sustained head injuries and contusions during the war.[39] At the Bekhterev's March 1946 conference, F.P. Maiorov presented his research into instances of war hysteria, based on 25 cases of hysterical reactions following concussion (*vozdushnaia kontuziia*).[40] Alongside these studies were a number of papers and studies of how best to provide care for patients and organize psychiatric services. The Institute had an additional role in organizing lectures, discussions and meetings with war invalids and their families, which disseminated research findings and suggested prophylactic treatments for depression.[41]

Individual case histories, written up as part of research projects, provide an indication of the manifestations of trauma observed by psychiatrists. M.M. Mirskaia, for example, conducted research into delayed or long-term psychiatric disturbances amongst people who had suffered head or brain injuries, most commonly the result of physical concussions (*kontuziia*). The project sampled 120 cases, the majority were men aged between 25 and 40, and almost certainly soldiers.[42] The case history of patient Sh-ik, a 39-year-old man, indicated the complexity of observed symptoms. Sh-ik was concussed on 5 November 1943. Initially his emotions and physical state were heightened and he experienced hearing loss. He was constantly hungry and thirsty. He would drink up to eight mugs of beer in rapid succession and smoke four or five cigarettes at the same time. This manic phase had passed by the time he was admitted to the institute on 15 November. He was sluggish, drowsy, suffering memory loss and his mental faculties had slowed. His speech would also be blocked by a tightening of his lips, teeth and tongue. He was emotionally withdrawn, remaining in bed for long periods of time, taking no interest in his personal hygiene. He became obsessed with ideas that, "nobody loved him, that he was unwanted, and that he was a hindrance to everybody."[43]

Another report described the symptoms recorded amongst soldiers who had fought in the Winter War with Finland. Patient P-v, a 25-year-old soldier, was admitted to hospital in January 1940. He had been engaged in a fierce battle between 25 and 31 December 1939, not sleeping during the entire period. After the battle, he fell into a deep sleep, experiencing nightmares about combat. When he awoke, he began behaving strangely and was unable to readjust.[44] Kr-ov, a 24-year-old soldier, was wounded in the neck and admitted to hospital, where medics observed his disturbed state. He confused dreams with reality, claiming that he had been awarded a medal by Stalin. At times he would become agitated and confused and ask about his medal and other gifts from the *vozhd'* (the leader, Stalin).[45] Twenty-three-year-old T-v had been injured by a grenade exploding in a dugout. Although his physical scars healed well, the mental scars went deeper. Obsessive fears of death and blood infection prevented him from sleeping. His behaviour became increasingly disturbed as sleep deprivation set in. He feared he might be punished and was concerned that he was being poisoned.[46] K-ov had lost a foot and several toes on his other foot to frostbite. The injury transformed his behaviour. He became withdrawn and had difficulties sleeping. By the time he arrived at hospital, he was depressed, suspicious and fearful that he would be shot for leaking military secrets in his letters home.[47]

Leningrad's psychiatrists offered explanations for the reactions they observed that were in keeping with the official organic and materialist frameworks for mental illness. They, like Soviet psychiatrists more generally, were working within ideological and theoretical frameworks which questioned how damaging the fear, violence and killing of war was for combatants. In his manual, Averbukh explained that *kontuziia* was the result of shock to the brain and functional changes in the central nervous system inflicted by the explosive force and sudden changes in atmospheric pressure, of modern shells, bombs and mines.[48] Other researchers argued that prolonged periods of heightened anxiety, stress and exertion gradually weakened soldiers' nervous systems, making them more susceptible to breakdowns or psychiatric disturbances.[49] The organic understanding of mental disability suggested relatively straightforward treatment. If psychiatric disorders were the product of stress and exhausted nervous systems, they could be remedied by rest and proper nutrition.[50] These explanations were consistent with the official medical history of the war and Moscow-based psychiatric research, for example, M.O. Gurevich's influential post-war psychiatric textbooks.[51] There was, however, less consensus on how to make sense of trauma than the official explanatory framework implied. The Bekhterev's researchers often found it difficult to square their observations with scientific and ideological realities. Elsewhere in the Soviet Union, psychiatrists criticized the use of the term *kontuziia*, because it was imprecise.[52] Leningrad's researchers were using a variety of other labels to describe traumatic reactions, including post-traumatic lesions, post-traumatic brain damage, internal injuries to the skull, and delayed effects of physical injuries. Veterans' families were not the only ones who struggled for an appropriate language to describe trauma.

According to Anna Krylova, the "cohort of Soviet psychiatrists who came to dominate the profession in the 1940s was unfamiliar with psychological explanatory frameworks"; as a result, psychological factors were excluded from treatment.[53] The Bekhterev's researchers, however, occasionally acknowledged the role of psychological factors in post-traumatic reactions. E.K. Iakovleva believed that psychiatric trauma was caused by contusions, but psychological factors on veterans' return could reactivate trauma. Anxiety about temporary invalidity, a reduction in work capacity, or general health, housing, family and everyday problems, alongside concerns about other people's reactions to them, could prompt emotional agitation. As a resolution, Iakovleva proposed psychotherapy and studying patients' personalities and behaviour from all perspectives.[54] The Bekhterev Institute's researchers were well aware of their predecessors' interest in trauma and previous analytical frameworks. Many of Leningrad's military psychiatrists could trace their careers back to before the Revolution. V.P. Osipov, for example, had been a student of V.M. Bekhterev in the late 1890s, and had directed the Military Medical Academy's psychiatric department during the First World War, studying and treating psychiatric casualties.[55] Vladimir Nikolaevich Miasishchev had directed the Bekhterev Institute since 1939, had worked there since 1919, and was a close colleague of V.M. Bekhterev.[56] Raisa Iakovlevna Golant, one of the Bekhterev Institute's leading trauma researchers, was also a former student of V.M. Bekhterev, and had been an employee of the Military-Medical Academy between 1917 and 1928.[57] These and other researchers were familiar with past research into the traumatic effects of war, even if they did not always agree with it.

In the introduction to the volume on nervous illness in the Great Patriotic War's official medical history, S.N. Davidenkov questioned pre-revolutionary research into hysteria, war neuroses and *kontuziia*. He argued that during the Russo-Japanese War and the First World War these conditions were often misdiagnosed. In his analysis, doctors frequently confused physical damage to the brain with psychiatric illnesses.[58] Other researchers adopted a similar position. F.I. Grinstein and A.Z. Rosenberg, for example, argued that older research describing unique forms of "war psychosis" lacked evidence.[59] Averbukh poured scorn on the idea that war generated its own forms of mental illness, arguing that peacetime syndromes adopted specific forms and nuances under wartime conditions.[60]

From the available evidence, it is hard to know whether the Bekhterev's psychiatrists genuinely believed the official explanations for trauma, or were parroting official mantras and ideological orthodoxies. Recent research has questioned the extent to which Soviet science was deformed and scientists constrained by a totalitarian ideology. Benjamin Zajicek has argued that Soviet psychiatrists made genuine attempts to diagnose, treat and explain the mental disorders within the scientific frameworks available to them.[61] Leningrad's leading researchers were establishment figures not dissidents. Vladimir Miasishchev, the Bekhterev Institute's director, was a party member, and between 1945 and 1948 a member of Leningrad's Nevskii district party committee. Between 1939 and 1948, Raisa Golant was a deputy of the city Soviet. Yet the Institute's research into war trauma proved relatively short-lived. Traumatized veterans and blockade survivors did not disappear, but their problems soon became lower priorities for researchers. This was not simply the product of an authoritarian state's desire to repress trauma, although there was perhaps an element of this. With the passing of a senior generation of research staff, interest in trauma diminished. Victor Osipov died in 1947, and Raisa Golant in 1953.[62] In March 1948, the USSR Ministry of Healthcare ordered an inspection of the work of the institute and its research.[63] In July 1948, the Ministry of

Healthcare ordered a restructuring of the institute, including the sacking of several brain physiology researchers, although these were subsequently overturned.[64] Within approximately five years of the war's end, the Bekhterev Institute was a very different institution, with different research plans.

Psychiatric research was hardly a guarantor of better care for Leningrad's veterans. Researchers were rarely able to make substantive contributions to treatment. The Bekhterev Institute was primarily concerned with theoretical questions, rather than practical clinical assistance. Of the 405 beds available in its wards, just 60 were reserved for treating disabled veterans with brain injuries or psychiatric problems.[65] Presumably only the most interesting cases were cherry-picked for closer examination. Nor was the city's official network of psychiatric hospitals up to the task. In 1946, Leningrad's psychiatric hospital No. 2 had 360 beds. In the course of that year, the hospital treated just 110 war invalids, a tiny fraction of the city's veterans.[66] Conditions in hospitals, particularly psychiatric institutions, were horrific. Even Leningrad's flagship hospitals for war invalids, located in the city centre, occupied dilapidated buildings, lacked basic sanitation and experienced shortages of basic equipment.[67] Faced with appalling conditions, few veterans wanted to pursue treatment if it identified them as victims or damaged goods. The overwhelming majority of psychiatric patients in the Soviet healthcare system were treated as outpatients at dispensaries. As of 1 January 1946, there were 3798 invalids from the Great Patriotic War registered with neuropsychiatric dispensaries in Leningrad, of which 167 were being treated for traumatic epilepsy, 781 for open head wounds and 1748 for the effects of internal head injuries, a label commonly applied to *kontuziia*-like disturbances. In practice, a significantly lower number were receiving regular treatment.[68]

Post-war psychiatric research provides valuable evidence that trauma never entirely disappeared from the official record. Psychiatrists, however, should not be granted an exclusive monopoly on observing, defining and discussing war trauma. Their findings, treatments and theories rarely penetrated beyond a small circle of experts. Many thousands of veterans returned from the front shaken by their wartime experiences, although they were never officially diagnosed as traumatized. As Maria Golubeva's and Olga Krymova's letters remind us, war's traumatic effects spread far beyond the medical profession. The Bekhterev's psychiatrists were not only the people thinking about "no longer normal" behaviour amongst veterans. Yet, most ordinary citizens usually lacked the vocabulary, knowledge and understanding to make sense of abnormal behaviour. Nevertheless, trauma was a social reality, manifesting itself in a variety of ways, contributing to a set of interrelated social problems, visible to Leningraders. Wider society was aware that veterans were often angry, irritable and aggressive, and experienced nightmares, flashbacks and survivor guilt. These symptoms were not recognized as trauma, but the capacity of war to damage soldiers' minds, as well as their bodies, was there for everybody to see.

Troubled veterans' preferred method of dealing with the difficulties of post-war adjustment was the bottle. Drink, just as it had done at the front, provided a means of escaping trauma.[69] In the absence of alternative medication or more widespread psychiatric care, vodka became a form of self-medication, the main means of numbing psychological and physical pain. Leningrad was a city awash with alcohol. Even in the most difficult months of post-war shortages, vodka remained freely available. One group of more abstemious veterans wrote to *Leningradskaia pravda*, the city's main newspaper, in September 1946 to complain of the proliferation of outlets selling alcohol in their neighbourhood, while bread remained difficult to find.[70] A hard-drinking culture amongst veterans had deep roots in Russian culture, and was bound up with notions of masculinity and male sociability. As Elena Zubkova has suggested, nostalgic drinking sessions amongst ex-servicemen congregating in cafes, bars and so called Blue Danubes served important social functions.[71] In the absence of official veterans' organizations, relaxing over a bottle, sharing the frustrations of civilian life, reminiscing about the war and temporarily recreating the comradeship of the "frontline brotherhood" was an important support mechanism. But alcohol always had the capacity to transgress the boundaries of acceptable behaviour. Excessive drinking and alcohol dependency were recurring features of the behaviour of troubled veterans, often not officially recognized as psychiatric casualties but who nevertheless failed to adequately reintegrate into civilian society.

Disorientated, confused and frustrated veterans could react in extreme ways to the challenges of readjusting to civilian life. Discharge from the army cut many veterans adrift from their wartime comrades and support networks. Their friends and families had often died during the war, or were still in evacuation. Their jobs and living circumstances were often at odds with their official status as returning veterans. Faced with the setbacks of demobilization, veterans very occasionally took, or attempted to take, their own lives. Those resorting to such drastic measures were not necessarily traumatized, but many were in states of extreme emotional turmoil or fragile mental health. Surviving archival evidence on suicide is fragmentary. Sometimes suicides are recorded in reports dealing with other issues but contain little analysis of the background to these tragic events.[72] Official interests in suicides after 1945 appear to have been much weaker than in the 1920s when all acts of suicide in the military and the circumstances behind them were systematically studied.[73] Occasionally, however, it is possible to glimpse signs of official concern. In June 1946, General-Lieutenant Shiktorov, Leningrad's police chief, compiled a detailed report analysing 77 suicides and 11 attempted suicides recorded between January and April 1946. The main reasons for suicide were given as drunkenness and the breakup of families and relationships. Family problems were seen as the product of war, particularly evacuation and lengthy separations, during which people formed new relationships. On 2 March 1946, for example, G.A. Zimin, a 39-year-old veteran hung himself in an attic. After his demobilization in November 1945, he returned to find that whilst he was at the front his wife had been having an affair, and that she had no desire to rebuild the marriage. In another case cited as typical, A.P. Slonov, a 27-year-old war invalid hung himself after a drunken argument with his sisters. However, only ten suicides (approximately thirteen per cent of the recorded cases) were amongst serving soldiers, war invalids and demobilized soldiers.[74] Suicides amongst Leningrad's veterans were extremely rare. There was no Soviet equivalent to the wave of mass suicides that swept Germany in the spring of 1945.[75]

Trauma was a contributing factor to many of the social problems which beset the post-war city. Many of the marginalized veterans who begged on city streets, who traded on the black market, and who committed petty crimes were not simply homeless and unemployed; they often bore the physical and mental scars of war. Psychological trauma and heavy drinking were recurrent features of criminal cases brought against veterans alleged to have committed violent crimes. Violence was not necessarily an aspect of veterans' traumatic reactions. However, traumatized veterans prosecuted for violence offences were more likely to have their symptoms noticed and described. Veterans who had suffered some form of head injury or had been diagnosed with *voennaia kontuziia* on the frontlines were likely to be referred for psychiatric assessment. Although courtroom psychiatrists were primarily concerned with establishing criminal responsibility (*vmeniaemost'*) and to check whether defendants were fit to stand trial, their reports offer valuable insights into veterans' psychological and psychiatric condition.[76]

In October 1945, Alexei Kravchenko became embroiled in a fight with a fellow disabled veteran, killing him in the process. For our purposes, the circumstances of the crime are of secondary importance to the discussion of Kravchenko's mental state during his trial. He had been called up for military service at the start of the war. He survived the carnage for four years, but suffered a catalogue of injuries. In 1941 he had lost four toes on his right foot to frostbite. In 1943 he was wounded in the shoulder, and in 1944 and 1945 he had suffered contusions. After the first instance, he began to suffer fits and occasionally lose consciousness. He also began to experience heightened emotions. He often reacted aggressively, and found relating to other people increasingly difficult. During the trial, it was revealed that following his second concussion he spent a month in a psychiatric hospital in Moscow. Before his medical discharge from the army, he had been disciplined several times for provoking fights. He also began to drink heavily as a means of self-medication. He described how everyday he drank at least 200 ml of vodka, estimating that he needed 300–400 ml before he started to feel intoxicated. On the day he was alleged to have killed his victim, he estimated that he had drunk 800 ml of vodka. He explained that alcohol helped relieve the pain he felt in his head, but that when drunk he became aggressive and hot-tempered. Remarkably he described how drinking prompted self-harming behaviour. On two separate occasions he had cut his own chest. There was no indication in the court record how serious these lacerations were, or whether Kravchenko was suicidal.[77]

Psychiatric examinations revealed that veterans accused of violent crimes were often suffering from mental health problems. Many of the accused had spent time in evacuation hospitals with head injuries during the war or in psychiatric clinics after the war. After having been shelled in July 1944, Gerasimov began to suffer convulsive fits. According to his descriptions of these attacks, it became difficult for him to breathe, his emotions became heightened, he became easily upset and would often breakdown in tears. These problems persisted after his demobilization in October 1945.[78] Other reports alluded to the after-effects of *kontuziia* and the influence of alcohol. One veteran who regularly consumed excessive quantities of alcohol required half a litre of vodka before he became drunk.[79] Psychiatrists described increased arousal, hyper-vigilance, irritability, angry outbursts, difficulty concentrating and alcohol abuse—all typical manifestations of trauma. Yet, all of these examinations, despite acknowledging psychiatric problems, concluded that the accused were sufficiently fit to stand trial and were responsible for their actions. Doctors were unwilling to exculpate ex-servicemen for their crimes on the basis of mental illness or trauma.[80] If veterans drew attention to trauma in the hope of leniency, they were to be disappointed. Mental trauma was given short shrift in Leningrad generally, but the notion that criminals may have been traumatized gathered even less sympathy.

War trauma left traces in one further area of Soviet life—the prosecution of war veterans for the political crime of anti-Soviet agitation. As the limits of public expression tightened after the war, blunt-speaking veterans often found themselves caught out by a political culture that increasingly sought to control public expression and behavior. Accusations of anti-Soviet agitation were frequently based on false denunciations, overheard conversations and trumped-up charges. Traumatized veterans, viewed as "no longer normal" because they behaved disruptively in public spaces, were especially vulnerable to denunciation. Accusations that veterans had voiced anti-Soviet sentiments in public may well have been an effective means of removing from circulation troublesome individuals, whose minds and bodies prompted uncomfortable reminders of war's horrors. The most vivid example concerns a series of supposedly anti-Soviet protests made by Iosif Martynov in 1952 and 1953. Martynov, a middle-aged war invalid, had been demobilized in September 1945. He had been injured and "concussed" a number of times. He had lost two fingers on his left hand, sustained nerve damage to his right arm, and injured the base of his spine. He was unable to find employment. He claimed that managers refused to hire him because they needed strong and healthy workers. On 21 April 1952, Martynov created a scandal begging on the platforms of Leningrad's Vitebsk station and at the station buffet. Several witnesses alleged that he had publicly slandered Stalin. In his account, Martynov claimed to be so drunk that he was hardly conscious. On 5 March 1953, coincidentally the date of Stalin's death, Martynov launched a barrage of anti-Semitic abuse in a housing administration office. That morning he had given blood, spending his fee on vodka. Already light-headed from the blood donation, it was not long before he was blind drunk.[81] Martynov was not a serious threat to Soviet power. He was an alcoholic ex-serviceman, no longer quite normal after a terrible war, unable to find his place in post-war Soviet society.

Traumatized veterans never entirely disappeared from public view in post-war Leningrad. Psychiatrists at the Bekhterev Institute studied and wrote about manifestations of psychological trauma, albeit within ideological and scientific explanatory frameworks that stressed Soviet psychological resilience. Yet, as remains the case today, many aspects of war trauma defied neat analytical categories. Experts and veterans' families alike often found it difficult to reach definitive conclusions why some veterans were "no longer normal." Irrespective of the science, veterans' psychological wounds were a medical and social reality. Most veterans proved remarkably resilient in the face of extreme violence, and were capable of drawing a line under the wartime chapter of their lives. It was not that Leningrad's veterans did not suffer psychological pain, but rather it was rarely recognized as trauma and rarely resulted in mental breakdown. The overwhelming majority of veterans found ways of coping with manifestations of trauma which didn't leave paper trails. No doubt the official narrative that Soviet society was fighting a war of survival against an invading fascist enemy offered a measure of protection against doubts that violence and killing had not been justified. The belief that the war represented a moment of supreme collective sacrifice and national rebirth may also have helped minimize trauma. These myths proved remarkably effective for the generations that had endured the war.[82] What was remarkable about Leningrad's veterans was not that some were traumatized, but how rarely their trauma broke through the surface of post-war society. Leningrad was, of course, a special case. The city's unique wartime experience may have helped ease veterans' transition. They were returning to a community which had been on the frontlines and understood the realities of war and its traumatic impact. Nevertheless, trauma was never quite as invisible as often assumed. Psychiatrists and ordinary Leningraders, although they used very different languages, were conscious that Red Army veterans were no more immune to war's mental aftershocks than they were to bullets or shells. What differed were social and cultural attitudes to trauma, which shaped popular and scientific responses to mental breakdown.

Notes

1. Tsentral'nyi gosudarstvennyi arkhiv Sankt-Peterburga (hereafter TsGA–SPb) f.7384/op.36/d.186/ll.76–7.
2. Gosudarstvennyi Arkhiv Rossiiskoi Federatsii (hereafter GARF) f.R–8131/op.31/d.36,641/ll.5–7.
3. GARF/f.R–8131/op.31/d.36,641/ll.16–17.
4. TsGA–SPb/f.7384/op.36/d.226/l.208.

5. Tsentral'nyi gosudarstvennyi arkhiv istoriko-politicheskikh dokumentov Sankt–Peterburga (hereafter TsGAIPD–SPb) f.24/op.2v/d.8230/l.1.
6. Population figures are based on those published in A.Z. Vakser, *Leningrad Poslevoennyi 1945–1982* (Saint Petersburg: Ostrov, 2005), 10; Nadezhda Cherepenina, "The Demographic Situation and Healthcare on the Eve of War," in *Life and Death in Besieged Leningrad, 1941–44*, ed. John Barber and Andrei Dzeniskevich (London: Palgrave Macmillan, 2005), 14.
7. TsGA–SPb/f.8557/op.6/d.1108/ll.46–7, reprinted in *Leningrad v osade. Sbornik dokumentov o geroicheskoi oborone Leningrada v gody Velikoi Otechestvennoi voiny. 1941–1944*, ed. A.P. Dzeniskevich (Saint Petersburg: Liki Rossii, 1995), 573–4.
8. Nadezdha Cherepina, "Assessing the Scale of Famine and Death in the Besieged City," in *Life and Death in Besieged Leningrad*, ed. Barber and Dzeniskevich, 64; Anna Reid, *Leningrad. Tragedy of a City Under Siege, 1941–44* (London: Bloomsbury, 2011), 417–18; Harrison E. Salisbury, *The 900 Days. The Siege of Leningrad* (London: Secker & Warburg, 1969), 514–17.
9. Salisbury, *The 900 Days*, 513.
10. Joanna Bourke, "Effeminacy, Ethnicity, and the End of Trauma: The Sufferings of 'Shell-shocked' Men in Great Britain and Ireland, 1914–39," *Journal of Contemporary History*, 35:1, January 2000, 57.
11. Ben Shephard, *A War of Nerves. Soldiers and Psychiatrists in the Twentieth Century* (Cambridge, MA: Harvard University Press, 2001), xxii.
12. Laura L. Phillips, "Gendered Dis/ability: Perspectives from the Treatment of Psychiatric Casualties in Russia's Early Twentieth Century Wars," *Social History of Medicine*, 20:2, August 2007, 334; Jan Plamper, "Fear: Soldiers and Emotion in Early Twentieth-Century Russian Military Psychology," *Slavic Review*, 68:2, Summer 2009, 259–83; Catherine Merridale, "The Collective Mind: Trauma and Shell-shock in Twentieth-century Russia," *Journal of Contemporary History*, 35:1, January 2000, 40.
13. Paul Wanke, *Russian/Soviet Military Psychiatry, 1904–1945* (London: Frank Cass, 2005), 17–29.
14. Wanke, *Russian/Soviet Military Psychiatry*, 30–41; Irina Sirotkina, *Diagnosing Literary Genius. A Cultural History of Psychiatry in Russia, 1880–1930* (Baltimore, MD.: John Hopkins University Press, 2002), 153–4.

15. Karen Petrone, *The Great War in Russian Memory* (Bloomington, IN.: Indiana University Press, 2011), 121.
16. Wanke, *Russian/Soviet Military Psychiatry*, 56; Merridale, "The Collective Mind."
17. Wanke, *Russian/Soviet Military Psychiatry*, 43–56.
18. *Voprosy psikhiatricheskoi praktiki voennogo vremeni*, ed. V.P. Osipov (Leningrad: Narkomzdrav SSSR, 1941).
19. V.P. Osipov, "Osnovy raspoznavaniia psikhozov i psikoticheskikh sostoianii v praktike voennogo vracha," in *Voprosy psikhiatricheskoi praktiki voennogo vremeni*, ed. Osipov, 6.
20. Osipov, "Osnovy raspoznavaniia psikhozov," 11.
21. V.A. Gorovoi-Shaltan, "Psikhonevrozy voiny. Postonovka voprosa i osnovnye istochniki," in *Voprosy psikhiatricheskoi praktiki voennogo vremeni*, ed. Osipov, 120.
22. Osipov, "Osnovy raspoznavaniia psikhozov," 5.
23. Catherine Merridale, *Ivan's War. The Red Army 1939–45* (London: Faber and Faber, 2006), 15, 232–4; idem, "The Collective Mind," 47–8.
24. Wanke, *Russian/Soviet Military Psychiatry*, 57–94; Benjamin Zajicek, "Scientific Psychiatric in Stalin's Soviet Union: The Politics of Modern Medicine and the Struggle to Define 'Pavlovian' Psychiatry, 1939–1953," (Ph.D Dissertation, University of Chicago, 2009), 113–67.
25. S.N. Davidenkov and V.A. Gorovoi-Shaltan (eds), *Nervnye bolezni: Osobennosti ikh vozniknoveniia, techeniia, preduprezhdeniia i lecheniia vo vremia voiny*, in *Opyt sovetskoi meditisny v velikoi otechestvennoi voine, 1941–1945 gg.*, ed. E.I. Smirnov, Vol.26 (Moscow: Medgiz, 1949).
26. GARF/f.R-5446/op.51/d.3528/ll.12–10.
27. Wanke, *Russian/Soviet Military Psychiatry*, 80.
28. Merridale, *Ivan's War*, 232–4.
29. Richard A. Gabriel, *Soviet Military Psychiatry. The Theory and Practice of Coping with Battle Stress* (New York: Greenwood, 1986), 47.
30. Anna Krylova, "'Healers of Wounded Souls': The Crisis of Private Life in Soviet Literature, 1944–1946," *The Journal of Modern History*, 73:2, June 2001, 316.
31. On the rivalry between Moscow and St. Petersburg Schools of psychiatry, see Julie V. Brown, "Heroes and Non-Heroes. Recurring Themes in the Historiography of Russian-Soviet Psychiatry," in *Discovering the History of Psychiatry*, ed. Mark S. Micale and Roy Porter (Oxford: Oxford University Press, 1994), 297–307; Wanke, *Russian/Soviet Military Psychiatry*, 15.

32. Wanke, *Russian/Soviet Military Psychiatry*, 46; Brown, "Heroes and Non-Heroes," 298.
33. E.S. Averbukh and V.N. Miasishchev, "Kratkii ocherk nauchnoi deiatel'nosti psikho-nevrologicheskogo institute im V.M. Bekhterev," in *Naucho-issledovatel'skaia deiatel'nost instituta za 50 let* (Leningrad, 1958), 3–5; Wanke, *Russian/Soviet Military Psychiatry*, 12, 46; Brown, "Heroes and Non-Heroes," 301, 303.
34. Averbukh and Miasishchev, "Kratkii ocherk nauchnoi deiatel'nosti," 10–11; Wanke, *Russian/Soviet Military Psychiatry*, 66.
35. V.N. Miasishchev and E.K. Iakovlena, "Ob organizatsii pomishchi pri psikhogennykh zabolevaniiakh," in *Konferentsiia, posviashchennaia voprosam psikhogenie, psikhoterapii i psikogigeny. 23–24 Marta 1946g. Tezisy dokladov*, ed. E.S. Averbukh (Leningrad, 1946), 19.
36. Catherine Merridale, *Night of Stone. Death and Memory in Russia* (London: Granta, 2001), 304; Merridale, "The Collective Mind," 48; Alexandra Wachter, "The Last Heroes of Leningrad. Coping Strategies of Siege Survivors in Soviet and Post-Soviet Society," (Ph.D Dissertation, Queen Mary, University of London, In Progress), Chap. 2—Trauma. On starvation's psychological effects, see *Nervno-psikhicheskie zabolevaniia voennogo vremeni (po materialam Leningradskikh konferentsii 1942–1943 gg.)*, ed. V.N. Miasishchev (Leningrad: Gosudarstvennoe izdatel'stvo meditsinskoi literatury, 1945).
37. On somatization, see Zajicek, "Scientific Psychiatric," 209.
38. Tsentral'nyi gosudarstvennyi arkhiv nauchno-tekhnicheskoi dokumentatsii Sankt Peterburga (hereafter TsGANTD–SPb) f.313/op.2–1/d.17/l.2.
39. For an indication of the variety of projects and conditions, see *Nauchnaia Deiatel'nost' psikhonevrologicheskogo instituta im. V.M. Bekhtereva za 1946 god. Avtoreferaty nauchnykh rabot*, ed. V.N. Miasishchev (Leningrad: Uchebno-proizvodstvennye masterskie Lenpoligraftekhnikuma 1947); *Nauchnaia Deiatel'nost' psikhonevrologicheskogo instituta im. V.M. Bekhtereva za 1947 god. Avtoreferaty nauchnykh rabot*, ed. V.N. Miasishchev (Leningrad, 1948).
40. F.P. Mairov, "Ob isterii u sil'nogo tipa nervnoi sistemy (po materialam voennoi travmy)," in *Konferentsiia, posviashchennaia voprosam psikhogenie, psikhoterapii i psikogigeny*, ed. Averbukh, 15–17.
41. *Nauchnaia deiatel'nost psikhonevrologicheskogo instituta za 1946 god*, ed. Miasishchev, 16–20.
42. TsGANTD–SPb/f.313/op.2–1/d.186/ll.6–8.
43. TsGANTD–SPb/f.313/op.2–1/d.186/ll.6–8.

44. TsGANTD–SPb/f.313/op.2–1/d.115/ll.2–4.
45. TsGANTD–SPb/f.313/op.2–1/d.115/ll.7–8.
46. TsGANTD–SPb/f.313/op.2–1/d.115/ll.8–10.
47. TsGANTD–SPb/f.313/op.2–1/d.115/l.2.
48. TsGANTD–SPb/f.313/op.2–1/d.17/l.3.
49. *Nauchnaia deiatel'nost psikhonevrologicheskogo instituta za 1946 god*, ed. Miasishchev, 7.
50. Wanke, *Russian/Soviet Military Psychiatry*, 54, 68.
51. M.O. Gurevich, *Nervnye i psikhicheskie rasstroistva pri zakrytykh travmakh cherpa* (Moscow: Medgiz, 1945); idem, *Psikhiatriia. Uchebnik dlia meditsinskikh institutov* (Moscow: Medgiz, 1949).
52. Zajicek, "Scientific Psychiatric," 117–18.
53. Krylova, "'Healers of Wounded Souls'," 318.
54. E.K. Iakovleva, "Psikhogenii i psikoterapiia u bol'nykh s posledstviiami zakrytykh travm cherepa," in *Konferentsiia, posviashchennaia voprosam psikhogenie, psikhoterapii i psikogigeny. 23–23 Marta 1946g. Tezisy dokladov, ed. E.S. Averbukh* (Leningrad, 1946), pp.9–10.
55. "Pamiati Viktora Petrovicha Osipova," *Voenno-Meditsinskii Zhurnal*, No.9, September 1948, 60–5.
56. "V.N. Miasishchev (K 60-letiiu so dnia rozhdeniia i 34-letiiu nauchoissledovate'skii pedagogicheskoi i obshchestvennyi deiatel'nosti)," *Zhurnal nevropatol'gii i psikhiatri imeni S.S. Korsakova*, Tom 53, Vyp. 12, December 1953, 979.
57. "Nekrologi. Pamiati R.Ia. Golant," *Zhurnal nevropatol'gii i psikhiatri imeni S.S. Korsakova*, Tom 53, Vyp. 12, December 1953, 976.
58. S.N. Davidenkov, "Vvedenie," in *Nervnye bolezni*, ed. Davidenkov and Gorovoi-Shaltan, 17–18.
59. TsGANTD–SPb/f.313/op.2–1/d.115/ll.1–20.
60. TsGANTD–SPb/f.313/op.2–1/d.17/l.2.
61. Zajicek, "Scientific Psychiatric," 51–2.
62. "V.N. Miasishchev (K 60-letiiu so dnia rozhdeniia)," 979; "Pamiati Viktora Petrovicha Osipova," 60–5; "Nekrologi. Pamiati R.Ia. Golant," 976.
63. Rossiiskii gosudarstvennyi arkhiv sotsial'no-politicheskoi istorii (hereafter RGASPI) f.17/op.132/d.40/ll.39–46.
64. RGASPI/f.17/op.132/d.40/ll.15–17.
65. *Nauchnaia deiatel'nost psikhonevrologicheskogo instituta za 1946 god*, ed. Miasishchev, 7.
66. TsGA–SPb/f.9156/op.4/d.508/l.1,10.

67. Robert Dale, "The Valaam Myth and the Fate of Leningrad's Disabled Veterans," *Russian Review*, 72:2, April 2013, 281–2. On the appalling conditions in psychiatric hospitals, see Zajicek, "Scientific Psychiatric," 69–74.
68. M.H. Genkina, "Meditsinskaia i sotsial'no-proiszvodstvennaia kharateristika invalidov otchestvennoi voiny s neiropsikhicheskimi narusheniami (v Leningrade), in *Organizatsionno-metodicheskie voprosy sovremennoi neiropsikhiatrii*, ed, E.S. Averbukh i V.N. Miasishchev (Leningrad, 1948), 49, 54. On psychiatric dispensaries, see Zajicek, "Scientific Psychiatric," 175–9.
69. Merridale, "The Collective Mind," 50.
70. TsGAIPD–SPb/f.24/op.2v/d.7702/l.52
71. Elena Zubkova, *Russia After the War. Hopes, Illusions and Disappointments, 1945–1957*, trans. Hugh Ragsdale (Armonk, NY.: M.E. Sharpe, 1998), 27–8.
72. TsGAIPD–SPb/f.24/op.2v/d.7480/l.18ob, 60.
73. Kenneth Pinnow, "Lives Out of Balance: The 'Possible World' of Soviet Suicide during the 1920s," in *Madness and the Mad in Russian Culture*, ed. Angela Britlinger and Ilya Vinitsky, (Toronto: Toronto University Press, 2007), 130–49.
74. TsGA–SPb/f.7384/op.36/d.276/ll.30–4.
75. Richard Bessel, "Hatred after War: Emotion and the Postwar History of East Germany," *History & Memory*, 17:1/2 Spring/Summer 2005, 195–216 (199–203); Christian Goeschel, *Suicide in Nazi Germany* (Oxford: Oxford University Press, 2009), 149–66.
76. Dan Healey, "Early Soviet Forensic Psychiatric Approaches to Sex Crime, 1917–1934," in *Madness and the Mad*, ed. Britlinger and Vinitsky, 150–71; Dan Healey, *Homosexual Desire in Revolutionary Russia: The Regulation of Sexual and Gender Dissent* (Chicago, IL: University of Chicago Press, 2001), 175.
77. Leningradskii oblastnoi gosudarstvennyi arkhiv v gorode vyborge (hereafter LOGAV) f.R–3820/op.2/d.2403/l.96, 109–11, 140, 145, 147–147ob, 150.
78. TsGA–SPb/f.8134/op.3/d.1025/ll.161–161ob.
79. LOGAV/f.R–3820/op.2/d.2468/ll.52–3.
80. Healey, "Early Soviet Forensic Psychiatric Approaches to Sex Crime," 157–60.
81. GARF/f.R–8131/op.31/d.39,030/ll.5–7, 8–10.
82. Merridale, "The Collective Mind," 52.

CHAPTER 7

Retreating into Trauma: The Fragebogen, Denazification, and Victimhood in Postwar Germany

Mikkel Dack

In the months that immediately followed the collapse of the National Socialist regime, amid the postwar setting of unprecedented death and destruction, a denazification questionnaire, or *Fragebogen*, was distributed by the four Allied military governments to millions of German civilians and returning soldiers.[1] This two- to-six-page survey required the respondent to provide detailed information about their past political affiliations and activities and had the purpose of purging German society of National Socialist and militarist elements. The *Fragebogen* was a cornerstone document of denazification; while pursuing Allied political objectives, it also had major psychological and sociological impacts on the predominantly devastated population.

Responding to the questionnaire forced Germans to revisit and reflect upon the intense physical and emotional traumas that they had endured during the war and under the Third Reich. An analysis of *Fragebogen* responses reveals the paradoxical ways in which Germans personally interpreted, described, and reinvented the traumas of war and hardships of

M. Dack (✉)
Syracuse University, Syracuse, NY

P. Leese, J. Crouthamel (eds.), *Traumatic Memories of the Second World War and After*, DOI 10.1007/978-3-319-33470-7_7

dictatorship, and how this instrument of denazification created an environment in which recovery from trauma was difficult, in part because inventing and perpetuating a "victim status" could be used as a powerful currency for economic and social gain. By using current psychological models and criteria related to trauma recovery and narrative identity, and by analyzing both the administration of denazification and the subsequent individual and societal response, it is shown that the *Fragebogen*, in its content, structure, and delivery, was an active agent in further fracturing German society and in creating conditions that delayed psychological and therefore community and national recovery from the war.

German suffering in the context of World War II (WWII) has always been a sensitive and at times controversial topic, and it has only been since the end of the Cold War that this subject has been able to be examined without, what Bill Niven describes as, a "distorted and manipulative representation of themes."[2] Both in and outside of Germany, significant opposition is faced when discussing German victims in relation to, or in isolation from, the Holocaust or to define as victims those who may themselves have acted, in one way or another, as perpetrators. At the center of this problematic victim-perpetrator dichotomy is the implicit assumption that the German people, as "perpetrators," have no moral right to claim ownership of suffering; that the violence that they collectively inflicted on "real" victims during the war outweighs any possible claim to sympathy.

In the past 20 years, there has been a significant increase in public dialogue about this politically charged topic and how to appropriately remember German wartime suffering. The entrance of German suffering and the politics of memory into the cultural mainstream has developed on the heels of a large body of scholarship, and not just within the field of history, but from all disciplines of so-called memory studies, including psychology, sociology, literary studies, and social anthropology.[3] Over the past 70 years, the historiography of post-WWII Germany has evolved from a single-framed story of western liberal triumph, focused entirely on themes of political reconstruction and large-scale social and economic change, to a series of intricate studies that deconstruct individual and collective experiences of recovery and remembrance, loss and neglect. Through an interdisciplinary lens of interpretation, the aftermath of the war has been dissected and analyzed, tracing the emotional, psychological, cultural, and material lives of Germans in the postwar years.

These publications vary widely in their perspective and understanding of German cultural representations of suffering, but one point most authors agree on is that the hardships of the war and of the immediate postwar period allowed ordinary German citizens to view themselves, in many cases quite correctly, as victims.[4] It is also generally accepted that Germans often used victim status to create a psychological disconnect between themselves and the National Socialist government and its crimes, constructing a narrative that depicted the regime as a criminal organization that had taken advantage of and manipulated the German people, dragging them into a long and destructive war.[5] As a result, to quote Robert Moeller, "the past about which Germans talked most was that of their own loss and suffering."[6]

Although created superficially mainly for economic purposes, "narrative distancing" by means of establishing victim identities was also common during denazification proceedings. Germans often reiterated stories of hardship and suffering, claiming victim or resistor status, with hopes to retain their position of employment or to pursue a new career that the military government authorities had deemed politically, economically, or culturally influential. Many Germans, even those who had never been party members or active in any Nazi auxiliary group, exaggerated their non-support for and opposition to the regime, deliberately creating cognitive and emotional distance between themselves and the Third Reich and constructing a personal narrative of victimhood. These internal dialogues, although created for positive economic purposes, had negative implications for the reconstruction of individual and national identity. As explained by Mary Fulbrook, "the very process of going through denazification tribunals helped to shape at least the outlines of a (sometimes overstated) 'community of the oppressed.'"[7]

It could be argued, therefore, that victimization and the experience of trauma became an important commodity during the Allied denazification campaigns: a valued means to solicit sympathy from the occupying forces, to excuse and dissociate oneself from the Nazi Party, and to exempt individuals from accountability and the consequences that they could possibly face. This resulted in the breaking and re-making of personal narratives for the purpose of postwar emotional and material recovery, a psychological activity that is examined further in this edited volume in chapters by Susan Derwin and Robert Dale.

German Suffering and Trauma

Despite the social and economic advantages that an individual could potentially gain from claiming victim status and dwelling on both past and present hardships, the truth is that many Germans *were* exposed to extreme and prolonged violence and multiple trauma-inducing experiences during and immediately after the war.[8] Every citizen was severely impacted by the unprecedented human loss and physical destruction produced by nearly six years of modern industrial warfare. By the time the armistice was announced, in May 1945, approximately 5.3 million German soldiers had been killed, another 4.4 million had incurred injuries, and more than a million had died, or soon would die, in prisoner-of-war camps.[9] During the Allied strategic bombing campaign, an estimated 600,000 German civilians perished, while another 900,000 were wounded, and 7.5 million rendered homeless. As many as 1.5 million refugees and expellees died as a result of their migration from Eastern Europe and hundreds of thousands of women had been the victims of rape by invasion and occupation soldiers.[10] In order to recover from such a devastating war, Germans in the early months of the Allied occupation were forced to confront legacies of unprecedented violence, including extreme anxiety and post-traumatic stress.

The *Diagnostic and Statistical Manual of Mental Disorders* (*5th ed.*) defines post-traumatic stress disorder (PTSD) as psychological distress triggered by the "exposure to actual or threatened death, serious injury, or sexual violation."[11] This exposure must result from a situation in which an individual directly experiences or witnesses the traumatic event, learns that the traumatic event occurred to a family member or close friend, or experiences first-hand repeated or extreme exposure to adverse details of the traumatic event.[12] Although the proportion of Germans who experienced such conditions cannot be calculated exactly, nor can their responses to real or perceived violence be measured, by considering the staggering statistics previously mentioned, as well as evidence found in historical literature and in postwar institutional studies on wartime suffering, it is reasonable to assume that millions of Germans were subjected to traumatic experiences during and immediately after the war.[13] German civilians, regardless of their affiliation with the National Socialist government, experienced acute psychological stressors that likely caused long-lasting emotional damage; they were, therefore, by the accepted psychological definition, and regardless of the nature and severity of their mental wounds, a traumatized people.

Despite the popular scholarly study of German wartime suffering, victim identity, and the process of *Vergangenheitsbewältigung* (coming to terms with the past), relatively little is known about the private thoughts and psychological state of German civilians in the months immediately following the war.[14] Research is hindered by the political and social chaos and uncertainty of the immediate postwar years and the strict control of information by the American, British, French, and Soviet military governments. As a result, historians have been forced to rely on a relatively sparse and scattered collection of Allied occupation reports and opinion polls, journal entries, newspaper articles, and latter-written memoirs. However, another historical source exists, one that provides a detailed account of the experiences of individual Germans during and immediately after the war, and allows for a deeper understanding of the complexities of the German psyche during the postwar period.

Der Fragebogen

The denazification *Fragebogen* was conceived as a joint Anglo-American initiative, drafted in the spring of 1944 by the Supreme Headquarters Allied Expeditionary Force (SHAEF) with the intended purpose of purging German society of National Socialism and militarism.[15] First distributed in early 1945, by the end of 1948, more than 16 million questionnaires had been circulated in the American, British, and French zones of occupation and millions more in the Soviet zone.[16] Although the requirements for filling-out a *Fragebogen* varied between zones, as a general rule if an individual was employed or hoped to be employed in a civil service position or as a manager in a private business, a questionnaire had to be completed. In the spring and summer of 1946, when denazification responsibilities were transferred to German authorities, the US version of the *Fragebogen* was shortened in length and renamed the *Meldebogen* (registration form), a form that nearly all German adults were required to complete. Caveats were printed at the top of every version of the *Fragebogen*, warning applicants that if they did not answer every question or if they submitted false information they would be subjected to judgment by a military tribunal.[17] These questionnaires acted as the cornerstone of all Allied denazification efforts, at least until the purge devolved into a watered-down and routine system of *Spruchkammern* (denazification civilian tribunals), which coincided with the prevalent issuing of statements of exoneration, the enactment of far-reaching political amnesties, and a popular German public sentiment of "forgive and forget."[18]

The original survey contained 78 questions that ranged from information on personal identity—"What is your date of birth?," "What is your permanent address?"—to questions regarding political affiliations and military history—"Have you ever been a member of the NSDAP?," "Have you rendered military service since 1919?"—to financial questions—instructing the respondent to list "sources and amount of your annual income since 1 January 1933."[19] But the *Fragebogen* was not a typical questionnaire in that it was composed of more than checkboxes and columned lists. The survey allowed for the inclusion of *Anlagen/Anhänge* (attachments/appendices) such as a *Lebenslauf* (résumé), within which respondents could comment on their answers to the standardized questions and provide justification for their membership in Nazi organizations. Respondents could also include character reference letters written on their behalf and statements of denunciation directed at co-workers, neighbors, and family members. Therefore, the denazification questionnaire contained not only one-word answers but extensive and often emotional-documented commentaries.

The significance of the *Fragebogen* campaign lies in the fact that it was not only the largest component of each of the four Allied denazification campaigns, but also the first international mass survey in history and the first example of a military occupation power using social sciences tools in order to bring about political and ideological change in a defeated nation.[20] The questionnaire program was also representative of the contradictory nature of Allied denazification, as the *Fragebogen* was used not only to root out Nazism from German political and economic systems and to punish "active" Nazis, but also to identify and in a sense reward those Germans who had, according to Allied criteria, remained either passive or resistant to the regime and who could potentially assist in the reconstruction of democratic principles and institutions. However, for the purpose of this chapter, the importance of the questionnaires lies in the simple fact that this was, for many Germans, the first instance in which they wrote anything down after the war and the first opportunity to not only reflect upon but also record the details of their recent past under the Third Reich.[21]

Of course one cannot expect the questionnaires to provide an honest account of the political lives of those living under the Nazi regime, as individuals who completed a *Fragebogen* were attempting to keep their jobs or to gain employment and therefore were motivated to embellish or exclude particular events and experiences. However, we also cannot assume that most of the written responses were fabricated. Germans were well aware of the extremely serious consequences that befell those caught falsifying their questionnaire (in many cases the punishment was probably worse than if the respondent had told the truth). After reading and analyzing hundreds of questionnaires, certain commonalities and trends emerge, such as the surprising inclusion of stories of suffering and loss, from which certain theories can be advanced regarding the psychological state of individual Germans, their self-constructed identities, and the way in which they processed and articulated real or perceived traumatic experiences. As such, the *Fragebogen* provides a unique look into war-related trauma and the private processing of mental debilitation in postwar German society.

While the creation of a German victim identity in the immediate postwar years has been studied at length, the existing literature concentrates almost exclusively on political and cultural continuities and the persistence of Germans in forgetting, manipulating, and substituting memories of the past. The various influences that the occupation authorities had on postwar German politics, economics, and popular culture have also been thoroughly explored in the relevant historiography, but the impact that American, British, French, and Soviet occupiers had on German identity and memory remains understudied. Therefore, by examining the denazification questionnaires not only is a valuable and previously unexplored historical source being brought to the surface for scholarly inquiry, one that has the potential to provide significant insight into the dynamic topic of postwar German memory, but it also allows for a new interpretation of how Allied efforts to "re-educate," "reorient" and "ideologically cleanse" the German people directly impacted individual and collective narratives of victimhood. Instead of focusing solely on German psychological resistance to political and ideological change, and the reluctance by individuals, families, and larger communities to confront their Nazi past and the crimes of the Holocaust, this research seeks to introduce the forgotten actor, the occupier, into the gestalt of the time and to analyze the major influences that the Allied authorities had on changing constructs of German identity, whether intentional or not.[22]

If the central tenants of modern trauma and narrative studies are consulted, it is shown that denazification inadvertently discouraged the individual from processing experiences of suffering and loss and perpetuated the development of victim identities. The *Fragebogen* program allowed for and encouraged Germans to retreat into trauma as a means to survive in the face of the Allied occupation and to cultivate an environment of deceit, disunion, low self-esteem, and helplessness.

Denunciation and Recovery from Trauma

According to Judith Herman's widely accepted model for trauma recovery, the survivor of a traumatic experience must create new intimate connections with the people in their lives and rebuild basic capacities for trust.[23] She argues that the survivor can only expect to recover psychologically within a context of healthy personal relationships, or "healing relationships," and with communal support. Furthermore, recovery from trauma is based upon the survivor's sense of personal empowerment, autonomy, and safety, and "no intervention that takes power away from the survivor can possibly foster recovery."[24] Remembrance and mourning, let alone reconnection with ordinary life, cannot be achieved until the survivor can trust and feel safe within his or her immediate community.

A similar dynamic is prescribed in Kai Erikson's model for disaster trauma recovery, which suggests that any trauma that has been endured collectively—as a culture, a nation, a family, or by any other group—can only be recovered from once communal bonds and networks of support have been restored.[25] Erikson maintains that a traumatic experience of any nature results in symptoms of vulnerability, helplessness, abandonment, and fear, and that without a "meaningful community" to turn to for support and without a conscious effort to avoid individual isolation, a survivor will have extreme difficulty recovering from their psychological injury.[26] According to Erikson, a loss of communal trust only perpetuates the trauma as it prevents the creation of an "emotional shelter."[27]

Such views regarding the role of community in the recovery from trauma have entered into orthodoxy and been integrated into the training of mental health practitioners for postwar and post-disaster humanitarian emergency efforts. Not only has the need for a community support system been included in the official mandate of the International Society for Traumatic Stress Studies (2002), but also recommended in the United Nation's Guidelines on Mental Health and Psychosocial Support in Emergency Settings (2007), a training manual endorsed by more than 200 non-governmental organizations.[28]

During WWII and in its immediate aftermath, much of the German population struggled to re-establish healthy and meaningful relationships within their communities, such as those prescribed by trauma recovery theorists. The process of re-forging communal bonds was undertaken in varying degrees through the shared experience of violence, the loss of family members, the destruction of one's home, and the sufferings endured under the occupation, as well as latent feelings of humiliation and helplessness, bonds that Frank Biess refers to as "postwar emotional communities."[29] However, such emotional solace was severely undercut by the widespread and accepted practice of political denunciations during Allied efforts to identify and punish former Nazis party members and sympathizers. Furthermore, it can be presumed that a personal sense of empowerment, autonomy, and safety, also identified as prerequisites for recovery from trauma, were largely absent during this same period as the early months of the occupation were defined by strict military government control of the population, commonplace discrimination, and recurring acts of violence committed against citizens, especially at the hands of Soviet soldiers and occupation authorities.

By the spring of 1945, German society was already familiar with government-encouraged denunciation. Under the Third Reich, the Gestapo relied heavily on political and racial denunciations from the German populace in order to secure its monopoly of information within the totalitarian government system and to maintain its image as an all-knowing and omnipresent secret police. Gestapo offices were often reduced to acting as mere clearing houses, processing the countless number of denunciation letters received by citizens.[30] According to Robert Gellately, there were so many voluntary denunciations that by the war's end the regime came close to having "files on the political lives and opinions of nearly every citizen."[31] Although the denunciatory atmosphere dwindled in the final months of the war, as citizens began to lose confidence in the regime, it was given new life by the Allied military governments.

Since the membership records of the Nazi Party and other affiliated organizations were not located and sufficiently organized by military government until early 1946, during the initial months of the occupation denazification officers in all four zones had an extremely difficult time evaluating *Fragebögen* and in deciding who to employ in civil servant positions.[32] As a result, denazification officers relied heavily on local informants to identify party members and enthusiasts and to recognize cases of *Fragebogen* falsification. Although the September 1944 SHAEF *Public Safety Manual of Procedures* clearly stated that the "objective criteria and standard procedures must be used to determine the 'degree of Nazism' of German officials rather than hearsay, denunciation, or rule of thumb measures,"[33] in the American, British, and French zones denunciations were encouraged by military government offices and consulted during denazification proceedings, so much so that the standardized "Fragebogen Work

Sheet," which documented all evidence collected for each individual case, included a separate section for the listing of denunciations.[34]

No matter the personal motivations of informants or whether their statements were accurate or not, German citizens submitted thousands of written denunciations to military government offices in all four zones of occupation. One British intelligence officer of German-Jewish birth stationed in Hamburg recalled the enthusiasm among the local population to denounce fellow citizens, writing that "the process of turning in Nazis was continuing all the time. There was plenty of evidence, in fact, too much. In this situation, denunciation was rife as ever. As soon as people realized I was [could speak] German, I was flooded with information."[35]

Items in the *Fragebogen* itself compelled denunciatory behavior from German respondents. For example, all versions of the questionnaire circulated in the American, British, and French zones asked for personal details regarding the Nazi affiliation of family members:

> Question 101: Have you any relatives who have held office, rank or post of authority in any [Nazi] organizations listed from 41 to 95 above?[36]

> Question 102: If so, give their names and addresses, their relationship to you and a description of the position and organization.

As noted in the "Evaluation of the Revised Fragebogen" section of the *United States Special Branch Denazification Manual*, the ultimate purpose of such questions was to determine whether the individual was falsifying their questionnaire, as denazification officers assumed that if one's spouse or close relative was affiliated with a Nazi organization so too was the respondent.[37] However, regardless of the intentions of the military government, these questions ordered all respondents to submit potentially incriminating information about family members, information that could result in dismissal from their position of employment or even imprisonment.

Furthermore, ample room was provided at the end of the *Fragebogen* for the individual to expand upon any of his or her answers to the standardized questions and to include a sworn statement regarding someone they personally knew was attempting to evade denazification. Letters of denunciation, of which tens of thousands were voluntarily included with the submission of questionnaires, were transferred to the denazification case record of the accused and filed under the title "Information Developed from Outside Investigation."[38]

For example, in December 1945, in the Bavarian town of Schlag, a group of concerned farmers sent a letter to the local Office of Military Government, United States (OMGUS), writing:

> A notable friend of the current Mayor Oswald, from Schlag, is the former Nazi Mayor Gigl … Gigl was an active Nazi in our opinion … he used to always say that National Socialism had penetrated his flesh and blood … we ask how long will Gigl be permitted to act as he does and how long will Oswald be permitted to support him? … One is surprised considering the financial situation of Gigl before 1933 and now. Today he is a rich farmer, before [1933] he was a poor man.[39]

In the neighboring town of Zweisel, in November 1945, a military government office received a letter attached to the *Fragebogen* of a candidate for a civil service position, stating:

> My son-in-law, Alois Grimm, has treated me badly. He promised to behave decently to my wife and me. We gave him our house, arable land, and 500 Marks. No sooner was he in the house when he began to act violent against me. My son-in-law was a strong supporter of the Nazi-Party, he collected much money and had the function of a *Blockleiter* … I cannot stand these maltreatments any longer … I have heard that the American Court of Justice has settled several such cases.[40]

In another case, Ludwig Loubl, a schoolteacher from Wolfersbach, attached a letter to his questionnaire that read: "The town clerk, Kathi Sigl, still has her job, though she is a Party Member and the daughter of the innkeeper Johann Sigl who himself was an ardent Nazi."[41]

With such a widespread practice of voluntary denunciation, an environment of distrust and anxiety was continued and reinforced in postwar German society. Germans who hoped to retain employment or to seek new opportunities in the workforce, an endeavor that was fundamental to individuals and families during the devastating economic climate of the immediate postwar years, were faced with the concern of being personally denounced. While attempting to rebuild and recover from the physical and psychological devastation of the war and the violent collapse of the National Socialist regime, Germans were not only required to function within an environment in which they possessed relatively little autonomy and where fear of the occupation authorities was commonplace for many, but also within a community that was socially fragmented and where personal and collective recovery from psychological trauma was inhibited by the prevalence of accusations, rumors, lies, and deceit. Although these conditions were common under the Third Reich, they were perpetuated by the military governments and their denazification *Fragebögen*.

The detrimental effects that this program had on the mental health of German citizens did not go unnoticed by the occupation authorities or by local community leaders. In a widely circulated memorandum written in May 1946 by the Control Commission for Germany (British Element), an official request was made for the Standing Committee on Denazification to take authoritative action to discourage political denunciations. In an anxious letter, the Chief of the British Legal Division expressed his concern about the "malicious denunciations" being made within the German legal community, explaining that "civil servants appointed with the approval of the Military Government were suffering from a feeling of insecurity as a result of the fear of denunciations made against them" and that "this practice of denunciation, which now threatens under the guise of denazification, is strongly reminiscent of Nazi methods."[42] Suspecting a wider prevalence of denunciations, the officer concluded that "there is fear that similar feelings are rife in other fields of German administrative business and industrial life."

Also in the spring of 1946, in a joint Pastoral letter written by leading members of the German Protestant Church, a petition was made to all four military governments, asking for the elimination of the denazification *Fragebogen*, or at the very least an alteration of its content. Later incorporated into the Church's "official position" on the Allied occupation, the letter commented that "the questions in the Fragebogen, not surprisingly, tempt [the respondent] in some instances to lie and encourages denunciation. This is not beneficial to the moral recovery of the people."[43] According to the Church, denazification "encouraged a wave of denunciation followed by mutual distrust and hatred among the people" and that attempts by the Allied powers to purge the German political and economic spheres had "deteriorated into a program of revenge."[44]

As prescribed by leading theorists of mental health and trauma recovery, in order for an individual to recover from a psychological injury, whether it be extreme anxiety or post-traumatic stress, an environment must be present in which communal bonds are strong, healthy relationships exist, and where personal feelings of trust, autonomy, and safety are nurtured. Within a postwar society of political and moral denunciations, the Allied authorities, in their efforts to categorize and punish the German population and purge it of National Socialist elements, discouraged such an environment. Instead, the military governments and their denazification *Fragebögen* perpetuated the fragmentation of families and local communities, encouraging Germans to turn on one another and to cultivate a culture of conflict and mistrust.

Constructing Narratives and Victim Identity

Narrative psychology, a burgeoning field of research concerned with the "storied nature of human conduct," maintains that our beliefs, behaviors, and self-identity stem from the stories that we have about ourselves, others, and the world; that we integrate our life experiences by constructing stories.[45] Social psychologist Theodore R. Sarbin, a pioneer of this now widely accepted viewpoint, argues that we are naturally inclined to organize our experiences into definable categories of interpretation and to create identities according to "narrative plots."[46] Sarbin contends that the process of recording one's experiences in writing is an act by which meaning and identity are constructed for the individual and communicated. Even if the written words are deliberately inauthentic they can be extremely convincing to the author, so much so that they can cause the narrative and the historical action itself to act as one and the same "semantic structure."[47]

This interpretation of the transformative and self-affirming nature of written language is maintained by leading cognitive psychologists, sociologists, and psycholinguists, who argue that writing assists in the construction of personal narratives and the establishment and reinforcement of identities. According to the renowned American sociologist Erving Goffman, the "individual" exists only within the narrative one *tells* one's self and the narratives one is *told* about one's self.[48] In other words, language practices, whether speaking, reading, or writing, shape and limit cognitive capabilities and solidify self-constructed narratives about ourselves in order to make sense of our perceived environment. Similarly, Frederick Wyatt argues that a story expressed vocally or in writing, while being told, begins to "recognize itself" and to establish a purposeful context and a "comprehensive, personal meaning."[49] Furthermore, when an individual omits or distorts memories, for whatever motive, a new coherent story begins to be constructed, one that can quickly acquire self-perceived truth and replace the actual events.[50]

If this line of reasoning is pursued, it can be argued that the denazification questionnaires, acting as the first instance in which many Germans documented pre-war and wartime experiences, played a significant role in the construction of early postwar personal narratives. Within an environment of unprecedented loss and destruction many Germans were in a state of disillusionment and emotionally challenged by the tumultuous times and therefore sought some sort of meaningful understanding and representation of the past 12 years and an explanation for the political collapse, the military defeat, and the extensive devastation of their lives. However, as maintained by Mary Fulbrook, the entire process of denazification blocked any "honest soul-searching" as Germans were preoccupied with fulfilling their basic needs for survival and in reinventing themselves politically and ideologically in the new postwar world in order to secure employment.[51] Instead of an emotional transition, marked by personal reflection, the holding of oneself accountable for past transgressions, and making a determined effort at political reorientation, denazification was treated simply as a means to an end. It represented an opportunity for Germans to replace individual memories of collaboration, coercion, and indifference with memories of suffering and victimhood in order to not only give meaning to past experiences but also to survive within the new democratic landscape and abide by its proclaimed rules.

The *Fragebogen* forced respondents to mentally organize recent experiences and encouraged them to reinvent themselves and reframe their past. Under the threat of military tribunal and amid a fear of being misjudged (or exposed) as an "active" Nazi, the questionnaire encouraged Germans to build politically approved narratives, whether fabricated or not, and to conceptualize their personal identity according to that narrative in order to secure employment. Millions of Germans were required to complete a *Fragebogen*, to document and elaborate upon their experiences during the Third Reich, and to define their political identities, ideological beliefs, and even moral character, all for the purpose of review by the military government authorities. Such a task surely had an intimate and fundamental impact on how the respondent internalized memories of the National Socialist period, including their private relationship with the regime and recent wartime and postwar experiences.

Of the thousands of questionnaires that I have personally reviewed, a majority of respondents in all four zones, although not asked directly in the survey, chose to include information concerning hardships and acts of violence that they had personally endured, or that someone close to them had, under the Nazi dictatorship. Often specific individuals were identified as the source of the respondent's misfortune, whether it was an intolerant boss, an intimidating relative, an unknown Gestapo officer, or Adolf Hitler himself. Economic and social conditions were also identified as sorts of "oppressors," such as wartime bombings or the fear of a starving family. In all such cases, the respondent situated himself or herself as an innocent victim of deceit, suffering, violence, prejudices, or ignorance. They often described themselves as the furthest thing from a Nazi enthusiast, as the only "real" victim in their workplace, and the recipient of extreme emotional stress. The motives for including such information are unclear, presumably they were meant to elicit sympathy from a faceless denazification officer reviewing a questionnaire or to persuade the military government that the respondent was not in fact an ideologically committed Nazi. Nevertheless, Germans, by and large, used the questionnaire to document traumatic events and to "voice" experiences of hardship, thereby confirming or creating narratives of victimhood.

If Cathy Caruth's work on trauma narratives is applied to this act of documenting individual and collective suffering, it can be argued that *Fragebogen* respondents were "asking to be seen and heard."[52] That the recipient of the story, the denazification officer as it were, was an active player in the construction of the respondent's personal narrative. Recent scholarship on the social psychology of narratives supports this view, that external communication is a powerful psychological tool for narrative building. Lars-Christer Hydén and Jens Brockmeier have argued that when recording one's past experiences, especially if these experiences involved incidences of personal suffering, communication moves beyond mere representation, taking on an expressive and "performative dimension" intended for a particular audience.[53] They maintain that narrating traumatic and disabling experiences allows for a process of "negotiation" and the "re-embodying" of one's identity, an opportunity for individuals to not only understand themselves but to "construct a self" and to do so within the public realm through external verification.[54] The immediate recipient, or audience, of such recorded stories and the relevant cultural, political, and economic contexts that are present at the time of communication directly influence the narrative identity that is being built; the respondents react to these external factors by constructing an identity, or self, that they think they "ought to be."[55]

Similar to the encouragement of denunciatory statements, specific questions in the *Fragebögen* distributed in the three western zones asked Germans to elaborate on personal experiences from their past and political activities that could be considered "acts of resistance" against the Nazi regime or instances in which they had been subject to persecution:

> Question 110: Have you ever been a member of an anti-Nazi underground party or group since 1933?[56]
>
> Question 114: Have you ever been dismissed from the civil service, a teaching profession or ecclesiastical positions, or any other employment for active or passive resistance to the Nazis or their ideology?

The Soviet *Fragebogen* contained a similar question, asking, "Did you take part in any illegal antifascist activities between 1933 and 1945?"[57] These questions were vague, allowing respondents to determine for themselves what was meant by "antifascist activities" and "passive resistance." It was quite common for individuals to identify themselves specifically as a "passive resistor" or as a victim of "political oppression," terms introduced in the questionnaire itself.[58] Of course, such claims were difficult, if not impossible, for denazification officers to verify. The records of underground anti-Nazi organizations were either non-existent or unattainable and while many employment records had been destroyed during the war, those that did survive gave little indication as to why the individual had been dismissed. Even if these records did contain such information, denazification officers did not have the necessary resources to investigate all cases. Furthermore, many respondents claimed that they had experienced undisclosed resistance or unreported persecution and that they had subverted their political or ideological beliefs; therefore, no documentation or witnesses could provide confirmation.[59]

The problems that such questions created for the denazification officers charged with reviewing *Fragebogen* responses is evidenced in the June 1946 revised manual on denazification law, intended for Special Branch officers stationed in US-occupied Bavaria, which outlined instructions for the evaluation of the questionnaire:

> Questions 110 to 116: These questions are intended to reveal those who remained in active or passive resistance to the Nazis. It should be borne in mind that almost everyone now claims to have been against the Nazis and to have joined the NSDAP under compulsion.[60]

By asking open-ended and ambiguous questions regarding individual acts of persecution and resistance, the military governments made denazification classification exceedingly difficult for their administrations and encouraged varying interpretations of the terms "victim" and "resistor" from the respondents. The questionnaire either allowed those Germans who had in fact experienced persecution at the hands of the Nazis, or some other identified "oppressor," to confirm their victim status, or allowed Germans to actively falsify their *Fragebogen* and to construct fictitious identities that could potentially be amalgamated with "real" experiences in order to produce a new narrative. Such manufactured identities would be further validated if the respondent completed the denazification process and was approved for employment, thereby, in a sense, giving the new narrative an official seal of approval. Regardless, both scenarios resulted in the individual focusing on traumatic experiences and using them for political and economic purposes.

The strict categorization inherent in denazification procedures further exacerbated the tendency of respondents to define themselves as victims of the regime. After reviewing a *Fragebogen*, denazification officers in the US and British zones placed the applicant into one of four predetermined categories, either "active Nazi," "nominal Nazi," "non-Nazi" or "anti-Nazi."[61] After denazification was handed over to German authorities in 1946, similar categories of affiliation were instituted, in which the vast majority of respondents were classified as either *Minderbelastete* (Lesser Offenders), *Mitläufer* (Followers), or *Entlastete* (Persons Exonerated).[62] The only category that did not mandate some form of punishment or sanction was *Entlastete*, which required the individual to have "not only showed a passive attitude but also actively resisted the National Socialistic tyranny to the extent of their powers and thereby suffered disadvantages."[63] In response to such a strict systematic procedure of categorization and emphasis on personal suffering, *Fragebogen* respondents were encouraged to make clear distinctions as to their Nazi identity, to define themselves as Nazi or anti-Nazi, perpetrator or victim. It is therefore not surprising that so many Germans went to considerable lengths to document traumatic experiences in their questionnaires and to depict themselves as some form of victim.

The vague and open-ended questions of the *Fragebogen*, asked within the strict system of categorization, were complemented by the opportunity to include an appendix, which could be used by respondents to expand upon the physical and psychological traumas that they had endured before, during, and after the war. For example, the 131 questions in the US questionnaire were immediately followed by a section titled "*Bemerkungen*" (remarks), where respondents could comment on any of the answers that they had given or to explain the professional and social contexts in which they had become affiliated with a particular Nazi organization. When respondents did make use of this section, their comments depicted personal instances of inflicted persecution, deceit, coercion, and suffering.

A former party member hoping to retain his job as a municipal tax inspector commented that "in 1943 I was considered an enemy of the Gestapo, charged with disseminating information and was constantly threatened to be punished in a concentration camp."[64] Another respondent explained that although he was a member of the *Schutzstaffel* (SS), he had once been a Freemason and therefore the threat of exposure and persecution was an everyday burden he was forced to live with.[65] Yet another applicant thought it relevant to share in his *Fragebogen* that his sister had died in the Łódź Ghetto as she had accompanied her Jewish husband there in 1941.[66]

Many more Germans reserved their emotional recounting of traumatic experiences for the allowable supplementary documents, such as the biographical datasheet, character reference letters, and denunciation statements. What resulted therefore were lengthy comments that not only proclaimed the respondents' political and ideological innocence, and in some cases acts of resistance, but also the hardships endured at the hands of others and violent acts committed against them and their families.

For example, in March 1946, an employee of the district court in the Franconian town of Münchberg appended a letter to his *Fragebogen*, declaring that despite extreme pressure from his superiors for many years he had refused to join the NSDAP and was therefore labeled a "traitor" by his colleagues.[67] He maintained that the only reason he eventually did join the Party, and later the SA, was out of fear of being harassed by the local Gestapo office and to retain his job in order to feed his family. Furthermore, he stated that his wife had been denounced by party members within the *NS-Frauenschaft* (National Socialist Women's League) and as a result was forced to work under "horrific conditions" in an armaments factory for the duration of the war.

Another civil servant, this time in Bremen, wrote that his four underage children had suffered tremendously during the war and subsequent occupation, and that any Nazi affiliations that he may have had in the past were now "more than compensated" by the "war damage" endured by his family, which included loss of income, personal health, and their home.[68] An applicant from Heidelberg wrote a long commentary to the local American military government office describing the hardships that his family had faced during the war. "My wife and children have been displaced to Gartow on account of the air raids. Our house and its surroundings were destroyed during battles between the 9th American Army and German troops here. They were forced to spend eight days in the woods, where my child contracted dysentery."[69]

Of course, we do not know the extent to which individuals fabricated or exaggerated traumatic experiences in order to construct a more politically acceptable past, one that would potentially improve their chances of obtaining employment under the purview of military government. However, regardless of economic and legal motivations, empirical research on memory has always been skeptical of the "truth content" of personal memories and that, according to renowned sociologist Harald Welzer, the relationship between experience and the memory of that experience is extremely complex and ambiguous.[70] Also, while we cannot assume that a majority of *Fragebogen* respondents concealed potentially incriminating information about their past, the fact that thousands of Germans were arrested and tried for *Fragebogen* falsification begs the question of how many others were simply not caught. However, even if one avoids making assumptions about the validity of such stories, it can still be inferred, according to narrative psychology, that the mere documentation of personal sufferings, the identification of specific oppressors, and the creation of a victim-victimizer dichotomy had a significant impact on the construction of personal narratives and the psychological strengthening of victim status.

In deconstructing the denazification questionnaire and interpreting the subsequent responses it is revealed that this instrument encouraged Germans to focus on traumatic experiences. Many of the *Fragebogen* questions were noticeably ambiguous, which allowed respondents to reconsider their relationship with the Nazi regime under new flexible definitions and to either solidify old stories or to construct new ones regarding victimhood. The strict system of denazification encouraged Germans to neglect or dilute their Nazi affiliations and to psychologically subscribe to ill-defined military government categories. Finally, the questionnaires were open-ended, allowing the respondent to rationalize their Nazi affiliations, seek compassion and sympathy from the military government by documenting traumatic experiences, and to rewrite their personal narrative as one of long-standing suffering and victimhood.

Conclusion

The long and divided path that has defined German *Vergangenheitsbewältigung* over the past 70 years has been riddled with memories of extreme violence and suffering, and although it is difficult to trace the healing or dissipation of individual and collective mental injuries, especially when one considers the trans-generational transmission of trauma, the German emotional condition has certainly improved. One paradoxical element of this complicated path toward postwar emotional recovery was the Allied denazification program and its cornerstone, the *Fragebogen*.

Although the questionnaire campaign did identify Nazis, many of whom were attempting to conceal their political past, and removed them from positions of influence, such measures came at a severe social and psychological cost. In the postwar setting of extreme devastation and despair, the German people were forced to revisit the physical and mental traumas that so many had endured during 6 years of war and 12 years of totalitarian government rule. A "culture of victimhood" had already begun to develop within the German population prior to the military surrender, but Allied-enforced denazification delayed recovery from personal trauma and reinforced German victim identity by encouraging the construction of politically approved postwar narratives.

The *Fragebogen* encouraged the practice of denunciation, pitting Germans against one another and further fragmenting personal relationships and local communities, emotional bonds that were necessary for recovery from war trauma. The questionnaire permitted Germans to invent themselves on paper, to rewrite history, and to reframe their past, allowing respondents to depict themselves as victims and to create, stress, and embellish the personal impact of traumatic experiences. Instead of processing and overcoming past experiences of war and violence, many Germans retreated into trauma, a withdrawal that was reinforced by the Allied authorities.

Notes

1. The civilian planners who drafted denazification procedures referred to the form by the German name, *Fragebogen/Fragebögen* (questionnaire/questionnaires).
2. Bill Niven, ed., *Germans as Victims: Remembering the Past in Contemporary Germany* (New York: Palgrave Macmillan, 2006), 4.

3. Despite W.G. Sebald's claim that after 1945 German writers avoided the topic of wartime suffering and that a discursive taboo prevailed surrounding depictions of Germans as victims, there has always existed a vast body of literature on this subject. For the scholarly critique of this traditional belief, see Aleida Assmann, *Der lange Schatten der Vergangenheit: Erinnerungskultur und Geschichtspolitik* (Munich: Beck, 2006); Helmut Schmitz, ed., *A Nation of Victims? Representations of German Wartime Suffering 1945 to the Present* (Amsterdam: Rodopi, 2008); Stuart Taberner and Karina Berger, eds., *Germans as Victims: In the Literary Fiction of the Berlin Republic* (Rochester, NY: Camden House, 2009); and Helmut Schmitz and Annette Seidel-Arpac, eds., *Narratives of Trauma: Discourses of German Wartime Suffering in National and International Perspective* (Amsterdam: Rodopi, 2011).
4. See, for example, Konrad Jarausch, "1945 and the Continuities of German History: Reflections on Memory, Historiography, and Politics," in *Stunde Null: The End and the Beginning Fifty Years Ago*, ed. Geoffrey Giles (Washington, DC: German Historical Institute, 1997), 13.
5. Ibid.
6. Robert G. Moeller, "Winning the Peace at the Movies: Suffering, Loss, and Redemption in Postwar German Cinema," in *Histories of the Aftermath: The Legacies of the Second World War*, eds. Frank Biess and Robert G. Moeller (New York: Berghahn, 2010), 139. This concentration had considerable consequences for the identification and remembrance of Jewish victims, especially during the early years of the German Democratic Republic when "official" victim status was reserved only for anti-fascists and communist party resistance fighters.
7. Mary Fulbrook, *German National Identity after the Holocaust* (Cambridge: Blackwell Publishers, 1999), 51. A similar perspective, although generating different conclusions, has been conveyed by sociologist Uta Gerhardt, philosopher Gösta Gantner, and historian Martina Kraus, all of whom argue that denazification and re-education projects acted as a *Ritualprozess* (ritual process); that the ritualized act of undergoing denazification proceedings resulted in the German people as a whole experiencing a positive and reformative sociocultural transformation. It should be noted that Fulbrook, Gerhardt, Gantner, and Kraus, when speaking of the German "collective

experience" of denazification, refer mainly to the US-zone tribunals (*Spruchkammern*), not the *Fragebögen/Meldebögen* and the personal act of recording memories.

8. Discussion of German wartime suffering has remained focused on WWII and its aftermath, specifically the Allied bombing campaign, the rape of German women at the hands of Soviet soldiers, and the flight and expulsion of ethnic Germans from Eastern Europe.
9. Rüdiger Overmans, *Deutsche militärische Verluste im Zeiten Weltkrieg* (Munich: R. Oldenbourg, 1999), 246, 292, 336; Percy E. Schramm, *Kriegstagebuch des Oberkommandos der Wehrmacht: 1940–1945* (Frankfurt am Main: Bernard & Graefe, 1961–1965), 1508–11.
10. Alice Förster and Birgit Beck, "Post-Traumatic Stress Disorder and World War II," in *Life after Death: Approaches to a Cultural and Social History of Europe during the 1940s and 1950s*, eds. Richard Bessel and Dirk Schumann (Cambridge: Cambridge University Press, 2003), 28; Ray M. Douglas, *Orderly and Humane: The Expulsion of the Germans after the Second World War* (New Haven: Yale University Press, 2012), 1.
11. American Psychiatric Association, *The Diagnostic and Statistical Manual of Mental Disorders*, 5th ed. (Washington, DC: American Psychiatric Association, 2013), 271.
12. Ibid.; The DSM-5 also states that the highest rates of PTSD are found among survivors of rape, military combat, and captivity.
13. The most popular of these postwar studies was a public opinion poll conducted by the Allensbach Institute between 1947 and 1955, in which two thousand Germans were asked about their wartime experiences. See Elisabeth Noelle and Erich P. Neumann, eds., *Jahrbuch der öffentlichen Meinung 1947–1955*, 2nd ed. (Allensbach: Verlag für Demoskopie, 1956).
14. For more recent scholarly work on German wartime suffering and trauma and its relation to memory culture, see Norbert Frei, *Vergangenheitspolitik: Die Anfänge der Bundesrepublik und die NS-Vergangenheit* (Munich: Beck, 1996); Mary Fulbrook, *German National Identity after the Holocaust* (Cambridge: Blackwell Publishers, 1999); Harald Welzer, Sabine Moller, and Karoline Tschuggnall, *Opa war kein Nazi: Nationalsozialismus und Holocaust im Familiengedächtnis* (Frankfurt am Main: Fischer, 2002); Susanne Vees-Gulani, *Trauma and Guilt: Literature of Wartime Bombing in Germany* (Berlin: Walter de Gruyter, 2003); Robert Moeller, *War*

Stories: The Search for a Usable Past in the Federal Republic of Germany (Berkley: University of California Press, 2001); Richard Bessel and Dirk Schumann, eds., *Life after Death: Approaches to a Cultural and Social History of Europe during the 1940s and 1950s* (Cambridge: Cambridge University Press, 2003); Aleida Assmann, *Der lange Schatten der Vergangenheit. Erinnerungskultur und Geschichtspolitik* (Munich: Beck, 2006); and Frank Biess and Robert G. Moeller, eds., *Histories of the Aftermath: The Legacies of the Second World War* (New York: Berghahn, 2010).

15. In February 1944, the German Country Unit was formed within SHAEF's Civil Affairs Division. This US-British body was charged with drafting plans for civil affairs operations in the SHAEF-administered areas of western and southern Germany, including denazification and the *Fragebogen* program, and to eventually constitute the main headquarters of military government in Germany.
16. Tony Judt, *Postwar: A History of Europe Since 1945* (New York: Penguin Books, 2006), 56. This number includes both military government questionnaires (*Fragebögen*) and US-zone German tribunal registration forms (*Meldebögen*). Although denazification questionnaires were also circulated in the Soviet zone, the exact number of those processed is unknown.
17. Completed questionnaires were cross-referenced with salvaged Nazi party and government records, the bulk of which were eventually archived at the Berlin Document Center.
18. After the passing of the "Law for Liberation from National Socialism and Militarism" on 5 March 1946, a network of 545 *Spruchkammern* was established in the US zone. These German-administered civilian courts were charged with organizing the quasi-judicial review of former NSDAP members and suspected Nazi sympathizers and militarists. However, due to the fact that these tribunals were severely understaffed and that at the time there existed not only a desperate need for skilled labor and low-level managers in the recovering German economy but also a general distaste for denazification among the larger population, the *Spruchkammer* system eventually failed.
19. "Military Government of Germany Fragebogen," 22 Aug. 47, Bundesarchiv-Koblenz (hereafter, BAK), Z 6II/25, Page 9.
20. Hajo Holborn, *American Military Government: Its Organization and Politics* (Washington, DC: Infantry Journal Press, 1947), 1–3.

21. My research has consisted of an analysis of responses and comments recorded in or appended to the questionnaires. I have interpreted the responses to the standardized questions, as well as the typewritten and freehand comments found in the supplementary pages attached to each individual survey.
22. See, for example, Frei, *Vergangenheitspolitik*, 54.
23. Judith Herman, *Trauma and Recovery: The Aftermath of Violence—from Domestic Abuse to Political Terror* (New York: Basic Books, 1992), 133.
24. Ibid., 133, 136, 155.
25. Kai T. Erikson, *Everything in its Path: Destruction of Community in the Buffalo Creek Flood* (New York: Simon and Schuster, 1971), 240, 259.
26. Ibid., 216, 234, 255–56.
27. Ibid., 240.
28. Stevan M. Weine et al., "Guidelines for International Training in Mental Health and Psychosocial Interventions for Trauma Exposed Populations in Clinical and Community Settings," *Psychiatry* 65:2 (2002): 156–64; Inter-Agency Standing Committee, *IASC Guidelines on Mental Health and Psychosocial Support in Emergency Settings* (Geneva: IASC, 2007). Further support for this view can be found in Nancy Baron, Soeren B. Jensen, and Joop de Jong, "Mental Health of Refugees and Internally Displaced People," in *Guidelines For Psychosocial Policy and Practice in Social and Humanitarian Crises*, eds. John A. Fairbank et al. (New York: Report to the United Nations, 2002): 243–70; Judith Landau and Jack Saul, "Facilitating Family and Community Resilience in Response to Major Disaster," in *Living Beyond Loss: Death in the Family*, ed. Froma Walsh and Monica McGoldrick (New York: Norton, 2004): 285–309; Froma Walsh, "Traumatic Loss and Major Disasters: Strengthening Family and Community Resilience," *Family Process* 46:2 (2007), 207–27.
29. Frank Biess, "Feelings in the Aftermath," in *Histories of the Aftermath: The Legacies of the Second World War*, eds. Frank Biess and Robert G. Moeller (New York: Berghahn, 2010), 41.
30. See Elisabeth Kohlhaas, "Die Mitarbeiter der regionalen Staatspolizeistellen: Quantitative und qualitative Befunde zur Personalausstattung der Gestapo," in *Die Gestapo: Mythos und Realität*, eds. Gerhard Paul and Klaus-Michael Mallmann (Darmstadt: Wissenschaftliche Buchgesellschaft, 2003), 220–35.

31. Robert Gellately, "Denunciations in Twentieth-century Germany," in *Accusatory Practices: Denunciation in Modern European History, 1789–1989*, eds. Sheila Fitzpatrick and Robert Gellately (Chicago: University of Chicago Press, 1997), 188.
32. OMGUS-7771 Document Center, *Who Was a Nazi? Facts about the Membership Proceedings of the Nazi Party* (Berlin: OMGUS, June 1947), 6.
33. "Public Safety Manual of Procedures, Military Government of Germany," Sept. 44, National Archives and Records Administration (hereafter, NARA), RG 331, SHAEF, Special Staff, Entry 56, Box 9, Page 41.
34. "Instructions on the use of the revised Fragebogen Action Sheet and Fragebogen Worksheet," 10 Jul. 45, NARA, RG 260, OMGUS, Civil Administration Division, Public Safety Branch, Box 442.
35. Frank Eyck, *A Historian's Pilgrimage: Memoirs and Reflections* (Edmonton: Brush Education, 2009), 299.
36. "Military Government of Germany Fragebogen," 22 Aug. 47, BAK, Z 6II/25, Page 9. These questions were preceded by a long list of Nazi auxiliary organizations, many of which mandated "automatic dismissal," such as the *Sicherheitsdienst* (SD) and *Schutzstaffel* (SS). The *Fragebögen* circulated in the Soviet zone also asked for information regarding the Nazi and military affiliations of family members. See, for example, "Personalfragebogen," 28 Aug. 46, BArch-Lichterfelde (hereafter, BAL), DO 105/19028.
37. "German Denazification Law and Implementations with American Directives Included," 15 Jun. 46, Archiv des Institut für Zeitgeschichte (hereafter, IfZ), OMGB, Special Branch, Page 127.
38. For example, "Fragebogen Work Sheet—Baum, Hildegunde," 24 Oct. 45, NARA, RG 260, OMGUS, Fragebogens, 1945–48, Land Hesse-Bergstrasse, Entry 313, Box 3.
39. "Bericht über den früheren Nazibürgermeister Gigl von Tramesried," 20 Dec. 45, NARA, RG 260, OMGB, Field Operations Division Records, Entry 731, Box 800.
40. Letter exchange, Joseph Hiller and American Court of Justice, 5 Nov. 45, NARA, RG 260, OMGB, Field Operations Division, Entry 731, Box 800. A *Blockleiter* was a NSDAP member responsible for the political supervision of a neighborhood or city block.
41. Letter, Ludwig Loibl to U.S. Military Government, Regen, 4 Aug. 45, NARA, RG 260, OMGUS, OMGB, Field Operations Division, Box 800.

42. "Denunciations of Officials and others persons approved by Military Government," 24 May 46, The National Archives of the United Kingdom (hereafter, TNA), Records of the Foreign Office (German Section), FO 937/134; "Denunciation of Legal Officials," 9 Apr. 46, TNA, Records of the Foreign Office (German Section), FO 1005/1387.
43. "Die Evangelische Kirche in Deutschland," 2 May 46, Evangelische Zentralarchiv, Entnazifizierung (Juli 1945–Febr. 1949), Vol. II, 7–2092.
44. JonDavid Weyneken, "Driving out the Demons: Denazification, German Churches, and Allied Policies in Occupied Germany, 1945–1949" (PhD dissertation, Ohio University, 2007), 229.
45. Theodore R. Sarbin, "Believed-In Imaginings: A Narrative Approach," in *Believed–In Imaginings: The Narrative Construction of Reality*, eds. Theodore Sarbin and Joseph de Rivera (Washington, DC: American Psychological Association, 1998), 15.
46. Ibid., 15, 29.
47. Theodore R. Sarbin, ed., *Narrative Psychology: The Storied Nature of Human Conduct* (New York: Praeger, 1986), 7.
48. Barbara Johnstone, *The Linguistic Individual: Self-Expression in Language and Linguistics* (New York: Oxford University Press, 2006), 57.
49. Frederick Wyatt, "The Narrative in Psychoanalysis: Psychoanalytic Notes on Storytelling, Listening, and Interpreting," in *Narrative Psychology: The Storied Nature of Human Conduct*, ed. Theodore R. Sarbin (New York: Praeger, 1986), 204. Some psychologists maintain that the construction of narratives by individuals who are processing difficult experiences tend to either "seek value and justification by constructing stories that depict their actions as right and good" or relieve themselves from responsibility by claiming loss of control. See Roy F. Baumeister and Leonard S. Newman, "How Stories Make Sense of Personal Experiences: Motives that Shape Autobiographical Narratives," *Personality and Social Psychology Bulletin* 20 (1994): 676.
50. Robert S. Steele, "Deconstructing Histories: Toward a Systematic Criticism of Psychological Narrative," in *Narrative Psychology: The Storied Nature of Human Conduct*, ed. Theodore R. Sarbin (New York: Praeger, 1986), 268–71. For more recent literature on narrative and identity, see Mark Freeman, *Hindsight: The Promise and Peril of*

Looking Backward (Oxford: Oxford University Press, 2009); Lars-Christer Hydén and Jens Brockmeier, eds., *Health, Illness and Culture* (New York: Routledge, 2008); Amia Lieblich, Dan P. McAdams, and Ruthellen Josselson, eds., *Identity and Story: Creating Self in Narrative* (Washington, DC: American Psychological Association Press, 2006); Robyn Fivush and Catharine A. Haden, eds., *Autobiographical Memory and the Construction of a Narrative Self: Developmental and Cultural Perspectives* (Mahwah, NJ: L. Erlbaum, 2003); Mark Freeman, "Rethinking the Fictive, Reclaiming the Real: Autobiography, Narrative Time, and the Burden of Truth," in *Narrative and Consciousness: Literature, Psychology and the Brain*, eds. Gary D. Fireman, Ted E. McVay, and Owen J. Flanagan (Oxford: Oxford University Press, 2003); and Jens Brockmeier and Donal Carbaugh, eds., *Narrative and Identity: Studies in Autobiography, Self, and Culture* (Amsterdam: John Benjamins, 2001).

51. Fulbrook, *German National Identity after the Holocaust*, 54.
52. Cathy Caruth, *Unclaimed Experience: Trauma, Narrative, and History* (Baltimore: The John Hopkins University Press, 1996), 9; Mary Cosgrove, "Narrating German Suffering in the Shadow of Holocaust Victimology: W.G. Sebald, "Contemporary Trauma Theory and Dieter Forte's Air Raid Epic," in *Germans as Victims: In the Literary Fiction of the Berlin Republic*, eds. Stuart Taberner and Karina Berger (Rochester, NY: Camden House, 2009), 169–70.
53. Lars-Christer Hydén and Jens Brockmeier, "Introduction," in *Health, Illness and Culture*, eds. Lars-Christer Hydén and Jens Brockmeier (New York: Routledge, 2008), 2.
54. Ibid., 6–7; Jens Brockmeier and Donal Carbaugh, "Introduction," in *Narrative and Identity: Studies in Autobiography, Self, and Culture*, eds. Jens Brockmeier and Donal Carbaugh (Amsterdam: John Benjamins, 2001), 15.
55. Lars-Christer Hydén, "Broken and Vicarious Voices of Narratives," in *Health, Illness and Culture*, eds. Lars-Christer Hydén and Jens Brockmeier (New York: Routledge, 2008), 38.
56. "Military Government of Germany Fragebogen," 22 Aug. 47, BAK, Z 6II/25, Page 9.
57. See, for example, "Personalfragebogen," 28 Aug. 46, BAL, DO 105/19028, Page 3.
58. See, for example, Fragebogen of Walter Korst, 19 Sept. 45, NARA, RG 260, Entry 313, Box 317.

59. See, for example, letter, Frau Maria Maser to Denazification Committee of the Municipality of Dortmund, 28 May 46, Archiv für Christlich-Demokratische Politik, CDU Parteigremien, 03-002-001/1.
60. "German Denazification Law and Implementations with American Directives Included," 15 Jun. 46, IfZ, OMGB, Special Branch, Page 171.
61. OMGUS, CAD, *Denazification, Cumulative Review. Report, 1 April 1947–30 April 1948* (Adjutant General, OMGUS, 1948), 2. All four military governments used a similar classification system.
62. Ibid., 54. The fifth and final category, which was rarely applied by regular denazification officers, was *Hauptschuldige* (Major Offenders). This category was reserved for individuals who had taken an active leadership role in the Nazi dictatorship or who had committed war crimes.
63. Ibid., 59.
64. Fragebogen of Ernst Albert Klingler, 16 Jan. 46, NARA, RG 260, Entry 313, Box 317.
65. Fragebogen of Oswald Heinrich Graf, 5 Jun. 45, NARA, RG 260, Entry 313, Box 318.
66. Fragebogen of Walter Korst, 19 Sept. 45, NARA, RG 260, Entry 313, Box 317.
67. "Permission for Reinstatement as Employee of Justice at the District Court (Amtsgericht) Münchberg," 21 Mar. 46, NARA, RG 260, Entry 313, Box 588.
68. Letter exchange, Siebold Poppina and Regierunsprasidenten, 12 Mar. 45, Friedrich-Ebert-Stiftung Archiv der sozialen Demokratie, Schumacher Bestand, Mappe 98.
69. "Application," 19 Jun. 45, NARA, RG 260, OMGUS, Civil Administration Division, Public Safety Branch, Entry 313, Box 356.
70. As summarized in Dorothee Wierling, "Generations as Narrative Communities: Some Private Sources of Public Memory in Postwar Germany," in *Histories of the Aftermath: The Legacies of the Second World War*, eds. Frank Biess and Robert G. Moeller (New York: Berghahn, 2010), 103. See also, Harald Welzer, Sabine Moller, and Karoline Tschuggnall, *Opa war kein Nazi: Nationalsozialismus und Holocaust im Familiengedächtnis* (Frankfurt am Main: Fischer, 2002); and Harald Welzer, *Das kommunikative Gedächtnis: Eine Theorie der Erinnerung* (Munich: C.H. Beck, 2002).

PART IV

Recollection

CHAPTER 8

Public and Private: Negotiating Memories of the Korean War

Sandra Kessler

In February 2014, pictures of elderly Koreans, North and South, reunited after more than 60 years of separation, saturated the international media. The images captured the emotional moments when long-divided family members met again at an official reunification gathering. Some tightly embraced their missed relatives and burst into tears; a 92-year-old South Korean man danced with his arms stretched out, beaming with joy. The majority of the 83 citizens of the Republic of Korea (ROK) who collectively traveled to the meeting place at the Geumgang Mountain resort in North Korea were in their seventies or eighties. Several of the aging attendants faced health troubles coping with the strenuous journey and unsettling situation; some had to be carried to the event under medical surveillance. Still, these participants invited to join their lost relatives among the 178 attending North Koreans were the lucky ones, chosen through a lottery system of approximately 71,000 South Korean applicants who have been on a waiting list to meet their kin residing in the Democratic People's Republic of Korea (DPRK). Time is working against the unconsidered candidates. As *New York Times* journalist Choe Sang-Hun points out in his online article "Amid Hugs and Tears, Korean Families Divided by War Reunite" dated 20 February 2014, an average of

S. Kessler (✉)
Johannes Gutenberg University of Mainz, Mainz, Germany

P. Leese, J. Crouthamel (eds.), *Traumatic Memories of the Second World War and After*, DOI 10.1007/978-3-319-33470-7_8

3800 list members pass away each year without being granted the wish to reunite with their families.

The reunification meetings are arranged through official channels and dependent upon the political atmosphere as well as the collaboration between the governments of the ROK and DPRK. The program was initiated in 2000 during the period of the "Sunshine Policy" introduced by the former South Korean president Kim Dae-Jung (1998–2003) that sought reconciliation and cooperation in inter-Korean relations.[1] In late 2010, the program for family reunions was interrupted by political tensions as North Korean artillery launched an attack on the border lands of the South Korean island Yeonpyeong. Relations between the two Koreas consequently deteriorated on this and other critical issues such as the conflict over the DPRK's testing of nuclear weapons leading to a temporary suspension of the reunions until 2014.

The organization of the reunification meetings is carried out in South Korea by the Korean Red Cross. While the meetings were paused, the tasks of the Red Cross were also limited. Its annual reports of the years 2010 and 2011 mention the supply of psychosocial support for affected family members, of letter exchange and occasional individual family meetings in third countries and of research on the whereabouts and possible deaths of family members.[2] These are demanding endeavors between the two states that have prohibited any official postal, email or telephone contact among their citizens since the end of the Korean War. Today, ordinary North Koreans face severe restrictions by the government and are not allowed to leave the country. Due to these constraints, divided Korean families are generally unaware if their relatives are still alive or where they reside. Their knowledge depends on the efforts of the Korean Red Cross, and the official reunions are currently their only chance for a temporary family reunion. Even these very occasional reunions only last for a scheduled time period, usually a few hours on consecutive days, with a predetermined agenda mainly accompanied by media and state representatives. Then all participants are required to return to their respective homes.[3] And yet these brief family sessions can be interpreted as the beginning of a healing process in which long-standing uncertainties are cleared and painful memories may be addressed and overcome.

Interviewing the War Generation in South Korea

In 2012, I conducted biographical interviews with a group of the aging Korean War veterans in South Korea. Narrating in retrospect, the elderly men were asked to recapture a much earlier phase in their lives, in particular, their time as young enlisted service members in the Korean military.

My research approach is cross-cultural. It focuses both on the sociocultural aspects of memory making in South Korea and on the processes of cross-cultural communication during the interviews, including differences of origin, age and gender between interviewer and interviewee. As a younger female cultural anthropologist from Germany without a personal military background, I interviewed the men as an out-group member. Furthermore, the research was carried out with various field helpers and contact persons whose relation to the interviewed men also influenced the setting of the interview and the content and extent of the narrations presented. Evidently, it is still unusual for Korean War veterans to talk openly about memories of the past, even within their own families. Some field helpers who arranged interviews for me with their family members heard of their relatives' war experiences for the first time. The transmission of Korean War memories between generations seems rare.

In this chapter, public and private narrations of the Korean War and the related trauma of war experience, relocation, family disruption, political suppression and state violence serve as empiric examples of memory making in East Asia. The analysis draws from public images of remembrance represented in South Korea's biggest war memorial and from the collected veterans' autobiographical narrations. By focusing on the conjunctive notion of family, I hope to show how elements of public and private narrations are interrelated and highly dependent on the audience and the degree of privacy in which they are presented. Individual narratives addressed toward a younger family member may elaborate on personal suffering or the depiction of operational areas. Meanwhile, to a certain extent, these life stories still adhere to the official historiography represented in public sites of remembrance, for example, stressing the positive effects of post-war South Korea's economic boom or referring to key moments in the war's history. To achieve an understanding of the ways in which South Koreans remember the war today, I will briefly retrace the events that led to Korea's current status as a divided nation, then analyze in greater detail particular instances of public and private remembrance.

Korean Partition

The Korean partition becomes most palpable in the inter-Korean border. In 2014, selected family members along with their supporting companions set out from South Korea and traveled by bus to the meeting point in North Korea. To do so, the South Korean group was allowed to collectively cross the Military Demarcation Line (MDL) that runs across the four-kilometer-wide Demilitarized Zone (DMZ) separating the two Koreas. Despite its name, the DMZ is vigilantly guarded by ROK and US military in the South and by armed DPRK personnel in the North. Since the ceasefire agreement that ended the Korean War on an interim basis on 27 July 1953, it has been prohibited to cross the MDL unless permission is officially granted by both Korean governments. Any such permission document, as the specialist of East Asian performance and visual culture Kim Suk-Young points out, is "nearly impossible to obtain."[4] The partition of the peninsula began in 1945, when Japan as former colonizer of Korea (1910–45) was defeated during the Second World War and consequently lost its territories to the Allies. The Korean peninsula was then divided along the 38th parallel, a pragmatically and hastily chosen line of demarcation that disregarded natural surroundings and social relations in the affected territories. The areas north of the 38th parallel fell under the military occupancy of the Soviet Union, the areas south to the USA.[5]

The political situation on the entire Korean peninsula was unstable and characterized by uprisings as well as leftist and rightist social movements. On 15 August 1948, after elections supervised by the United Nations (UN) had been upheld, the South proclaimed the ROK with its first president Rhee Syngman as representative for the entire peninsula. Shortly after, on 9 September 1948, the North proclaimed the DPRK headed by Kim Il-Sung with the same representative status.[6] The tense situation escalated on 25 June 1950, when the army of the DPRK crossed the 38th parallel and expanded into the ROK.[7] By the end of August 1950, the South Korean army and the allied UN forces were pushed back to a corner of the Southern peninsula around the city of Pusan (Pusan perimeter). The majority of the Southern territories were controlled by North Korea.[8] UN forces under US command reacted by engaging in the conflict with greater numbers and consequently shifted the war tide with their amphibious Incheon Landing on 15 September 1950. By the end of the year, ROK and UN forces had pushed back the DPRK army over the 38th parallel, marching further north. As a consequence, the People's Republic of China (PRC) entered the conflict siding with the DPRK.[9] Their armies fought back the UN command toward the middle of the peninsula where battles continued until the armistice agreement put an end to the hot period of Korea's Cold War. To this day, North and South Korea have not agreed on a peace treaty and officially remain in a state of war, while even the armistice agreement has repeatedly been canceled. The country's division was reinforced by the establishment of the DMZ, not far from the original dividing line at the 38th parallel that had anticipated the current territorial separation.[10]

Even after the downfall of the Soviet Union in 1991, the DMZ has remained a strongly visible remnant of the Cold War. For many Koreans, the border symbolizes a "mnemonic scar of war" they "wish to eradicate from the geopolitical map."[11] Kim Suk-Young explains the highly symbolic weight the inter-Korean border obtains for Korean citizens. She considers even its very existence a form of national trauma: "[One] of the reasons that the DMZ figures so prominently as national trauma is because so few Koreans are able to cross it. Those who have, have done so often in highly dramatic ways—as defectors, spies, political emissaries, separated family members, war prisoners, participants in cultural exchanges, environmental activists, and tourists."[12] The elderly participants' border-crossing by bus described at the start of this chapter is therefore a rare, an emotionally charged and an emblematic act, which, if it takes place at all, is only open to a limited number of citizens.

Despite its heavy guard and scattered landmines, the DMZ has recently caught the attention of pacifists and environmentalists alike who not only reinterpret the silent buffer zone as a symbol of peace between two hostile Korean nation-states, but also focus on its unique ecosystem as a stretch of land that has almost been untouched by civilization for over half a century.[13] Yet, the southern side of the MDL has not only developed into a "wildlife habitat" and "sanctuary of birds"[14] but also attracted tourists from many parts of the world. The tourist route is constantly busy with organized tours. Commonplace features such as souvenir and coffee shops cater to the groups' needs as in any other tourist district. Yet, despite the much visited tourist highlights and the developing wildlife around those areas, the DMZ remains a fortified border. Two opposing states face each other across the heavily armed divide and are still engaged in outplaying each other with national images in a Cold War fashion. Both, the ROK and the DPRK, fly huge ensigns on flagstaffs high up in the air on each side of the border, attempting to surpass the opponent in size.

These concordant efforts to display national triumph over the adversary state are similar in style but cannot disguise the contrast between the two Koreas. Compared to the restricted, isolated and impoverished communist regime in the North, South Korea's difference is exaggerated. The ROK seems to have risen like a phoenix from the ashes: the poor agricultural nation before the war, with its devastated areas and demolished cities during and directly after, has developed into an economic power house and a democratically ruled East Asian country that has politically integrated into the world community. Apparently, South Korea has surpassed North Korea in every respect. The rapid economic and social changes during the post-war years have repeatedly been termed "The Miracle on the Han River" to the point of a "jaded cliché."[15]

Remembering 6.25

After the Korean War, the ROK underwent grave economic and social changes as a developing nation. In an environment where public commemoration of the war and its outcome mainly served political and economic goals, citizens were forced to make sacrifices for their own survival and the benefits of upward mobility. Hence, suppressing criticism toward the official historiography and "forgetting" violent memories that opposed the unilateral public presentation of the incidents were some of the adjustments South Koreans had to make to keep at bay the severe penalties imposed by state institutions.

During the post-war years, the ROK government's overall goal was to stabilize the state, mainly by developing a strong economy and military. The authoritarian regimes under military rule had declared anticommunism as "one of the state's primary guidelines."[16] According to Cold War antagonism and the rhetoric of the time, fuelled by periodic assaults from North Korea, another outbreak of the Korean War seemed constantly possible. Public remembrance, memorials and commemoration ceremonies of the war were portrayed as a dichotomy of good versus evil, South versus North Korea, implying the DPRK's continual readiness to launch another attack on the ROK.[17] In South Korea, the term for what foreign audiences are commonly acquainted with as "Korean War" is *yug-i-o*, which translates to "six-two-five" (6.25). The South Korean name for the conflict marks the outbreak of the war, 25 June 1950, and reflects the official view of events. Publicly remembering the Korean War by the date of its outbreak has left little room for doubt about who is to blame for all of the miseries caused by the subsequent war: the belligerent communist North whose armies crossed the 38th parallel on the mentioned day, initiating the tragic struggle and the damage and loss that followed. The term 6.25 also reminds ROK citizens that the war has technically never ended as no peace treaty has been signed.[18] During the Cold War, this "continuous war paradigm"[19] shaped South Korea's self-image as a developing state under siege, confronted with its threatening North Korean neighbor. This official remembrance is a restrictive one; it leaves out the circumstances and reasons for the civil conflict, which originates in Japanese colonial rule as well as the increasing inner-Korean social and political tensions during the subsequent occupation by the allied forces. According to Kim Dong-Choon, the public remembering of 6.25 has been a main pillar of the political and social system in South Korea. This perspective on the conflict is fundamental to strong anticommunism.[20] The narrative of 6.25, particularly in the rhetoric of the Park Chung-Hee dictatorship (1961–1979), put the DPRK's invasion at the center of the story. It stressed the aggressors' brutality in order to keep traumatic memories active and prevent mental wounds from healing.[21] By declaring North Korea as sole aggressor, the Cold War narrative suppressed all deviant memories of war, so that mass killings and atrocities committed by South Korean citizens, police or military as well as by US forces became part of a collective amnesia.[22] These were topics that could not possibly be addressed openly.

Especially during the military dictatorship (1961–1987), contemporary witnesses who voiced alternative experiences of the Korean War and its aftermath—mainly survivors of war crimes committed by ROK or US forces as well as bereaved family members of deceased victims—were harshly persecuted as traitors of their home country. By offering opposing memories, they questioned the official historiography and with it South Korea's power structures, including the state police and the military. As a consequence, the victims were suspected of subversive activities, regarded as supporters of communism and hence declared a threat to national security. Once a person was stigmatized as "Red," the accusation infected and endangered not only the particular individual and his or her direct family members but also more distant relatives and friends due to the guilt-by-association system. In addition to state violence, imprisonment and torture, further disadvantages through social discrimination and marginalization were inherent to the guilt-by-association system. It was active in South Korea until the early 1980s, while the systematic repression of bereaved families lasted until the end of the decade. Out of fear, many counter narratives of the Korean War remained unspoken and were buried in silence.[23]

In the more liberal political atmosphere of the 1990s, memories that had been repressed under the preceding regimes slowly started to unfold.[24] In this setting, ambiguous incidents related to the US military's involvement in the Korean War, such as the killings at No Gun Ri, became known to the public and challenged the dominant interpretation of the war events. These "subversive accounts"[25] also shed light on civilian casualties inflicted by

South Korean and US military troops during the Korean War and put into question the disparate relationship between the two countries. In 2005, the Truth and Reconciliation Commission of the Republic of Korea (TRCK) started to investigate "the other war,"[26] as former standing commissioner Kim Dong-Choon puts it. Critical incidents such as mass killings belonged to this "other" side of the Korean War that had been excluded from public discourse. Subject to the official institution's mission were investigations and truth-finding processes about war massacres as well as cases of repression, discrimination and human rights abuses during the authoritarian rule in post-war South Korea. Also the anti-Japanese independence movement and the history of overseas Koreans were targeted by the TRCK.[27] Kim names truth verification as a precondition for the victims to restore their honor and to be able to conduct memorial services for the dead.[28] Through the findings of the TRCK, bereaved families that had been discriminated against in the past were now given a public voice and South Korean society was finally confronted with the silenced aspects of its history.

The War Memorial of Korea in Seoul

One remarkable institution that publicly displays South Korea's national history is the War Memorial of Korea (WMK) in downtown Seoul (Fig. 8.1). The building stands in Yongsan district on the former grounds of the Korean Army Headquarters, across from the Ministry of National Defense and next to the US Eighth Army base stationed in Korea.[29] The memorial and museum, along with its outdoor exhibitions of sculptures, memorial stones and heavy war machinery comprises a total space of 116,589 square meters.[30] The building hosting the indoor museum stands at the center of the site. Its massive outward appearance of gray, solid stone walls and pillars is shaped symmetrically and surrounded by open exhibition areas. The architecture amid the wide open spaces sets the construction apart from the contrasting urban neighborhood and inner-city traffic. Conceived in 1988 during the democratic presidency of Roh Tae-Woo, the memorial opened its doors in 1994. It is a state-sponsored public museum and entry is free of charge.[31] The spacious and prestigious setting of the WMK close to government and military institutions already indicates the importance that the government ascribes to the public remembrance of war and the display of national history. Kristin Hass compares the WMK to the Korean War Veterans Memorial in Washington, DC. The US equivalent is placed within the National Mall, surrounded by other state monuments and located close to the White House: "[The Korean War Veterans

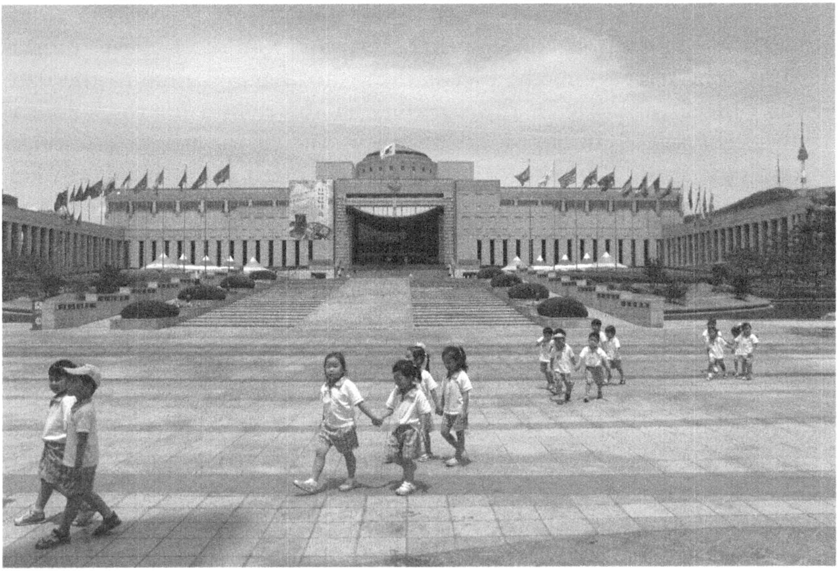

Fig. 8.1 The War Memorial of Korea, Seoul (Photo by the author.)

Memorial in Washington, DC] remembers that it was important to make a grand gesture to memory—the memorial occupies a great deal of the most sacred symbolic real estate in the United States."[32] The significance of public war memory is emphasized by both memorials' central locations in the USA and South Korea.

South Korean citizens reacted to the memorial's conceptual and geographical alignment with military and state institutions with protests. Built shortly after having overcome the military dictatorships, critics saw the WMK as a representation of state authority and celebration of a patriotic state narrative that was imposed unwillingly upon citizens. The visitors, so the critical voices said, felt insecure and daunted by the colossal WMK.[33] Also, the memorial was originally planned to exhibit only the Korean War which was recognized by public criticism as a reminder of the continuous war paradigm of the past restrictive anticommunist regimes.[34] In response to the protests, the WMK has aligned the Korean War with other historical Korean conflicts that stretch back to ancient times. Still, the Korean War representation obviously dominates the site, since more than half of the exhibition grounds concern the conflict which is furthermore located at the very center of the memorial complex.[35]

The Korean War exhibition inside the museum begins with a video installation showing a contemporary exhumation of soldiers' mortal remains. The next room then leads the visitor back in time to the date of the official outbreak of the war, linking the reason for the soldiers' death to the initial conflict. From there on, the visitor follows a selected chronology of the war's history presented through major incidents, key events and battle tactics that cover the timeline of the "hot" period of the conflict. On the whole, the exhibited Korean War events are similar to the 6.25-narrative that rehearses the idea of a South Korean defense against an unjust war of aggression by North Korea. Starting with the key date in South Korea's master narrative of the Korean War, 25 June 1950, the following dates mentioned are accompanied by displays of arms and machinery from the period. Meanwhile, the museum refuses to detail any effects of the conflict on the individual in war-time Korea. Although the printed memorial tour guide of September 2013 carries the title "The War Memorial of Korea: Telling the Moving Story of the People of Korea,"[36] the tragedies imposed on the civil population are hardly shown in the museum.[37] They are represented in universal pictures and dioramas of refugees that demonstrate the results of the war, not its brutality. Clearly, the emphasis on "the Moving Story of the Korean people" refers to North and South Koreans alike and therefore evokes cohesion. Sheila Miyoshi Jager and Jiyul Kim indicate the WMK's "tacit forgetfulness" of the war's viciousness is achieved through "focusing on universal themes of war-time suffering, dislocation and poverty."[38] In a way, the portrayal of the social effects of the war seems interchangeable with the aftermath of most other armed conflicts. Most North Korean atrocities are omitted. This may be understood as recognition or acknowledgment of the need to forget and forgive the opponents' misdoings. Yet, alongside this lack of evidence for the many war crimes committed by the North Koreans, the museum also misses the chance to come to terms with South Korea's own critical aspects in history. As Tessa Morris-Suzuki criticizes, "[the museum] remains equally silent on the subject of massacres or maltreatment of prisoners by Southern forces and their United Nations allies."[39] Although the WMK reacts to current political affairs in its exhibitions[40] and notwithstanding many parts of its display have been introduced since the opening in 1994, concrete findings of the TRCK concerning war crimes committed by ROK and US forces are left out. Instead of catching up with recent history writing, the idea of familial belonging is stressed on the memorial's grounds.

War between Brothers

The overall theme of overcoming the war as a family tragedy is highlighted in the "Statue of Brothers" in the memorial's outdoor exhibition (Fig. 8.2). The stone sculpture depicts two men of different sizes standing on a dome through which runs a jagged gap. Bridging the divide, both men embrace each other, with the smaller leaning toward the bigger. A sign explains to the visitor that the statue depicts a family's older brother, a South Korean officer, and his younger brother, a North Korean soldier. Both, so the sign reads, "meet on the battlefield and express reconciliation, love and forgiveness." The national origins of the two brothers can be easily differentiated by their military uniforms; physical contrast is equally apparent in their body features and body language. The stronger and taller man wears the ROK uniform. According to the memorial's inscription, he also holds a higher military rank: He is an officer, his counterpart is not. The officer seems well-equipped, shouldering a gun and wearing a helmet. His posture is erect with his head tilted toward the smaller man in his arms. The latter, unarmed but wearing the DPRK's uniform, hugs the bigger one in apparent desperation. The soldier's entire body is shifted, clinging to the other's upper body and looking him in the eyes from below. By doing so, the North Korean is stepping forward, almost stumbling. Although his gesture appears feeble, it is he who is taking the step toward the South Korean officer, bridging the gap between them. As Jager and Kim have pointed out, the dome that the two male statues stand on resembles an ancient tomb mound of the Silla Kingdom. Because the kingdom was able to unify the peninsula in the seventh century, the tumulus-shaped dome not only portrays a shared historic past but also carries ideas of "hope, birth, and national renewal."[41]

Metaphorically sharing a common history and belonging to the same family, namely the Koreans, what divides the two brothers is not only the fracture between them but also the ideological background expressed by their different uniforms. In this disparate relationship, South Korea appears altogether superior: militarily, as the South Korean brother is armed with a gun, protected by a helmet and also higher in rank; economically, as he is well fed and displays strong arms; in terms of age, as according to the sign the South Korean man is older just as the ROK was founded before the DPRK, implying its political sovereignty; and lastly, morally, as the stronger brother does not misuse his powers but offers a forgiving embrace to the weaker. The North Korean soldier's diminutive features and despairing body language leave no doubt as to who is in power in this

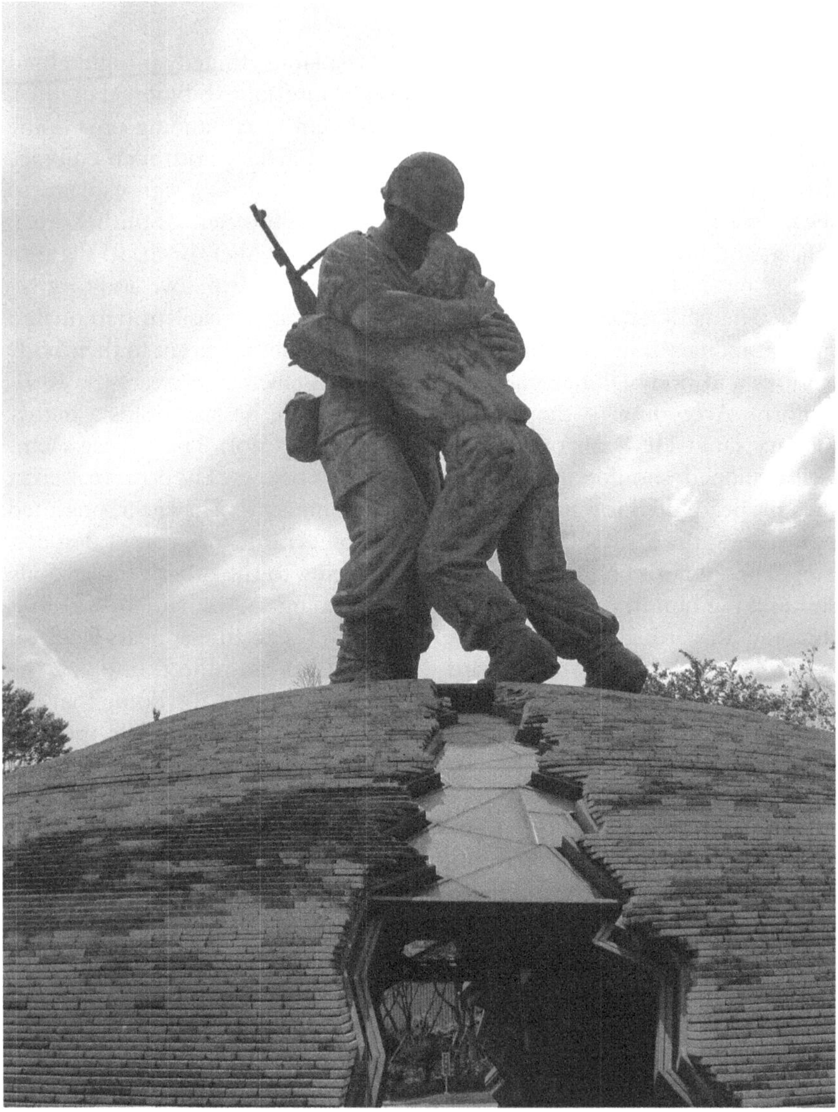

Fig. 8.2 The Statue of Brothers (Photo by the author.)

fraternal yet alienated relationship: the ROK. Despite the attempt of displaying brotherly love and affection based on a common past (implied by the dome) and shared bloodline (they are kin) leading to the reunion that the embrace suggests, the statue reflects antagonisms associated with Cold War dichotomies. The employed imagery shifts from the "good versus evil" rhetoric to a "stronger versus weaker" equivalent; and by doing so it reproduces the familiar opposition between the two Korean states. The evident contrasts in size and shape are sooner observed than the metaphor of the shared origin based on the dome-shaped tomb. Clearly, in the depiction of the WMK, Korean reunification will be achieved through South Korea's terms and conditions. It is the stronger ROK that absorbs the weaker DPRK.[42] The reunion does not occur at eye level but is based on a disparate status. The "Statue of Brothers" can thus be interpreted as a moderate version of former Cold War symbolism. It does not overcome, merely adjusts, the earlier forms of the official state narrative. Detached from current social and political realities, which allow very few aging individuals the opportunity to reunite with their relatives temporarily in an officially arranged and controlled setting, the imagery implies a shared future by restating South Korea's superiority.

Since its opening, the WMK has become a popular destination for school trips.[43] During one of my visits to the memorial in late June 2012, the exhibition areas were crowded with groups of children from the approximate age of five who visited the WMK together with their supervisors. Commenting on the extraordinarily huge number of children present, a museum employee stressed the relation between collective trips and the recently passed commemoration date of the beginning of the Korean War. Through organized trips to the WMK, South Koreans absorb particular historical images at an early age; they are introduced to and grow up with the official war narrative and interpretation of the past. Official commemoration sites and textbook knowledge become some of the principal sources for the young generations' understanding of the nation's history as the aging war generation passes away, as fewer witnesses who could voice their experiences remain.

Veterans remember the Korean War

My experiences in doing fieldwork with the war generation in South Korea showed that even in 2012 many contemporary witnesses were reluctant to talk about their private memories of the times. Interviews with Korean War veterans about their experiences of the conflict were often denied even when requested by the veterans' close acquaintances or relatives who wanted to support my research. Despite the personal appeal that usually opens doors in South Korean society effortlessly, the veterans responded hesitantly. Some of the appointed meetings were canceled at short notice and not rescheduled; some veterans referred directly to the official historiography of the war by giving me the advice to study library books instead of oral narrations, because there, as they pointed out, more was to be found than their own stories could tell. One of the men came to the interview with a history book, others with printed lists of battles that they later referred to as corner points in their life stories; some reassured themselves with the company of befriended veterans who could also share their experiences, just in case their own stories "were not enough."

The strength of group cohesion in Korean society partly explains why veterans did not want to come alone to the interviews. Although the topics of conversation involved loss and sadness, the atmosphere of the group interviews was rarely tense. Moreover, the elderly men seemed to appreciate each other's company at these apparently unusual events. Overall, the group situation helped reduce insecurity on their part and fuelled a willingness to narrate their life stories. A negative side effect, which is hard to prove in qualitative research but probable, could be that individual memories burdened with guilt or shame remained unspoken within this expanded group of listeners. If more than one veteran was interviewed, the men were peer group members, for example, of the same veterans' association. Through the recommendation by a familiar person or family member, who often also interpreted during the interviews, an additional member of the veterans' circle of friends or relatives was present. When I instead offered to bring a professional interpreter to the meetings, my contact person objected, explaining that an outsider's presence was not desired during the interviews. The mutual contact functioned as mediator between interviewer and interviewee and established a basis of trust between the parties. Consequently, the mediator's advice of working without an out-group interpreter was given priority. In the following, two narratives resulting from my fieldwork will be analyzed in extracts.[44] Both address the intergenerational narration of war experiences within their families.

Letters from Grandfather to Grandson

Veteran A, born in 1930 and a retired civil servant, had been asked by another veteran to join the latter in his interview situation. Both men and our mutual contact person from the Korean Veterans Association were present for the interview that took place in a Seoul hotel coffee shop. In South Korea it is quite common to meet or dine in hotel facilities, but the setting often also indicates an official occasion or a business meeting and, in this case, the interview was regarded as such.

Although Veteran A had been invited to the interview belatedly, it was he who began to recount his memories first. Veteran A was older than the other ex-serviceman, so according to Korean social hierarchy his voice was given priority. In contrast to his fluent mode of narration, the interviewee made it clear that his willingness to talk about war-time experiences was far from ordinary: "Really, you know, I have not even told my friends. Because you ask me, I will tell you about it. You don't say such a thing light-heartedly […]. There are hardly any people who do something like that." After the interview, he handed me a summary of letters written to his grandson during the latter's compulsory military service. Between 1 June 2005 and 15 February 2006, the veteran wrote regularly every two weeks, recapturing his own involvements in the military. The content mirrors the veteran's autobiographical experiences in the months of letter writing 55 years earlier during his time as a service member in the Korean War. The accurate and extensive summaries of the original letters complement his oral narration in style and content. Like the memories presented in the interview, the letters to his grandson mainly follow a report-like structure, retrace the warfare of the time and link the greater historical events to the military missions carried out by Veteran A himself. The letters are rich in facts, not feelings, but also contain some personal appeals to the grandson. The following extract from a letter written on 1 January 2006 describes the veteran's retreat from North Korea:

> 01.01.1951 to 15.01.1951: With the turn of the year, the Korean War went to a new phase. The fighting on the Odae Mountain, on the Daegwan and Jindu peaks was a remaining attack and defense battle. When both sides, South and North Korea confronted each other, it came to fierce fighting. Our unit went from the Taebaek Mountains to Gangneung, so along the highway distance between Seoul and Gangneung in Western direction. We reached Gusan-Ri, Seongsan-Myeon, from where Gangneung is 10 km […] away.

Here, even among family members, the war is not portrayed as social reality but as warfare, retold almost from a bird's eye perspective. There is an accuracy expressed in time, location and distance that seems detached from feelings or possible suffering. To achieve understanding from his grandson, he relates past to present, which becomes obvious in the reference to the highway distance. By sharing his experience in retrospect, in other letters the veteran also combines official dates and data of the retraceable course of history with his correlating individual place and position. What is presented is precise and therefore verifiable data about the course of war; the focus is on outside action without giving psychological insights. An almost official, non-critical report emerges that bears traces of pride and nationalism. Considering that the veteran had worked for Seoul's city office for approximately 40 years before retiring, a patriotic approach to the nation's past could be expected. The narrated events are less controversial than personal opinions or critical assessments could have been. For cross-cultural analysis, considering the audience during the interview is essential: while the setting was rather formal, the listeners were not only a younger female foreign researcher but also two other acquainted ex-service members. During the interview, the three men at times exchanged expert knowledge about the names of Korean military medals and the commanders in charge during Korean War missions. Clearly, the academic purpose was one aspect of the gathering; another was the reunion among men who chatted over similar life experiences or shared knowledge. Age, gender and social position determine one's status in Korean society, and the status directly translates into communication by language choice and social behavior. In our group, the veteran was the eldest person, and therefore obtained the highest social status. Due to Korean social norms, revealing possibly shameful or discordant memories would have been uncharacteristic for the setting as it would have implied a loss of face for Veteran A and could have disrupted group harmony.[45]

The letters must be interpreted against the background of social hierarchy that has its roots in Confucianism, too. In Korean family ranking, the son and grandson are the male heirs and representatives of the family; they need to be educated accordingly. The relationships between family members are constituted as a vertical hierarchy, drawing from filial piety, authority and benevolence.[46] The elders provide guidance and advice to the young who in return are asked to follow respectfully and obediently. In addition to the presumable aim of connecting with his grandson over similar experiences, namely the military service, cultural standards clearly request the grandfather to function as role model for his offspring. He closes the quoted letter with a personal appeal to his grandson's integrity by praising his willingness to contribute to the nation: "Military service is a sacred service. It is owed to the soldiers that parents and brothers can live in peace." In an earlier letter from October 2005, Veteran A had already stressed the honor of the task. He pondered: "When I was younger than you are now, I spent one year in battle. [...] It is somehow strange and terrible that I now recall those times. However, I am proud of it." The male bonding takes place through the letters that are, as evidence from the civil world, intimate and educating at the same time, albeit sent along familial hierarchy. Certainly, the grandson's service term was neither the time nor place to record self-doubts or criticism, to write about possible fear or despair. After all, the letters arrived at a national military base and, as a comment made by the veteran suggested, were eventually read by fellow service members. The letters may have been intended to encourage the group of young men.

Unheard Memories

In stark contrast to Veteran A, during the interview with Veteran B, a retired shop owner also born in 1930, I witnessed an open conversation between a grandfather and a granddaughter about the struggles lived out during the Korean War and post-war times. Here, the audience was exclusively female: the granddaughter in her early twenties to whom the war was an unknown chapter in her family history; the veteran's wife, who also added to her husband's memories; and I. This in-depth interview can be characterized as a familial talk about the war, in which my researcher's role was that of a participant observer. The setting was private; it took place in the veteran's family home. Being a university friend to the granddaughter, my role as researcher was less apparent as in the official gathering with Veteran A.

In his narration, Veteran B also mentions exact locations but these serve to support the narrative and are not its main focus. As a young man, he was severely wounded in battle and found it hard to cope with his physical and mental impairments during and directly after the war. He was therefore ashamed to return to his wife and family. It is striking how elaborately Veteran B speaks of his life at this time as seemingly doomed. Forced to serve in the North Korean army, he deserted when the chance arose. The interviewee describes his misery, fleeing at night in the rain, wearing only his undergarments so as not to be identified as a deserter. His flight put his family in danger as their home was subsequently raided late one night by soldiers searching for him. After hiding in the mountains, Veteran B entered the South Korean army when power shifted. Wounded by a gun shot in battle, he held out alone and waited for help, unsure if it would ever arrive. In his desperation, he disobeyed the military command to leave no weapons behind when he withdrew. Without embellishment, he indicates the hurt and distress he experienced after a bullet hit his leg:

> How big was my pain! […] I was crawling along so slowly. While I was crawling, I later could not lift my head anymore and could not move anymore either. I had no strength left, I was losing more and more blood, and I was about to die. I probably had not eaten in 24 hours. Also during the night, no one came. That's why I went beneath a pine tree, took off my jacket and covered myself with it. If I had to die, I would die here, because I could not move. […] 'I know I will die, but why am I still not dead? Had I just a weapon to kill myself!' When I was wounded, I left my weapons behind. My hand grenades and so on. I just had my body.

His narration is rich in detail but void of any heroic or patriotic characteristics. In his despair, Veteran B even considered suicide. During the interview, he directly confronted his granddaughter with his past weakness: "What do you think? You hear of this for the first time, don't you?" Veteran B's narration stresses personal suffering and creates an image of individual tragedy connected to the events of the war. Here, the memories focus on an experiential level instead of warfare and historiography. Veteran B tells an intimate story of his life that may emerge due to the private setting and the confidential relationship to his listeners, primarily his granddaughter, whom he constantly addresses during the interview. The cultural hierarchy is less strict in this relationship and the good rapport between him and her even enhances the frankness in his account.

Veteran B's narration is also non-critical toward the government. He contrasts his former suffering to the social upward movement in the post-war years during which his family became quite successful as small business owners. Speaking positively about state support and economic growth in the ROK, the veteran's biographical narration complements the official post-war social history. His oral accounts are in line with public remembrance that emphasizes the idea of the "Miracle on the Han River," evolving triumphantly out of a destructive situation. Despite apparent differences that partly arise from a discrepancy in audiences, both narrations reflect the official remembrance of war and post-war South Korea. Veteran

A achieves this by concentrating on warfare and facts, Veteran B by stressing personal tragedy that later converts to economic success and rehabilitation. In the letters sent by Veteran A, more private elements of his memories are found in his self-reflection and the encouragement toward his grandson. Veteran B's narration is on the whole more intimate, as he recounts his individual circumstances and lines of thought during war and after. Accordingly, both interviews contain aspects of public and private memory making. Depending on the nature of the relationship, family members may be spared the details to save their integrity or they may be let in on tragic events to enhance an intimate familial relationship and feelings of knowing and belonging. Hierarchy between speaker and audience is a key factor to Korean narrations and indicates the extent to which narrations of war and trauma are shaped by the context in which they are presented.

Conclusion

Memories may emerge and be communicated or silenced depending on the circumstances. The phenomenon of forgetting and suppressing brutal memories from collective memory and public discourse is not a uniquely Korean experience. The memory theorist Aleida Assmann argues that this model has been commonly employed throughout history and can be traced back to ancient Greece. According to her, forgetting was a method employed to achieve closure after a period of internal violence and to mark a new era in which a divided society could grow together again.[47] She also links her findings to wars' particular nature: "Especially after civil wars, forgetting was prescribed as a potent remedy against socially dangerous and explosive forms of remembering to foster a speedy integration."[48] The Korean War that today is commonly characterized as civil or fratricidal war[49] has long been portrayed in a 6.25-narrative stressing North Korea's guilt and erasing misfit memories. Social anthropologist Heonik Kwon stresses that war and occupation, especially when repetitive power shifts occur, lead to "distorted intimate human relations of trust."[50] In regard to the national and international dimensions of the fratricidal conflict and against the backdrop of Cold War conjunctions, the histories of the Korean War become comparable to those of the Vietnam War. In both countries, the wars have strongly impacted the social sphere, disuniting village life, local alliances, and family relations. As Kwon elaborates, the wars' effects targeted not only military personnel but also caused "relational trauma"[51] as communal and family structures were targeted in their morality and spirituality.

In South Korea, the work of the TRCK has contributed to restore bereaved families' honor and helped to rewrite the "forgotten" parts of the Korean history. But despite the grass roots engagement of the commission, much memory work has been left undone. While not coming to terms with updated critical findings by the TRCK, public remembrance portrayed in the country's prestigious WMK stresses the peaceful although one-sided idea of familial reunification with North Korea. The "Statue of Brothers" with its personifications of the ROK and DPRK as reunited relatives refers to the idea of a nation family that includes all Koreans, irrespective of current political and geographical belonging. At the same time, the statue contains an emotional appeal addressed to the individual who may suffer under the actual separation from his or her relatives. Thus, the WMK combines and initiates both public and private memory making. Indirectly, as was shown in my analysis, it reiterates persistent former notions of the Korean War in a softened version of Cold War dichotomies. As public memorials try to address the individual with the interpretation of history they represent, the individual in return constructs personal autobiography by positioning one's life events in the greater course of history. These traces can be found in the interviews that follow the official historiography of war events (Veteran A) and highlight the benefits of post-war development in the ROK (Veteran B).

Looking at non-Western, specifically Korean, ways of handling past disturbances, cross-cultural analysis should not only consider the social and historical backdrop the memories are narrated against but also focus on the interpersonal dynamics during the interview situation. Here, especially the hierarchical structures and family relations between the veterans, the researcher and the mediator indicate the extent to which the narrations are elaborated and which topics addressed. According to Yang Sungeun and Paul C. Rosenblatt, Koreans would not communicate shameful acts due to their ambition to spare family members from the shame they would share if the family knew of the act.[52] This relates directly to the Korean familial hierarchy encountered in the interviews: If a "person of higher status is morally responsible for those he or she supervises" and a child's failing automatically indicates the failing of the child's parents,[53] the narrator will most likely avoid mentioning critical aspects in his narration toward family members or befriended veterans, especially if the latter are younger or lower in social or military rank. On the one hand, this finding complicates cross-cultural fieldwork that already addresses themes that are hardly ever spoken of openly, in this case war memories of veterans in South Korea. Yet, on the other hand, as the interview with Veteran B shows, if interpersonal relationships between the interviewer, the interviewee and their mutual mediating person—in this case the veteran's granddaughter—are close enough, they may overcome predominant cultural standards. The constellation in group interviews as well as the role of the mediator in the process of collecting life narratives on traumatic events can therefore be considered a helpful expansion of the perspectives on cross-cultural communication of trauma.

Notes

1. James D. Bigley et al., "Motivations for War-related Tourism: A Case of DMZ Visitors in Korea," *Tourism Geographies*, 12:3, August 2010, 374; accessed 19 March 2014, doi:10.1080/14616688.2010.494687.
2. "Korean Red Cross Annual Reports," accessed 31 March 2014, http://www.redcross.or.kr/eng/eng_introduce/introduce_publication_annualreport.do?action=detail&brdctsno=37543&pagenum=1.
3. James A. Foley, *Korea's Divided Families. Fifty Years of Separation* (London and New York: Routledge, 2003), 120–2.
4. Suk-Young Kim, "Documenting the 'Flower of Reunification': Lim Su-gyeong and the memories of Korean border crossing," *Memory Studies*, 6:2, April 2013, 205; accessed 11 March 2014, doi:10.1177/1750698012473699.
5. Bruce Cumings, *The Korean War. A History* (New York: Modern Library, 2010), 103–4; Suk-Young Kim, "Staging the 'Cartography of Paradox': The DMZ Special Exhibition at the Korean War Memorial, Seoul," *Theatre Journal*, 63:3, October 2011, 382.
6. Ying-Feng Yang, *Der Alleinvertretungsanspruch der geteilten Länder. Deutschland, Korea und China im politischen Vergleich* (Frankfurt: Peter Lang, 1997), 73–4.
7. While the official American position has held that North Korean together with Soviet forces attacked South Korea with a surprise offensive that had not been provoked, historian Bruce Cumings also considers previous incidents possibly connected to the assault. He also stresses the fact that concrete evidence of the entangled events is still inaccessible, closed up in archives of the engaged parties (Bruce Cumings, *Korea's Place in the Sun. A Modern History* (New York and London: Norton, 2005), 260–4).
8. Cumings, *Korea's Place in the Sun*, 267–9.
9. Cumings, 275–88.

10. Kim, "Staging the 'Cartography of Paradox'," 382.
11. Kim, 383.
12. Kim, 383.
13. Kwi-Gon Kim, *The Demilitarized Zone (DMZ) of Korea. Protection, Conservation and Restoration of a Unique Ecosystem* (Heidelberg: Springer, 2013); Kim, "Staging the 'Cartography of Paradox'," 381–3.
14. Kim, *The Demilitarized Zone (DMZ) of Korea*, 2–4.
15. Kim, "Staging the 'Cartography of Paradox'," 392.
16. Heonik Kwon, "Legacies of the Korean War: Transforming ancestral rituals in South Korea," *Memory Studies*, 6:2, April 2013, 165; accessed 22 April 2013, doi:10.1177/1750698012473687.
17. Yoo-Seok Oh, "Formen südkoreanischer Erinnerung an Krieg und Nachkrieg," in: *Der Koreakrieg. Wahrnehmung—Wirkung—Erinnerung*, eds. Christoph Kleßmann and Bernd Stöver (Cologne: Böhlau, 2008), 179.
18. Dong-Choon Kim, *Der Koreakrieg und die Gesellschaft* (Münster: Westfälisches Dampfboot, 2007), 9–22.
19. Sheila Miyoshi Jager and Jiyul Kim, "The Korean War after the Cold War. Commemorating the Armistice Agreement in South Korea," in: *Ruptured Histories. War, Memory, and the Post-Cold War in Asia*, eds. Sheila Miyoshi Jager and Rana Mitter (Cambridge, MA, and London: Harvard UP, 2007), 242.
20. Kim, *Der Koreakrieg und die Gesellschaft*, 17–21.
21. Jager and Kim, "The Korean War after the Cold War," 242; Tessa Morris-Suzuki, "Remembering the Unfinished Conflict. Museums and the contested memory of the Korean War," in: *East Asia Beyond the History Wars. Confronting the Ghosts of Violence*, ed. Morris-Suzuki et al. (London and New York: Routledge, 2013), 132.
22. Dong-Choon Kim, "The Truth and Reconciliation Commission of Korea: Uncovering the Hidden Korean War," *The Asia-Pacific Journal*, 1 March 2010; accessed 31 March 2014, http://www.japanfocus.org/-Kim-Dong_choon/3314.
23. Kim, "The TRCK"; Hunjoon Kim, "Seeking Truth after 50 Years: The National Committee for Investigation of the Truth about the Jeju 4.3 Events," *The International Journal of Transitional Justice*, 3, 2009, 411 and 421; accessed 27 July 2012, doi: 10.1093/ijtj/ijp014.
24. Suhi Choi, "Standing between intransient and transient memories: The statue of MacArthur in South Korea," *Memory Studies*, 6:2, April 2013, 9; accessed 11 March 2014, doi: 10.1177/1750698012454872.

25. Choi, "Standing between intransient and transient memories," 9.
26. Kim, "The TRCK".
27. Kim, "The TRCK"; "Truth and Reconciliation. Activities of the Past Three Years," TRCK; accessed 31 March 2014, http://www.adoptionjustice.com/download/reports_&_papers/T&RCommissionKoreaReport.pdf.
28. Kim, "The TRCK".
29. Hong Kal, *Aesthetic Constructions of Korean Nationalism. Spectacle, politics and history* (London and New York: Routledge, 2011), 63; Jager and Kim, "The Korean War after the Cold War," 242.
30. Oh, "Formen südkoreanischer Erinnerung,“ 187.
31. Jager and Kim, "The Korean War after the Cold War," 234; Kal, *Aesthetic Constructions of Korean Nationalism*, 63; Hong Kal, "Commemoration and the Construction of Nationalism: War Memorial Museums in Korea and Japan," *The Asia-Pacific Journal*, 6 September 2008; accessed 31 March 2014, http://japanfocus.org/-Hong-KAL/2880.
32. Kristin Hass, "Remembering the 'Forgotten War' and Containing the 'Remembered War': Insistent Nationalism and the Transnational Memory of the Korean War," in: *Transnational American Memory*, ed. Udo J. Hebel (Berlin: Walter de Gruyter, 2009), 278.
33. Sheila Miyoshi Jager, *Narratives of Nation Building. A Genealogy of Patriotism* (Armonk: M.E. Sharpe, 2003), 120.
34. Hass, "Remembering the 'Forgotten War,'" 272–3.
35. Oh, "Formen südkoreanischer Erinnerung,“ 188; Roy Richard Grinker, *Korea and its Futures. Unification and the Unfinished War* (New York: St. Martin's Press, 1998), 30.
36. In June 2012, the tour guide was titled differently. Back then, the slogan "Watch, Feel, Experience. The War Memorial of Korea" stressed the entertainment value of the exhibitions that is conveyed through various multimedia installations and replicas of weapons that the visitors may experience and shoot on the museum grounds. With this equipment, an effort is made to recreate an "authentic" feeling of war. Although these tools and sites still remain in the memorial, the tour guide of 2013 used a more emotional appeal, possibly bearing in mind the sixtieth anniversary of the armistice agreement between both Korean states.
37. Oh, "Formen südkoreanischer Erinnerung,“ 188.
38. Jager and Kim, "The Korean War after the Cold War," 244.
39. Morris-Suzuki, "Remembering the Unfinished Conflict," 132–3.

40. Examples of current reactions within the memorial's exhibitions are the commemoration of the sunken ROK navy ship "Cheonan" near the maritime border to North Korea on 26 March 2010 in the building's entrance hall, visited by the author in 2012, as well as a special exhibition hosted in 2010 about the recent developments inside the DMZ (Kim, "Staging the 'Cartography of Paradox'").
41. Sheila Miyoshi Jager, *Brothers at War. The Unending Conflict in Korea* (London: Profile Books, 2013), 447–8; Jager and Kim, "The Korean War after the Cold War," 249.
42. Jager, *Brothers at War*, 447–8; Jager and Kim, "The Korean War after the Cold War," 248–9.
43. Jager and Kim, "The Korean War after the Cold War," 243.
44. All interviews were fully recorded and then transliterated by Korean native speakers. Subsequently, the transliterations were translated in writing from Korean to German. The interview excerpts quoted in the following chapters are English translations of the German templates made by the author.
45. Youn-ja Shim, Min-Sun Kim and Judith N. Martin, *Changing Korea. Understanding Culture and Communication* (New York: Peter Lang, 2008), 36.
46. Insook Han Park and Lee-Jay Cho, "Confucianism and the Korean family," *Journal of Comparative Family Studies*, 26:1, spring 1995.
47. Aleida Assmann, "From Collective Violence to a Common Future: Four Models for Dealing with a Traumatic Past," in: *Other People's Pain. Narratives of Trauma and the Question of Ethics*, eds. Martin Modlinger and Philipp Sonntag (Bern: Peter Lang, 2011), 45.
48. Assmann, "From Collective Violence to a Common Future," 47.
49. Bruce Cumings, "The Korean War. What Is It that We Are Remembering to Forget?" in: *Ruptured Histories. War, Memory, and the Post-Cold War in Asia*, eds. Sheila Miyoshi Jager and Rana Mitter (Cambridge, MA, and London: Harvard UP, 2007), 274.
50. Heonik Kwon, "Korean War Traumas," *The Asia-Pacific Journal*, 20 September 2010; accessed 26 February 2015, http://japanfocus.org/-Heonik-Kwon/3413.
51. Kwon, "Korean War Traumas".
52. Sungeun Yang and Paul C. Rosenblatt, "Shame in Korean families," *Journal of Comparative Family Studies*, 32:3, summer 2001, 371.
53. Yang and Rosenblatt, "Shame in Korean families," 366.

CHAPTER 9

Endless aftershock. The Katyń Massacre in Contemporary Polish Culture

Maria Kobielska

Nearly 70 years after its end, World War II remains a compelling reference point for questions of self-definition and cultural identity. The war has become a laboratory within which various versions of past events can be re-shown and re-told, using new, often politically motivated perspectives, but also incorporating pop-cultural and media discourses. Illustrative examples from recent years include on the one hand, the German mini-series *Unsere Mütter, unsere Väter* (*Generation War*, 2013), and on the other, Tarantino's *Inglorious Basterds* (2009).

In Poland, this "memory boom" has in recent years been able to pay particular attention to previously unmentionable events and interpretations. This is a result not only of the political change of 1989, but also of the quickly evolving possibilities of mnemonic media, and a reflection of the extensive "memory work" performed by many conflicting parties on Polish identity. The untold story of Polish complicity in persecutions of Jews has now resurfaced, for instance. One of the most attended museums in Poland shows the tragic Warsaw Uprising as a heroic and at the same time exciting adventure. Finally, the theme of Poles being persecuted by the Soviets, officially banned before 1989, is central within the flourishing of contemporary public recollection. This intricate tangle of memories,

M. Kobielska (✉)
Jagiellonian University, Faculty of Polish Studies, Cracow, Poland

P. Leese, J. Crouthamel (eds.), *Traumatic Memories of the Second World War and After*, DOI 10.1007/978-3-319-33470-7_9

both creative and iterative, serves varied purposes. Sometimes versions of historical events emerge in the working through the difficult pasts, on other occasions they amount to a repetitive fixation. Moreover, events can be recast according to a variety of generic codes: not only as tragedy or farce, but also as tiring nightmare and striking horror.

Cultural Memory and Trauma

This chapter deals with present-day Polish memory culture in response to the Katyń massacre—the mass execution of Polish officers carried out by NKVD in 1940, which is one of the core events of the twentieth century Polish collective memory. Katyń is used in politics, explored in literature and other cultural texts, and revealed in commemorative celebrations. My intention is to explain why and how this traumatic event has achieved such a prominent position within Polish society, and to explore the mechanisms of its representation.

Aleida Assmann's *Cultural Memory and Western Civilization* defines "cultural memory" as a specific construct: plural, dynamic and political at the same time. Cultural memory is a constant process of transformation and reconstruction since it uses various media, serves the purposes of different groups, and frames the experience of different individuals.[1] Assmann shows how the boundary between the individual and that which transcends the individual (e.g., community, media, or culture) blurs in any analysis of memory practices. What is remembered is constantly being shaped and modified in interactions between individual memories and the collective reiterations of culture, media and politics.

I am particularly interested here in analyzing these entangled memory practices, which are expressed, transformed and reconstructed by and through cultural texts. I consider cultural memory—which manifests itself via a variety of media and is shaped by diverse politics—within its social setting, trying to determine which moments are important for the development of collective recollection. Past events, which, in a special way, serve as present centers of cultural memory and key topics of memory texts, are for this reason of particular interest.

The association between "cultural memory" and "trauma" is crucial for an understanding of this problem. One argument here is that there is an analogy between individual, collective and cultural memories: in reactions toward, as well as in attempts to understand and process, traumatic experiences. Traumatized cultural memory acts out the painful experiences of the group which can also be worked through within it, although this does not always or necessarily happen. In particular, the main reactions to such experiences, such as silence, the inability to articulate, and, conversely, the pressure to speak, leading to compulsive repetition, occur in a variety of cultural texts, for example in literature, as rhetoric figures of aposiopesis or as amorphous logorrhea. The trauma I am interested in is thus not individual, nor is it necessarily related directly to actual events, as in the cases of survivors or victims' relatives. It is indirect, processed, non-conscious, but collectively constructed, linked to repressed and banned memory, consisting in a set of elements such as cultural texts, visible in close-up. This is not the trauma which hurts individual lives, but a social structure which prevents the common memory, expressed within culture, from fully confronting the past of the group, processing it and no longer being haunted by it (which would not, of course, mean forgetting).

The Katyń massacre plays a central role in Polish cultural memory after 1989, as do the Warsaw Uprising (1944) and the introduction of Martial Law (1981). Each of these events is intensively and constantly retold and reinterpreted, often within incompatible discourses and various visions of the past. Memory culture thus constantly generates different ways in which these experiences are articulated and expressed, and is also influenced by fluctuations in the politics of memory. Each of these events can be described in terms of traumatic experience of the collective Polish community, serving as a frame for thinking about the past; each of these events is also commonly constructed as the core of a specific trauma complex. Nevertheless, the traumatic core of Polish memory has not yet been fully acknowledged by scholars, except in the recent, important work of Lech Nijakowski[2] and Adam Ostolski,[3] who deal mainly with collective memory rather than cultural memory. Other recent work[4] by Polish scholars concentrates on the impact of one medium, such as film or visual arts, on memory culture. Among the three traumatic historical events in question, the Warsaw Uprising has lately drawn the most attention. By contrast, the only detailed account on the memory of Katyń is still *Remembering Katyń* (2012), edited by Alexander Etkind, a collection of essays produced outside Poland, which has not been preceded or followed by any similar Polish project.

Etkind's collection maps the legacy of the events at Katyń "through the interconnected memory cultures of seven countries—Belarus, Poland, Russia, Ukraine and the Baltic States" and explores "its meaning as site and symbol, event and idea, fact and crypt."[5] These essays together provide a detailed historical description of how different meanings are constructed within each of the nations represented. The tension between historical truth and performative memory practices, necessarily linked, but in violent conflict when it comes to the "Katyń lie" (see below), is essential to the authors' perspective. They analyze the political discourses and counter-discourses of Katyń, the production and evolution of "memory hardware," and, above all, the circulation of the "Katyń term" (metonymical and metaphorical) in Eastern Europe: its spread from the representation of a Polish past to other national pasts, where it serves a variety of different social and political requirements. The aforementioned mapping consists thus in describing tensions, clashes, meetings, dialogues and changes within the discourses of Katyń. Taking into account the rhetoric of memory, the "forms and strategies of representation as well as questions of audience and reception,"[6] are thus critical for any competent analysis of a particular memory culture.

For this reason it is my intention to investigate how the apparatus of memory functions publically. What follows is, then, an examination not only of images, figures, models and mechanisms, but also of the wider field of cultural memory, of Katyń's consequences for Polish memory culture as a whole. In this respect the cultural processing of the Katyń massacre can serve as a laboratory of broader procedures of collective remembering and reveal its hidden structure, which has profound consequences for what can be called contemporary Polish identity. If, as Etkind states, "remembering Katyń has been a literal re-membering for Poland,"[7] a ground for connecting and unifying members of the community, the next step should be a consideration of what conditions and limitations are founded by these means.

The first critical question is, then: what are the mechanisms by which Katyń has taken up such a prominent position within recent Polish culture? I start with a brief description of the events at Katyń and their importance, then propose a map of present-day Polish cultural memory connected to the Katyń murders. This mapping includes a discussion on populist representation via a public campaign from 2010; an interpretative reading of the film *Katyń* (2007) by Andrzej Wajda; and a case study of a widely known poem by Zbigniew Herbert.

Katyń: Circumstances and Consequences

The circumstances of the event and the political forces of the 1940s defined the future mnemonic configuration of the Katyń murders. In September 1939, Poland was invaded not only by Nazi Germany, but also, two weeks later, on 17 September, by the Soviet Union, as a result of the Molotov-Ribbentrop Pact, which included the secret protocol that divided the territory of Poland into Nazi and Soviet spheres of influence. Thus, the eastern part of pre-war Poland came under the military occupation of the Soviet Union, and suffered various campaigns of repression.

Polish soldiers and policemen were then imprisoned, deported to the territory of Russia and other Soviet Socialist Republics and interned in camps. After 8 months, by the end of May 1940, over 20,000 members of the Polish Officer Corps were already dead. They were executed (by firing squad) on the orders of the Soviet Politburo, signed personally by Stalin. The executions took place in April and May in several places in the Soviet Union, among which the best known location is the forest near the village of Katyń; other places include Kharkiv and Miednoye. The execution was kept secret, so the fate of the officers was not known either to Polish officials or their families.

A year later, in June 1941, the non-aggression pact between Nazi Germany and the Soviet Union was broken by Hitler's Operation Barbarossa. The Eastern Front was opened; consequently, the Nazis invaded the Soviet Union and occupied the territories where the executions were carried out and the mass graves of the Polish officers remained a secret. Meanwhile, Stalin joined the Allies and signed the agreement with the Polish government in exile, which announced the willingness of both parties to fight together against Nazi Germany and the formation of a Polish army on Soviet territory. It was soon revealed that very many of the officers supposed to stay under Soviet rule were missing. Moreover, their whereabouts remained unknown over the following two years, during which time the strength of the Soviet Union among the Allies was growing as a result of its huge military efforts on the Eastern Front.

In April 1943 Berlin Radio, a tool of Nazi propaganda, announced the discovery of mass graves of Polish officers in the Katyń forest, and accused the Soviets of carrying out the massacre in 1940. This essentially truthful, but carefully controlled story was presented so as to cause great unease among the Alliance, and it partly worked. The Soviet Union denied the accusations and claimed that the victims were executed by the invading Germans in the summer of 1941, and when Polish officials insisted on opening an investigation, Stalin accused them of collaborating in Nazi propaganda and broke off diplomatic relations with the government. This in turn had a huge impact on the subsequent history of Poland: the diplomatic position of the government in exile was weakened; the future collapse of Polish pre-war political tradition was prepared.

This was the beginning of the falsification of the events at Katyń. Following the end of World War II, when the pro-Soviet government was established in Poland, and over the 40 years of The People's Republic of Poland, any public mention or commemoration of Katyń was banned, and if any mention did slip into the public sphere, Nazi Germany was consistently blamed for the crime. Soviet responsibility for the massacres was not officially confirmed until the 1990s, and only then was it possible to consider any kind of commemoration, or any official Polish monument in the Katyń forest.

Understandably, the ban was counter-productive. It provided the Katyń massacre with great symbolic power and for the general public marked its importance in the history of the Second World War. Moreover, the years of falsification meant that anything other than adulation of the Katyń martyrs was condemned out of hand. Hence the newly coined term "the Katyń lie" (*kłamstwo katyńskie*), which is a calque of the "Auschwitz lie" (*kłamstwo oświęcimskie*), a phrase popular in Polish to indicate Holocaust denial. When denial of the Soviet responsibility for the Katyń murders is implicitly compared to Holocaust denial, the Katyń massacre is being given a symbolic moral "equivalence" to the tragedy of the Holocaust. Moreover, from 1998 the Polish law criminalized not only the denial of the Holocaust and other genocides, but also of "crimes perpetrated against persons of Polish nationality and Polish citizens of other ethnicity, nationalities in the period between 1 September 1939 and 31 December 1989"[8]—which of course includes the Katyń murders. The Institute for National Remembrance, then established, has the task to investigate such crimes. The Institute has both a legal and historical function, and is a prominent voice in national debates on the politics of memory.

Still, termination of the Russian investigation in 2004 could not fully satisfy the families of the victims (associated in the so-called Federation of Katyń Families) or Polish officials, as it ruled out the possibility of the judicial rehabilitation of the dead and refused to classify the act as a war crime. Wider political histories and interests continue to direct the memory struggles over the Katyń murders, which have become one of the most important themes of the politics of memory since the transformations of 1989. As Donald Tusk, the Polish Prime Minister, stated in 2010, in his speech at the commemoration ceremony in the Katyń cemetery: [9]

> The truth about Katyń became a founding myth of Independent Poland; consequently, all of us Poles are one big Katyń family, not only those who lost their loved ones.

This sentiment represents well the official state politics of commemoration concerning the Katyń massacre. The recollection of Katyń serves as a foundation for the wider national community, and as a *raison d'être* for Polish independence. Every Pole is in this way said to be personally connected to the victims of the massacre. It is worth emphasizing that the term "family" is especially significant in this context—it is not, for instance, common citizenship that brings the Poles together, but family ties. A hierarchy of values is simultaneously created: presumably, conservative values, in which the concept of family plays a leading role.

To sum up, state politics and international relations have meant that the events at Katyń have not been officially acknowledged or commemorated for nearly 50 years. The forbidden memory of these events has nevertheless been working beyond state control throughout this time. The symbolic strength of the event has increased. The present-day general public views on Katyń, as well as contemporary Poland's legal framework, have been shaped by this "secret" history. The symbolic and political use of a traumatic event as the basis of a national identity effectively means that the uses of Katyń as a memory can never come to an end: it continually serves as a founding myth on which to build political alliances and support for various patriotic causes. All these circumstances constitute what can be called the continuing aftershock of the massacre in contemporary Polish memory culture.

This complicated set of circumstances has produced an equally complex traumatic response: the non-acknowledgement of the truth as well as the shocking extent of deaths, have made the Katyń massacre, to use Cathy Caruth's term, a "crying wound"[10] in Polish identity and history. My argument here is that, given the extended delay in recognition, commemoration and reconciliation with the events of 1940, it is too late for Polish culture to deal with the untold Katyń trauma.

This view is based on my analysis of a wide variety of cultural texts, which, I believe, nearly exhausts this particular "memory field."[11] These texts include a dozen documentary films, as well as the first and so far the only feature film, *Katyń* (2007). Among the other sources are works of prose, including a novel by Włodzimierz Odojewski, and a huge amount of poetry, professional as well as amateur; a design of the Katyń Museum which is to be opened in 2015, and social marketing campaigns aimed at commemorating the victims and honoring their memory. The majority of these texts concentrate on endlessly acting out the massacre, persistently using the same clichéd images, copying several basic stories and schemes that form a kind of a catalogue of representational rules within the memory field. These similarities, as I will show, are striking and significant.

State Memory: "Katyń 1940. We remember"

This catalogue of Katyń "signifiers" is observable where culture, politics and marketing meet—namely, in a commemorative social campaign using the slogan "Katyń 1940. We remember." The project, which could be also called an "image campaign" of the Katyń massacre, is especially worthy of examination as an example of the affirmative politics of memory led by a public institution, the National Centre for Culture. The campaign demonstrates too how various media can be used to communicate an officially sanctioned meaning, to propagate and strengthen a particular interpretive memory of past events. The campaign led by the NCC was organized in two stages: the first stage was inaugurated on 11 April 2007, the agreed anniversary of the Katyń murders, under the patronage of the then Minister of Culture and National Heritage, Kazimierz Michał Ujazdowski. In this stage, the project was linked to and profited from the forthcoming release of Wajda's *Katyń* and its advertising campaign. The second stage of the NCC campaign was organized in 2010 to commemorate the 70th anniversary.

The NCC is a state cultural institution, founded in 2006 with the task of popularizing of Polish culture, history, heritage and language within the country. The extensive activities of the NCC aim particularly at tradition and national heritage, and their purpose is to influence the formation of contemporary patriotism. The same goals were implicit in the Katyń campaign. In the initial press release, the organizers pointed out that the death of the Katyń victims was a heroic sacrifice, the memory of which should be preserved in an expression of civic allegiance:

> The time has come, after almost 70 years, to re-establish the memory of the Great Poles who made the ultimate sacrifice to defend their motherland. (…) With this project, the NCC wants to bring back the heroes of these events to the society. The heroes, without whom there would be no independent and free Poland.

In describing the campaign's objectives the idea of a syncretic, modern patriotism is set out: [12]

> It is our aim not only to convey historical knowledge, but also to stimulate reflection on the shape of contemporary, modern patriotism. A patriotism that is civic, authentic, and spontaneous. A patriotism that is able to draw strength from the heroes of the past.

The NCC proposes, then, an identity constructed on the basis of memory, structured according to the interpretation of Katyń set out above. This patriotic attitude, based on past events, is intended to be "modern:" intentionally shaped, constructed using sophisticated media techniques, following distinct patterns, becomes not only authentic, but also apparently spontaneous. Yet taking into account the politics of the NCC, the attitudes which would supposedly result from its successful influence on society seem more calculated than spontaneous. On the one hand, the department plans and runs a carefully defined politics of memory and identity; on the other hand it tries, consciously or not, to create a bottom-up movement which is free, voluntary and somehow "authentic."

Among the various strands of the campaign, the exhibitions or educational competitions, publications, website, merchandise and much more, the visual and audio-visual works that were widely distributed in the mass media and on billboards in urban spaces, and which consequently became particularly recognizable, are of special interest.[13] Contemporary mass communication, as Bartosz Korzeniowski writes, means that "the past signifies differently, its traces in memory can be decoded in a new way, there are thus other possibilities to re-read them."[14] According to Korzeniowski, the iconic turn intensifies the visual media presence in human space, as well as "widening the range of various memory media," which subsequently opens up new possibilities to shape memory, to re-model it more broadly than ever. It also influences the memory practices of individuals and groups in a more efficient way. These posters and videos show that although the campaign took advantage of new media in shaping the cultural memory of Katyń, it nevertheless copies old themes, reproduced previously in countless poems, diaries, testimonies and other works of art.

One of the posters showed a crumpled sheet of paper covered with children's writing. This was a letter to "Dear Daddy," expressing anxiety and love. Old-fashioned glasses suggested a time lapse and a board stating "I remember. Katyń 1940" revealed the meaning of the picture.

This was one of the letters which were found during the exhumation and then preserved, mainly by families. The personal belongings of the officers often become props recognizable as marks of the Katyń victims, while the theme of letters and diaries is commonly used in Katyń films and books as a semantically capacious narrative tool. The wording is particularly significant here: using the first-person singular, "I," defines the role for the campaign recipient, "the remembering subject." Such a formulation does not allow any imaginable objection or indifference (unlike, for example, the imperative "Remember!" in response to which one can still refuse the order). The content of the memory of this "remembering subject" is precise: the unique event, the Katyń massacre, should be the foundation of identity.

The poster's effect exploits the figure of an orphaned child. The child had written a heart-touching letter to "Dear Daddy," and the father, in turn, had the letter in his possession when murdered. The letter is supposedly found later, during the exhumation—hence the damage to the paper (though of course it is not a real picture of any particular document excavated from a Katyń grave). The poster thus uses the set themes of the Katyń memory by imagining a relic of a victim, and by invoking the figure of an orphaned child to generate a powerful emotional response. The touching statement built by these elements encourages the recipient to take on the role assigned to him or her by the message as one who can say "I remember."

A second poster's background showed a birch-tree forest, easily recognizable as an execution site. It also featured concentric circles made of the words of one of the Katyń poems. An inscription "Katyń" and dates showing the 70th anniversary of the massacre ("1940–2010") were written in the middle in the colors of the Polish flag, red and white. The forest, which witnessed the shooting, is one of the main clichés of the Katyń memory, present in almost every book or film on the subject. The meaning of the circles is vague: they can remind one of a gun sight—the spectator would thus look through it on the Katyń forest, taking the position of the perpetrator. If associated with annual rings of trees, they can also indicate the time lapse (underlined by the dates). These elements are even more pronounced in a short TV piece that was a part of the investigated campaign. The third possibility is linked with film language: the circles form a distant depth point, and the word "Katyń" is placed on this background in a way reminiscent of the caption "The End" in the closing frames of a film. Once more, it would evoke the victims' fate, and simultaneously the special meaning of the word in cultural memory. "Katyń" means the massacre, the death, the end, not only one of the execution sites.

The video in question illustrates even more cogently mnemonic mechanisms of filling attractive, appealing form with tried and tested themes. The film was prepared using highly developed computer animation techniques, which is a novelty in the range of the Katyń memory media. Nevertheless, the content is not surprising: the petrified clichés, the images of a train and the forest as a witness, are re-used here once again. The fast journey of a train creates a disquieting and uncanny effect, intensified by the music and the fantastic shape of the locomotive, decorated with the red star, the emblem of the Soviet Union, shown from the frog perspective and then from the bird's eye-view. The train is covered with thorns and throws sparks, evoking the feeling of danger. A black-and-white, leafless and barren forest is its destination, while some kind of a climbing plant appears to enlace and constrain the trees. It is red and prickly and may be associated both with the barbed wire in the fences of the camps, and with the thorny crown of Christ. Finally, the board stating "Day of Remembrance for Victims of the Katyń Massacre. 13 April 2010" reveals the meaning of the dreadful images (and indicates the organizers of the anniversary, together with the Ministry of Culture and National Heritage and the NCC). The train, which is headed east, is carrying, by implication, the Polish officers into the Soviet Union, where they will be executed. Evocations of horror and the effective exploitation of propaganda techniques meet here to create a devilish image of the USSR, which is presented as the incarnation of an extreme evil. These visual elements produce the basis for an obvious figurative meaning within the cultural memory of Katyń. The classic themes of forest and train are undertaken in a new visual form; the perpetrators are identified and demonized, as the red plant, whose color is linked with the symbol of USSR. Neither the perpetrators nor the victims are directly shown, but their existence is suggested within a non-human vision of totalitarian violence. The intentions of the "image campaign" are presented in an intense, concentrated form in this attractive, modern commemorative text.

Yet the memory texts on the Katyń massacre avoid addressing it directly. They commonly use ellipsis and metonymy—the trauma is not called by its own name or shown in its own form, but by the names or in the forms of something closely associated with it. Consequently, the images of the letter, the train and the forest stand for the entirety of the Katyń murders. The film reveals further "rules" of the memory field, such as fitting the events of Katyń 1940 into various narrative schemes, and explaining its sense mythologically. The death of the officers is more or less explicitly linked with the sacrifice of Christ. Consequently, the messianic narrative of Poland's fate is once again revived.

The perseverance of these ideas and images reinforces the strictly enforced governance and regulation of Katyń memory. There are hardly any texts or practices in this field that oppose the accepted rules, or that form any kind of oppositional provocation. The most original attempts are still subjected to some of the established principles, while the majority of texts multiply and copy the tried and tested ways of remembering and expressing remembrance. I will explore the most notable examples in the following sections of my analysis.

Canonical Memory: Wajda's *Katyń*

Andrzej Wajda's *Katyń* (2007), first and so far the only feature film on the subject, is of particular importance as it attempts to establish a canon of national mythology around the Katyń massacre. It plays a crucial role in the field of contemporary Katyń cultural memory, having both summarizing and rule-imposing power within it. The special position of Wajda in Polish culture is also an important factor. He was considered to be the best choice as the director of *Katyń* for personal reasons (as his father was killed in Kharkiv), not only because he is an internationally lauded director, but also due to the widely acknowledged themes of his work. Wajda's films create an expressive, potent vision of national Polish identity, character, myths and symbols. To quote Tadeusz Lubelski, a leading authority on Wajda's work, "the essential themes of national history of the last two hundred years take shape through the images in his films,"[15] and within them are deconstructed, problematized and rethought in a variety of ways. It is essential, therefore, to ask how trauma is expressed in Wajda's film, and to consider the ways in which it may or may not be processed. Moreover, it is important to understand how the film is supposed to fulfill the essential task of telling the historical truth, how it opens up possibilities for new Katyń memory projects to come, and how it shapes national Katyń mythology.

The plot of the film is structured around 17 September 1939, showing the agreement between the Soviet Union and Nazi Germany, the cooperation of their armies, and the arrest of Polish officers. Subsequent scenes present their life in the Kozielsk camp between the autumn of 1939 and April 1940, during which time the officers were taken away to the execution site in Katyń; these moments are interspersed with episodes from the life of their families, left in Cracow under Nazi occupation and in former East Poland, now under Soviet rule.

After the scenes showing transportation of the captives (who hoped their situation would improve), the action moves to 1943, to Cracow, still under occupation, when Nazi propaganda puts out news about the discovery of the Katyń graves, announcing a list of victims. These reports promote the Nazis' objectives, but their story is essentially a truthful one: it is the Soviet Union that is responsible for the massacre. The film does not refer to the political problems concerning Katyń before 1945, concentrating instead on the prolonged pain, uncertainty and hope of the women from the family of a heroic officer Andrzej.

In the second part of the story, when Cracow is liberated from the German occupation and when the Red Army are seen by many solely as new invaders, the Katyń lie is the center of the film's attention. The characters protest against the deception and while some consequently suffer from various forms of repression, others meet a tragic fate. There is an unavoidable conflict between those who seek to reveal the truth about the massacre, and those who have chosen to accept the new Polish reality. The film ends by returning to April 1940 to show in detail the last moments of the arrested officers, their executions, and finally their mass burials.

In the following part of this essay, I consider *Katyń* with reference to the notion of trauma and its manifestation, and I investigate the potential role of the film in the process of working through trauma. *Katyń* is a historical drama film, trying to show all the aspects of its topic, depicting the personal histories of many characters and lacking a central plot, it attempts to create a kind of a panorama. It assumes that there is the possibility to represent trauma and to express it by means of cinema. As Wajda says himself:[16]

> the domestication [of the past] requires showing it in a material, concrete form. This can be done by means of theatre, painting or literature, but it's the cinema that does it literally. The ghosts must materialize in front of us and give us their story. [...] They are looking at us from the screen, speaking directly to us as humans.

Consequently, the last sequence of the film gives a close-up account of the massacre, revealing all the details in an effort to show events exactly as they happened, so as to, paradoxically, produce the truth. This brutal, naturalistic (and prolonged) scene is designed to expose the death of the officers, showing their last moments, words (of prayers), falls, injuries, blood, bodies and piles of corpses in mass graves. The realism of these images is matched by the sophisticated composition and rhythm of the scene and completely satisfies the spectators' awkward (if not perverse) curiosity about the massacre. As the authors of *Remembering Katyń* state, "the execution scene in *Katyń* aspires to recreate the past in its certainty, to access the knowledge available only to the deceased and to the perpetrator."[17] Is the film successful in its implicit task of placing the viewer in the position of the witness?

This disturbing willingness to show every detail of the execution stands in contrast to the incapacity to express the traumatic experience, as postulated primarily in psychoanalysis. According to the classic definitions, the traumatized subject cannot respond adequately to the traumatic event, which leads to medical disorders, and to endless echoes of the traumatic past. The trauma cannot be understood, and expressing it cancels its horror and uniqueness; thus any representation of particular traumatic events always seems incomplete and improper.[18] In these terms, the last scene of Wajda's film, expressing as it does the possibility of "showing" the Katyń massacre, makes it non-traumatic, fails to recognize it as extraordinary, and fails to acknowledge the perpetual lack it produces or the suffering which cannot be fully experienced. What is more, taking the characters' perspective into account, such a realistic representation of the execution cannot express the individual trauma of the victims, nor the trauma of their families, which resulted not least from a lack of knowledge and prolonged uncertainty. The film brings everything to life, makes it understandable, but simultaneously and paradoxically, it hides a horror with which it is impossible to cope. Thus, *Katyń* fails to confront the traumatic; instead, it smoothes over the trauma, familiarizes it, relates it lucidly, bringing it into the wider field of collective cultural memory.

This mnemonic structure makes it more difficult for Polish culture to deal with the collective trauma of Katyń, to discuss the past, let alone to see the Katyń memory in terms of its potential dynamic and diversity (that is to say, multidirectionally in the sense proposed by Michael Rothberg, as a "subject to ongoing negotiation, cross-referencing and borrowing, as productive and not privative.")[19] The construction of characters instead creates an image of unblemished heroism (the Katyń victims and their families), inflexible, respectable, and unyielding in their patriotism and religious faith. The principle characteristic of these heroic protagonists is not their individual psyche, but rather their collectivity: the group within which attitudes are commonly shared.

The officers from the Kozielsk camp are shown as members of a community, sharing determination, dignity and sense of honor (so, for example, when one of them collapses, others force him to fight the breakdown by rosary prayer). The heroic image is completed with a proud, constant attitude toward death—the officers fight their fear, once more thanks to religion (the executed men recite succeeding verses of the Lord's Prayer). Their mothers and sisters, the Katyń widows and their children, are similarly unyielding. They never hesitate nor resent their fate, they stay loyal to their loved ones even after their death, and after 1945 they heroically fulfill their duty by condemning the Katyń lie and by utterly rejecting the new political order.

Surprisingly, the image of the perpetrators is not very important in Wajda's film. He is rather more interested in a particular, black-and-white portrayal of Polish society. Consequently, the characters who are somehow linked to the post-war Polish state, who encourage "the Katyń lie," play the roles of villains. For instance, the survivor from the Kozielsk camp, who managed to come back to the country with the so-called Berling's army, which was subordinated to the Soviets, is told by his killed friend's mother that he "should rather be dead" than survive for the price paid, and subsequently commits suicide.

One is thus obliged to act heroically and any other choice is judged in this context. There is no place for hesitation or moral collapse, and the members of the Katyń families fulfill this heroic ideal. The acceptance of the conditions of post-war Poland, engaging with the new state, is also seen as a form of collapse. *Katyń*, which initially seems to provide a panoramic view of Polish social history from the perspective of the story of the massacre, actually simplifies this task, attributing simplistic merely good and bad motivations and decisions to its characters. A seemingly complicated, profound vision is actually black and white, as the film produces a reduced, monumentalized version of the past, according to which there is only a choice between the absolute loyalty toward the group and fraternizing with the enemy. Such a project prevents any working through of the many traumas within the collective past and produces instead an illusory, superficial form of identity. Witold Mrozek, a researcher investigating the Polish politics of memory, states that *Katyń* could be called "a film of national remembrance,"[20] aimed at a mass public (the whole nation), an instrument of patriotic education and state politics, which uses national mythology and simultaneously creates a mythological history of the homogeneous national community.

Katyń thus builds a canonical form of memory, fixing rigid norms and standards of remembering, and of belonging to the community at the same time. It occupies a special position on the Katyń memory field, shaping the collective imaginary past, and creating the image of the Katyń massacre as a crucial event in recent Polish history. Its role is absolutely constructive, it does not question the schemes, work through the traumas or even capture the possible nuances of the story (what could strengthen its persuasive effect). It puts together pieces of the Katyń cultural memory and standardizes them into a well-defined and accessible shape. Moreover, *Katyń* could even be defined as a "memory text" in the narrow sense of the term proposed by Jan Assmann, according to whom cultural memory is institutionalized, ritual, traditional and symbolic, working as a mythical pre-history of the community.[21]

Metonymic Memory: Zbigniew Herbert's "Buttons"

The final part of this chapter considers the best known poem within Poland connected to Katyń, "Buttons," published by Zbigniew Herbert in 1992, and translated into English by Alissa Valles.[22] Herbert is among the most respected of twentieth century Polish poets, whose importance lies particularly in his role as a keeper of memory and conscience: ethically radical, adamantly resisting totalitarian powers, constantly clarifying the difference between right and wrong.

Andrzej Wajda stated in an interview published on the release of *Katyń* that the massacre "did not find its place in Polish literature;"[23] the only poem he mentions as a "Polish art tribute to Katyń victims" is "Buttons," appreciated by him as a work of genius. Wajda omitted many texts of course, but this poem still deserves special attention, not only as a work of art, but also as an important element in the cultural memory of Katyń. Consequently, my aim is not a full, close reading of the poem, but rather an analysis of how and why it became such an important point of reference.

The poem is dedicated "In memory of Captain Edward Herbert," the poet's cousin and one of the Katyń victims. The buttons that gave the poem its title were actually found during the exhumation of mass graves in the Katyń forest and other execution sites. In the poem they provide definite proof of the massacre and at the same time symbolize the memory of the victims. While the truth about Katyń cannot be revealed, the buttons replace the missing witnesses and substitute as banned commemoration symbols:

> Only buttons witnesses to the crime
> proved unyielding outlasted death
> and as sole memorial on the grave
> rise up from the depths of the earth

The scenery of Herbert's poem is a forest, a site of execution and mass burial of the victims. After the World War II, Eastern and Central Europe has been marked with numerous spots of this type: non-sites of memory,[24] topographic objects, where acts of mass violence, torture, execution and death took place, which yet remain dispersed, unmarked, indeterminate and non-commemorated. The case of the real Katyń graves is slightly different—the sites were actually demarcated and commemorated, but in a false, deceitful and totalitarian way (not least by the placement of inscription boards stating that Nazi Germany was responsible for the massacre).

However, Herbert creates his vision using only images of nature, thereby creating a parallel to the story of the Katyń memory, to the pain caused by its suppression and the impossibility of fitting justice and commemoration. He refers here to Holocaust iconography where nature plays a double role: either it is a witness to the crime, standing on the side of the victims (as in the memory site of Belzec, where old trees, growing there during the time when the camp existed, were intentionally and purposefully preserved[25]), or it is a cruel and silent observer, indifferent to suffering and hiding it. Herbert uses both models: nature is indifferent, while other non-human actors, the buttons, bear witness.

Their real, tangible presence is used metaphorically in the poem. First, the tiny, inappreciable objects become a visible, solid, material sign, the "sole memorial on the grave." Secondly, the inanimate souvenir or memorial acquires an ability to act: to be a witness, to testify, to appeal for God's attention (which is also their duty). Finally, the buttons "from coats and uniforms" substitute the murdered army; they are, like the soldier-victims, "unyielding:" they speak the truth about their death as a paradoxical "mighty voice of muted chorus."

In this optic, they work as metonymy for the Katyń massacre as a whole and for its suppressed, banned, but lasting memory. This simple poetic technique has been repeated in many works, where, as mentioned earlier, the surviving personal belongings of the officers are shown or recalled. Objects found in graves, such as fragments of clothing, but particularly awards and orders, documents, books and notes, holy medals, crosses and rosaries, sometimes stored by the families, become souvenirs, but at the same time a necessary sign of the victims' death (and respectively of their bravery, nobility, social status, and piety). The buttons in Herbert's poem are the best known prop of this kind, to the point that they are recognizable as an emblem of the Katyń victims. Wajda's film also uses this motif: one of the officers says to his camp companion: "buttons is all that will be left of us." This clear allusion to the well-known poem, spoken by an imaginary victim, legitimates the interpretation of the buttons as the only trace and testimony of the victims' death.

It is also noteworthy that the "Katyń 1940. We remember" campaign reinforced the power of this emblem, as buttons became its symbol, represented on the posters and in leaflets. Replicas of uniform buttons also became trinkets in the commemorative campaign, for instance, they were given out in the streets during educational events, and attached to religious and patriotic newspapers. The organizers' commentary clearly indicated the source of inspiration for the idea, quoting another verse of Herbert's poem: "buttons are memory signs because—as the poet wrote—'they are a testimony'."[26]

A new perspective in which to read Polish cultural memory in its entirety, one already indicated by the way "Buttons" was used in the discourse of Katyń memory, emerged after the 2010 Polish Air Force Tu-154 crash at Smoleńsk airport, where all of the dignitaries who were supposed to attend the ceremony of the 70th anniversary of the Katyń massacre, including the President of Poland, were killed. This event powerfully confirmed and strengthened the paralytic effect of Katyń's memory, reinforcing its position again as a frozen, traumatic moment.

As the authors of *Remembering Katyń* suggest "the crash would bring in its wake a new wave of encounters with the memory of Katyń"[27] and was soon labeled as "Katyń-2" both in the individual comments of mourners (including public figures such as Lech Walesa) and in media coverage of the event. There were several reasons for the subsequent linking of the Smolensk and Katyń tragedies. The extraordinary coincidence of space and time—the President was traveling to the anniversary ceremonies of the massacre in the place where his compatriots were murdered—was strengthened by the fact that he was himself a promoter of Katyń commemoration and of the sacrificial discourse around it, as were many of the other victims of the plane crash, who were themselves important figures in Polish politics and the public sphere. The incredible fact of the crash doubled the grief; it was noted too that the victims of 10 April 2010 were representatives of the Polish elites, a fact often emphasized also in relation to the officers murdered in 1940, and, in an attempt to find the meaning of the event, the death of the former was called by some commemorative martyrdom. The revelation of these continuities could not possibly remain only a part of the mourning discourse, the next step was to refuse to accept the crash as accidental and to demand "the truth about Smolensk." According to some, this truth meant that "Smolensk" was yet another Russian attack on Poland, a stance giving rise to numerous conspiracy theories, but also inspiring political quarrels, investigations of the possibility of the "Smolensk assassination," and ultimately creating powerful dividing lines across Polish society.

The uses of Herbert's poem serve as a slight, but meaningful example of the parallel mechanisms which connect the politics of collective, the traumatic memory of Katyń and of Smolensk. Surprisingly, the very name of Smolensk, a Russian city about 30 kilometers west of Katyń, also appears in the poem: Herbert does not use the words "Katyń forest" but instead refers to Smolensk:

> a bird flies over a cloud sails past
> a leaf descends mallows grow lush
> a mist drifts in the Smolensk forest
> and up in the heights a deep hush

The passage is astonishingly well suited to the circumstances of the crash, not only because of the place name, but also the foggy weather on 10 April. It was consequently cited over and over again during funeral ceremony epitaphs, and widely reproduced. The ghostly return of the traumatic past reaches its peak in a macabre intertextual outburst: "Song on Buttons" by Przemysław Dakowicz is an obvious allusion to Herbert's "Buttons."[28] In Dakowicz's poem, the rusty brass buttons of the uniforms and the contemporary plastic buttons of the clothing of the crash victims whisper to each other in the ground of the Katyń forest. This confirms the special role of Herbert's poem as a particular source of the ready-to-use themes expressing cultural memory. Dakowicz turns Herbert's simple synecdoche into a metaphor, the buttons are personified, which not only creates an analogy between the tragic deaths of 1940 and those of 2010, but also suggests an alliance between the victims of both: their common ideological attitude, their sacrifice, and the mnemonic myth that joins them all.

Consequently, when the memory of Smolensk uses the clichés of the Katyń memory, the constructed cultural images of the massacre and the plane crash unite. The characteristic of the former is contagious in its associations with the latter. Both, for instance, can be seen as a planned attack on Poland (as in the various Smolensk conspiracy theories). What is more, the use of the patterns of the Katyń memory does not involve their transference or reconstruction; they remain fixed and petrified just as they have been described, and the mechanism of remembrance of the Smolensk crash seems to be equally paralyzed.

Conclusion

The cultural memory of Katyń, when seen in relation to Assmann's theory, can be understood as a dynamic process only insofar as it absorbs mnemonic texts and practices, and develops their presence within the new media. Of course the context of the Katyń memory has changed: from official silence before 1989, it has become recognized and acknowledged, but simultaneously is being exploited and manipulated for political interests. Nevertheless, the Katyń memory profile is fixed and, to a large extent, formed within clandestine mnemonic activity before 1989. The interaction between its elements does not involve any creative transformation of themes and motifs; they limit their scope to a simple repetition of what was already said and shown. Although there are no longer official sanctions and regulations concerning the memory of Katyń, as was the case before 1989, the discourse surrounding it is still governed by strict rules. The catalogue of these rules reveals both the hidden history and the contemporary conditions of remembering the massacre within Polish culture: it includes some almost obligatory emblems, as well as the law of metonymy and narrative schemes (of patriotic and religious origin) constructing the Katyń cultural memory. The strength of these regulations is crucial in the shaping of this memory field: the rules are virtually never contested or challenged by any mnemonic texts. The mainstream of Katyń memory continues to assemble and replicate the tried and tested ways of remembering.

This points to a different interpretation of the mechanisms of Katyń memory than those put forward by Etkind and his fellow authors. *Remembering Katyń* assumes a dynamic re-working through particular subsequent "memory events" (Wajda's film, or the 2010 crash of Lech Kaczynski's plane) whereby an established memory template is revised and transformed. These memory events "generate new memories bearing the structural imprint of old ones."[29] In my view, by contrast, there is an unusual constancy to the Katyń memory: new events do not so much serve to transform the original memory event as to strengthen the old imprint.

A partial explanation for this mnemonic paralysis is trauma's influence. The traumatic experience of Katyń cannot be worked through by means of secondary, simplified texts and practices. Such accounts attempt to act out the horror "as it happened," but without understanding it or considering its aftermath. The final scene of Wajda's *Katyń* is exemplary in this respect, while the metonymic strategies of other texts discussed in this essay display the same impulse.

After 1989 the traumatic, collective memory of Katyń, prolonged in the 40-year period of enforced lies about the perpetrators, was almost impossible to process. Poland's image of the past remains haunted by these specters, images of Katyń continue to paralyze the nation's cultural memory in endless, compulsive recollections and re-activations of past suffering. The only conclusion to which such memory pattern can lead is identifying the bearers of Katyń memory with the victims of Katyń, thereby producing a national community of "those hurt and harmed in Katyń," while this harm becomes a source of various claims. These claims are founded on the traumatic past, the aftershock of which seems never to end, which within contemporary Polish culture and politics is preserved and revived constantly.

Notes

1. Cf. Aleida Assmann, *Cultural Memory and Western Civilization: Functions, Media, Archives* (Cambridge: University Press, 2011).
2. Lech Nijakowski, *Polskie polityki pamięci. Esej socjologiczny* (Warszawa: WAiP, 2008).
3. Adam Ostolski, *Trauma i pamięć publiczna. Spuścizna II wojny światowej w pamięci zbiorowej współczesnej Polski* (unpublished manuscript of doctoral thesis, University of Warsaw, Faculty of Philosophy and Sociology, 2011).
4. Cf, Izabela Kowalczyk, *Podróż do przeszłości. Interpretacje najnowszej historii w polskiej sztuce krytycznej* (Warszawa: SWPS Academica, 2010).

5. Alexander Etkind et al., *Remembering Katyn* (Cambridge: Polity Press, 2012), 2.
6. Ibid., 8.
7. Ibid., 14.
8. Act of 18 December 1998 on the Institute of National Remembrance—Commission for the Prosecution of Crimes against the Polish Nation, art. 55 [online]. http://ipn.gov.pl/__data/assets/pdf_file/0008/49292/1-24338.pdf.
9. Andrzej Przewoźnik, Jolanta Adamska, *Katyń. Zbrodnia—prawda—pamięć* (Warszawa: Świat Książki, 2010), 629.
10. Cathy Caruth, *Unclaimed Experience. Trauma, Narrative, and History* (Baltimore and London: Johns Hopkins University Press, 1996), 4.
11. Jeffrey K. Olick, *The Politics of Regret. On Collective Memory and Historical Responsibility* (New York and London: Routledge, 2007), 93.
12. The cited press release is available online on the official campaign site: http://www.pamietamkatyn1940.pl/116.html.
13. The described posters and spot are available to download from the official campaign site: http://www.pamietamkatyn1940.pl/135.html.
14. Bartosz Korzeniewski, "Medializacja i mediatyzacja pamięci—nośniki pamięci i ich rola w kształtowaniu pamięci przeszłości," *Kultura Współczesna* 2007/3, 13.
15. Tadeusz Lubelski *Wajda* (Wrocław: Wydawnictwo Dolnośląskie, 2006), 6.
16. Andrzej Wajda, "Zaklinacz duchów," *Film* 2007/9, 39.
17. "Massacre on screen," in *Remembering Katyn*, 53.
18. Cf. Agata Bielik-Robson, "Słowo i trauma: czas, narracja, tożsamość," *Teksty Drugie* 2004/5, 23–34.
19. Michael Rothberg, *Multidirectional Memory: Remembering the Holocaust in the Age of Decolonization* (Stanford: Stanford University Press, 2009), 3.
20. Witold Mrozek, "*Film pamięci narodowej. Najnowsze kino polskie w dyskursie polityki historycznej*," in *Kino polskie jako kino narodowe*, ed. Tadeusz Lubelski, Maciej Stroiński (Kraków: Korporacja Ha!art, 2009), 295.
21. Cf. Jan Assmann, *Cultural Memory and Early Civilization: Writing, Remembrance and Political Imagination* (Cambridge: University Press, 2011).

22. Zbigniew Herbert, *The Complete Poems: 1956–1998* (New York: Ecco Press, 2007), 477.
23. Wajda, “Zaklinacz”, 39.
24. Cf. Roma Sendyka, “Pryzma—zrozumieć nie-miejsce pamięci,” *Teksty Drugie* 2013/1-2, 323-244.
25. Cf. Jacek Małczyński, “Drzewa—żywe pomniki w Muzeum-Miejscu Pamięci w Bełżcu,” *Teksty Drugie* 2009/1-2, 208-214.
26. Quoted from the official campaign site [online]. http://www.pamietamkatyn1940.pl/161.html.
27. “Coda: Katyn-2,” in *Remembering Katyn*, 132.
28. Przemysław Dakowicz, *Piosenka o guzikach* [online]. http://wierszeosmolensku.blogspot.com/2010/11/przemysaw-dakowicz.html.
29. *Remembering Katyn*, 10.

PART V

Representation

CHAPTER 10

War Rape: Trauma and the Ethics of Representation

Marzena Sokołowska-Paryż

In October 2013, a student of the Academy of Fine Arts illegally installed a statue of a pregnant woman being raped by a Red Army soldier in the Avenue of Victory in Gdańsk. The police were called in, the statue was promptly removed, yet the incident captured the attention of news media both in Poland and abroad. The artist, Jerzy Bohdan Szumczyk, explained his intentions in a statement released to the Polish Press Agency: "I wanted to direct public attention to the monuments that surround us. [...] Among all the erected monuments there are too few commemorating victims. I wanted also to postulate the need to speak openly about rape in general."[1] This was an art work in service of a commendable cause, yet what ultimately counts is the final effect. In Arthur Danto's words, "[we] build memorials so that we shall never forget,"[2] and the question that arises in the case of the *Komm Frau* statue is *who* precisely *must we never forget*—the female victims or the male perpetrators? The artist's declared purpose to commemorate women victims of wartime was thwarted by the shockingly naturalistic rape scene, with the woman's suffering visually subjugated by male aggression. The victim was completely dominated by the towering soldier figure. It is a striking contradiction that this statue proved by its blatant "re-enactment" of rape that "rape cannot be visualized [...]

M. Sokołowska-Paryż (✉)
University of Warsaw, Poland

P. Leese, J. Crouthamel (eds.), *Traumatic Memories of the Second World War and After*, DOI 10.1007/978-3-319-33470-7_10

because rape makes the victim invisible. It does that literally first—the perpetrator 'covers' her [...]. Finally, rape cannot be visualized because the experience is, physically, as well as psychologically, inner. Rape takes place inside."[3] The statue showed less the victim than the victimization of women, that is rape as "dominance, power, and contempt, a rejection of the woman's right to self-determination."[4] Viewers were forced to become involuntary spectators of "a second violation," the victim "re-raped" by the "graphic representation of sexual violence."[5]

Though the artist asserted that he did not wish to re-ignite national antagonisms, *Komm Frau* was a clear indictment of the Soviet soldiers as the barbarian-rapists of the Second World War (the woman being conspicuously pregnant). The choice of the location right next to a Soviet WWII tank, a relic monument from the Communist period, created a clash of two diametrically opposed political discourses, the tank "speaking" of the Soviet victory over Nazi Germany, and the statue "speaking" of the "Rape of Gdańsk", which, in turn, became (too) easily generalized as "Rape of Poland" and "Rape of Europe" in the public debate that ensued. The Ambassador of the Russian Federation in Poland issued a formal protest: "The vulgar statue on the city's main street insults not only the feelings of Russians, but of all clear-headed people who remember to whom they owe their liberation from the Nazis."[6] The Polish media response was immediate and unequivocal, with journalists, historians and politicians more or less explicitly accusing the Russian diplomat of arrogantly falsifying history, his alleged "liberators" being, from the Polish point of view, invaders on route to Germany, bringing about the Soviet occupation of Poland, as well as other Eastern-Europe nations, that was to last for the next four and half decades.

Komm Frau and the heated debate it provoked perfectly encapsulate the issues at the heart of my discussion on the ethics of representing rape in the war film, first and foremost, the disconcerting over-indulgence in "the pornography of pain,"[7] to be understood as a preference for showing atrocity and neglecting the psychological consequences of sexual victimization, as well as the foregrounding of the perpetrators at the expense of the victims who become "invisible", though present on screen. As Tanya Horeck has rightly and emphatically asked, "What are the ethics of reading and watching representations of rape? Are we bearing witness to a terrible crime or are we participating in a shameful voyeuristic activity"?[8] Furthermore, though equally important, there emerges the problem of the widespread practice of embedding war rapes within the frames of an overtly political discourse which metonymically equates the victims with their nations, for as Kirby Farrell has emphasized, "People not only suffer trauma; they use it, and the idea of it, for all sorts of ends, good and ill. The trope can be ideologically manipulated, reinforced, and exploited".[9] The conventional expectation of war films is adherence to historical truth. This is because the war film, in comparison to other genres, is the one that "carries with it [the] almost sacred trust to preserve history."[10] I would argue that the vast majority of war films taking up the subject matter of rape are historically truthful only with regard to the fact of such rapes occurring but not to the women's traumatic experience, as they offer practically no insight whatsoever into the psychological consequences of sexual violation in wartime. Paraphrasing Elie Wiesel's famous remark on the representation of the Holocaust in literature, it can be said that a war film about rape is either not a war film or not about rape.[11]

Sarah Projansky writes that "despite [the] 'timelessness' [of rape] [as a key aspect of storytelling throughout Western history], the structure of rape narratives varies historically, depending on cultural and national contexts."[12] The war films selected for my discussion represent different national cultures, were produced in different times, and take up the subject of war rape in different historical contexts. I have deliberately chosen war films produced before and after the second-wave feminist revolution in order to show that their patterns of representation of war rape remain disconcertingly similar, apart from the post-1970s tendency to "eroticize" sexual violence in wartime by means of naturalistic re-enactments. Thus, one may well consider the metaphorization of war rape, as well as the prioritization of the male protagonist over the female victim, as transhistorical and transnational phenomena in the realm of the war film.

It is impossible to provide the overall number of women raped in all the wars fought in the twentieth century, though the estimates in particular cases of mass rape (Nanking, Berlin, Bangladesh, Bosnia, Kosovo, Rwanda) are staggering.[13] There can be no doubt that "the twentieth century in Europe [and beyond] was not only a century of extraordinary brutality, [but it] can also usefully be thought of as 'the century of sex,'[…],"[14] necessitating "new questions […] about old topics—from the complex relationships between prejudice, ideology, and faith to the role of emotions like fear, hatred, exhilaration in the act of killing […]."[15] The scale of the atrocities requires not only in-depth investigation and documentation, but also a critical analysis of how these atrocities have been ideologically manipulated in popular culture. One should ask whether war films, rather than commemorating rape victims with empathy and bespeaking the truth about women's trauma in wartime, do not actually promote, as a conventionally "male genre,"[16] "a rape culture" that encourages rape in part by giving men permission, even encouraging men, to watch women sexually and that acknowledges the male gaze as sexually assaultive."[17] Secondly, one must also raise the question about the role of war films in perpetuating stereotypical associations with gender by depicting, to borrow Joshua S. Goldstein's words, "male soldiers [in] a masculine and dominant position relative to a feminine and subordinate enemy."[18]

War Rape: Acknowledgment and Understanding

Susan Brownmiller's *Against Our Will: Men, Women, and Rape* is generally considered to have been the ground-breaking book of the 1970s second-wave feminist campaign launched to break the silence surrounding the subject matter of rape. Her chapter on the sexual victimization of women in the historical contexts of the Great War, the Second World War, Bangladesh and Vietnam was aimed to counteract the hitherto popular thinking that rape belongs to the "package" of suffering brought about by war.[19] The term "rape trauma syndrome" (RTS) was introduced in 1974, defined as "the acute phase and long-term reorganization process that occurs as a result of forcible rape or attempted forcible rape. This syndrome of behavioral somatic and psychological reactions is an acute stress reaction to a life-threatening situation."[20] It would take some time before RTS gained the recognition it deserved: "only after 1980, when the efforts of combat veterans have legitimated the concept of post-traumatic stress disorder, did it become clear that the psychological syndrome seen in survivors of rape, domestic battery, and incest was essentially the same as the syndrome seen in survivors of war."[21] War rapes were—and continue to be—perceived as a distinctive category of sexual violence, in acknowledgment that "to understand the effects of rape in wartime, one must consider the additional trauma that women may have experienced: death of loved ones, loss of home and community, dislocation, untreated illness, and war-related injury," not to mention that "having already suffered the trauma of rape, women who then become pregnant face further emotional and psychological trauma."[22]

The statement that women are "probably the greatest single group" to be "defiled, debased, and dehumanized for the aggrandizement of others" in the time of war[23] is not surprising in a book published in the 1990s, a decade marred by media reports of the scale of rape, mutilation and death of women in the current military conflicts: "It was the Balkan wars [...] that exposed the issue of mass rape to international visibility [...]. The term 'genocidal rape' began to be widely employed to convey the centrality of sexual assault to the wider campaign of group destruction. Although rejected by some [...], the concept gained further credibility with events in Rwanda [...]."[24] The decade proved a turning point for many reasons, as not only "for the first time in international history, victims have appeared as witnesses before international courts; perpetrators, both direct and indirect, have been successfully prosecuted; and sexual violence has been tried as a crime of genocide, a war crime and a crime against humanity," but also the shock of Bosnia and Rwanda put previous and subsequent military conflicts under close scrutiny: "mass media documentation in diverse geographical locations has since revealed both the gravity and extent of wartime sexual violence; truth and reconciliation commissions have heard harrowing victims' narratives; and books, documentaries and films have captured the unceasingly common horrors of rape, forced impregnation and sexual slavery."[25]

Since the 1990s, there have appeared numerous studies of war rape analyzed from various scholarly perspectives (historical, sociological, anthropological, medical, psychological, legal), as well as powerful documentary productions empathically involved in bringing to light the trauma of sexual violence in wartime and giving voice to the victims. In the recent decade, however, another trend has become discernible in rape trauma studies, represented most notably by Sarah Projansky, Sabine Sielke and Tanya Horeck. Their works underscore the need of focusing on the ethics of "telling" and "showing" rape in literature and film: "[if] for second-wave feminism the primary objective was to put rape on the agenda [...], what is at stake [now] is [...] how we speak about rape and to what end."[26] Regardless of the time and place of production, war films perfectly exemplify the disheartening view that "rape is often remembered not to honour the traumatic personal experiences of women, but rather to celebrate or exalt a masculinized war narrative of victory and defeat. [...] official narratives of both past and present forms of wartime sexual violence are compellingly political, despite the crime itself and the impact on victims being irrefutably private."[27]

(Mis)Representations of War Rape

If in interwar or immediate post-Second War films, rape could only be implied but never explicitly shown, the changes in cultural norms regarding the presentation of nudity and sexual violence on screen since the 1960s/1970s have resulted in a tendency to depict rape as naturalistically as possible. In Audrius Juzenas's *Ghetto* (2006), Bruno Dumont's *Flandres/Flanders* (2006), or Brian De Palma's *Redacted* (2007), the rape scenes border on pornography, primarily because it is "the [male perpetrator] [who] controls the film fantasy and also emerges [...] as the bearer of the look of the spectator, transferring it behind the screen to neutralise the extra-diegetic tendencies represented by woman as spectacle. This is made possible through the processes set in motion by structuring the film around a main controlling figure with whom the spectator can [or must] identify."[28] It is this framing "male gaze" that too frequently forces the audience of the war film to adopt the awkward position of the voyeur in a spectacle that renders Eros and Thanatos indistinguishable: "Thrusting the sexual appendage (the penis) deep into the body of the victim can be perversely linked to thrusting the killing appendage (a bayonet or knife) deep into the body of the victim."[29]

Joanna Bourke emphatically states that "rape is not a metaphor for the ruin of a city or nation [...]. It is the embodied violation of another person."[30] It remains, however, an inherent paradox of war films that the explicitness of rape scenes goes hand in hand with the tendency to "translate tales of violation onto nationally specific cultural symbologies and conclusive narratives. As such, they both form and interfere with the cultural imaginary. Like news about crime, they may even offer a lesson, some higher concept."[31] In other words, war films 'undo' the trauma of rape by contextualizing "[the] out-of context experience"[32] and by substituting "[the] absence [of the] event that [cannot] come to existence, in spite of the overwhelming and compelling nature of the reality of its occurrence"[33] with a presence—the graphic visualization of rape. In effect, rape is not only familiarized but also transfigured into an almost sublime event. Adapting Kirby Farrell's words, one can say that it is never the aim of the war film to show the "psychic ruin" of women but to "make terror and loss heroically [or tragically] meaningful."[34]

War films are conventionally about nations or ethnic/religious/tribal groups. The focus is thus placed on victims and perpetrators representing the belligerent sides in the conflict. It is commonly assumed that "the winning side is the side that does the raping," whereas "documentation of rape in warfare is something the other side totals up, analyses and propagandizes when the smoke has cleared up after defeat."[35] This metaphorization of rape as the violation of an entire community serves principally to create an ethical distinction between the enemy and the defeated, the barbarian rapist-aggressor versus the conquered yet noble victim: "Gender plays a role in ethnonationalism. The nation is often gendered female and the state male. [...] Rape of 'our' women sometimes becomes a dominant metaphor of the danger to the nation from enemy males. [...] [This construction] also provide[s] 'opportunities for heroism.'"[36] The political distinction between "us" and "them" counteracts the possibility of showing women's victimhood in war time from a transhistorical and transnational perspective. Helke Sander attempted such a perspective in *Befreier und Befreite/Liberators Take Liberties* (1991/1992) by including the following introduction to her documentary: "This is about war-time rapes cases. As I know the Berlin conditions better than any other conditions, this film is about what happened there. Everybody knew about it but no one talked about it, as it is in Kuwait and Yugoslavia today."[37] According to Atina Grossmann, representations of war rape must abide by certain rules in order to remain truthful and moral: "even as we struggle to name sexual violence and to create a community among women in order to combat it, we must understand it as both an intensely personal, and *a public, politically and historically constructed event*" (emphasis mine).[38] She follows with an accusation that "[the] eagerness to integrate German women into the international transhistorical sisterhood of victims of male violence leads to a problematic historical slippage and displacement in which German women seem to become the victims primarily of National Socialism and the war [...] (and not also agents, collaborators, or beneficiaries) of National Socialism."[39] One could venture the opinion that this harsh criticism of the documentary was provoked by Sander's decision to combine rape victim testimonies with images of war-ravaged Berlin, which endowed the victims' stories with an overt national meaning: "The intersection of [the victims'] memories with the visuals leads to an indictment of the soldiers whose entry into the city is purely sexualized. Within this constellation, the shelled-out buildings stand for women's mutilated and battered bodies and the allusion to the city as a defenceless feminized space suggests that Berlin, and by extension Germany, was raped and humiliated."[40]

It must remain an open question whether it is possible to achieve, in documentaries or popular war films, a more universal take on war rape as "transhistorical, transpolitical patriarchal violence."[41] Such an experiment was undertaken by Bruno Dumont in *Flandres/Flanders* (2006), though it is highly debatable to what extent the attempt was successful. The plot revolves round a group of young men of an indeterminate nationality who are conscripted and sent off to an unspecified war. The landscape suggests the Middle East, but there are a few disconcerting details. One review, by posing more questions than giving answers, is indicative of how difficult it is to decipher the precise historical and/or geopolitical context of the military action: "Which war, though? Afghanistan? Iraq? It's never clear. [...] And why are these men being called up? [...] A trench? Surely, trenches are not used in modern warfare in the Middle East? Could this detail resonate with the title, a suggestion that the film is about a new Flanders field, a Flanders field of the mind, a world war fought just as hard on the home front by civilians as well as those in uniform?"[42] In this unidentified war zone, the European male soldiers encounter a female fighter (soldier?) and they brutally rape her. Despite the deliberate vagueness shrouding the conflict, the woman is clearly constructed as the "Other" by means of the occidental male gaze. She is raped because she represents an ethnicity and culture that is the "enemy" of the Western world and because she has adopted the conventionally masculine role of a warrior. Dora Apel's conclusion regarding the meaning of a Great War photograph of German soldiers standing over the corpse of a raped Russian female soldier applies equally well to Dumont's film where "rape may [also] be understood not simply as a wartime abuse but as a punishment for a different sort of hostilities, that is, for the transgression of gender boundaries."[43]

Flandres/Flanders is a controversial film, not only due to the shocking explicitness of the rape scene, but also owing to its use of the rape-revenge format which reverses the roles of victim and perpetrator: the female victim is transfigured into a perpetrator of violence and the rapist becomes the woman's victim as she carries out her revenge for the violation of her body, which is private (to punish her own suffering), public (to punish the sexual subjugation of women) and metaphorical (to punish the invasion of her land). Nonetheless, considering the character of the pre-war relationship between the main character Demester and his sexual partner Barbe, other interpretations of the war rape offer themselves. The sexual act is mechanical and brutal, without love or even desire. Setting together the pre-war sex scenes and the war rape scene, Bradshaw is right in concluding his review that this may not be a war film in any sense of the term: "Flanders looks as if it is about Afghanistan and Iraq, and yet it is not, and fascinatingly, may not be about war at all, but is rather a meditation or hallucination on the subject of male sexual aggression, tricked out in military costume."[44]

Though in times of military conflict women are raped not only by soldiers of the invading armies but also by their own countrymen, such cases are seldom the subject of war films for they fail to "highlight a nation's victimhood or heroism."[45] Even if such a theme appears, the intent is to show the rapist as the "Other" within the community. A good example is Mikhail Kalatozov's *Летят журавли/The Cranes are Flying* (1957), where a Russian woman is raped by her own countryman; here rape is a means of exposing the man as a coward evading his patriotic duty to fight. Rape is also used/abused as an anti-war argument. In Chris Noonan's and John Duigan's TV series *Vietnam* (1987), the rape of a Vietnamese woman accentuates the difference between brutal and primitive American soldiers and honorable and compassionate Australian soldiers, and allows to make a very strong anti-American statement, depicting Australian involvement in the Vietnam war as a grave mistake, in both political and ethical terms. Brian De Palma's *Casualties of War* (1989) and *Redacted* (2007) are the most telling examples of the exploitation of actual rape cases to make a political statement against American military involvement in Vietnam and Iraq.[46] Rape is too frequently included in war films to show the devastating impact of war upon the soldier, shifting the attention from the victim to the rapist: "To understand the crime, however, one needs to see things from the perpetrator's eye, [...] it tends to suggest that there is a dark area of male sexuality which can emerge all too easily, especially in war, when there are no social and disciplinary restraints. Much also depends on the military culture of a particular national army. [...] the practice of collective rape can even become a form of bonding process."[47] The title of Brian De Palma's anti-Vietnam War film has little to do with the Vietnamese as victims of American aggression but, considering the centrality of the male characters, the eponymous "casualties of war" are soldiers who become rapists under the duress of combat. Furthermore, as Joanna Bourke aptly notes, not only "the invention of Post-Traumatic Stress Disorder (PTSD) allowed men who had participated in atrocities to portray themselves as victims of trauma" (384) but also "the most common reason given for rape in wartime drew attention not to male power and solidarity but male fears and vulnerability."[48] In most war films, the rape victim is of secondary importance, or, as in the case of the 1979 film adaptation of Günter Grass's *The Tin Drum* (*Die Blechtrommel*, dir. Volker Schlöndorff), she has no significance whatsoever. The gang rape of Lina appears to serve the sole purpose of underscoring the absurdity of Alfred's death. While she is being raped by Red Army soldiers, Alfred tries to swallow his Nazi pin so that it does not fall into enemy hands and betray his political allegiances. His desperate attempt to save his own life ends with him choking on the pin which, in turn, provokes a Soviet soldier to shoot him. This is what the viewer remembers from the scene, what happens to the woman in the aftermath of the rape is not given any prominence in the plot.

Male Trauma and Female Victims

Sidney Lumet's *The Pawnbroker* (1964), Reg Traviss's *Der Feind im Inneren/Joy Division* (2006), and Wojciech Smarzowski's *Róża/Rose* (2011) are not classic war films if we adopt a very restrictive definition of the genre. However, though the action of the films is set in the post-Second World War period, they are all films primarily about war and its repercussions for the protagonist in the present. In each film, the traumatization of the male protagonist is the result of his inability to save the woman from being raped and killed. These films create a gender-based hierarchy of suffering where the female victim is relegated to the function of the instigating factor of the man's trauma. The woman is downgraded to a fleeting character in the flashback, the central concern being the male protagonist's inability to cope with having been "the witness of his own impotence."[49] It is morally unsettling that in these cinematic representations of war rapes the violation of the female body is of lesser importance than the violation of the male psyche.

The plot of *The Pawnbroker* is centered on Sol Nazerman, a Holocaust survivor unable to come to terms with the rape and murder of his wife in a concentration camp, which he was forced to witness. In this film, "images are wounds that will not heal."[50] The film consistently uses the traumatic flashback defined as "an intrusive, anachronic image that throws off the linear temporality of the story. [...] This brutal splicing of temporally disadjusted images is the cinema's rendition of the frozen moment of the traumatic impact: it flashes back insistently in the present because this image cannot yet or perhaps ever be narrativized as the past."[51] The purpose of the traumatic flashbacks is to let us see what Nazerman saw as a prisoner and thus understand the manner in which he treats his Harlem customers, his inability to forge any lasting relationships of friendship and love, and his alienation from the community. The present is a mirror of the past: "through sublimal flash cuts that gradually lengthen into painful scenes, the linear narrative is thickened with the weight of the past."[52] When a prostitute uncovers her breasts as a symbolic offering of her body to Nazerman, a flashback interrupts the storyline, showing Nazerman's wife, Ruth, sitting half-naked on a bed, awaiting her doom as the SS-guard slowly approaches her. It is an indisputable fact that female prisoners of concentration camps were raped or forced into prostitution, but in Lumet's film the only reason why we see Ruth about to be raped is because this is what her husband witnessed, with "the cinematic technique eloquently express[ing] Nazerman's fractured state of mind."[53] The rape victim is therefore significant only insofar as she is "framed" by Sol's trauma; it is his survival guilt that brings her into "being" in the plot of the film.

Der Feind im Inneren/Joy Division is a hybrid film, combining the war story with the spy thriller. The purpose is to create an intersection of the past and present and foreground the interrelated themes of loyalty and betrayal. The action is set in the reality of the Cold War, the protagonist is a KGB agent sent to London in search of a traitor. Yet, it is Thomas's past that resurfaces as the most important part of the film, set in the final days of the Third Reich. He was a German youth conscripted into the *Volkssturm* to make the last stand against the overwhelming forces of the Red Army. He saw the death of his comrades, his parents were killed in a bombardment, and his sweetheart Melanie was repeatedly raped by Soviet soldiers. Similar to *The Pawnbroker*, Traviss's film consistently uses the traumatic flashback. It is Melanie to whom Thomas continuously returns to in his mind, for she saved his life by offering herself to drunken Soviet soldiers. It is not always the case that the traumatic flashbacks are "a precise return to a specific memory, [where the image is] eidetic and entirely veridical,"[54] for Thomas often "remembers" what he could not have possibly seen. Psychological plausibility is not, however, the aim of the film. At the core of the intertwined plots we have a protagonist struggling to regain his identity shattered by shame and guilt, the combined signifiers of "masculine trauma."[55]

The emotion of shame is "directly about the self, which is the focus of evaluation" whereas in the case of guilt "the self is not the central object of evaluation, but rather the thing done."[56] Thomas's shame derives from the fact he had no time to become a man and soldier, being only 14 at the time of the defeat of Germany. His emasculation is augmented by the fact that he was protected by women, first by Melanie who saves his life, then by Astrid who gives him civilian clothes, and finally by a Russian female soldier who takes him under her care. Shame devastates the self because it is "accompanied by sense of shrinking or of 'being small' and by a sense of worthlessness and powerlessness."[57] As Thomas says to a fellow-agent, one cannot understand the meaning of loyalty without committing betrayal. He joined the ranks of those who had humiliated and murdered Melanie because "a situation of guilt with all its anxiety can be sought as a refuge from a pressing sense of shame."[58] As a 14-year old, Thomas was unable to protect the people he loved. It is only in the role of a KGB agent that he is able to reassert his masculine identity.

Róża/Rose is likewise exemplary of this aggravating tendency to transfer the viewer's attention from the female victim to the male survivor. The film opens with a symptomatic scene where the rape and murder of a Polish woman by Germans during the Warsaw Uprising is shown through the eyes of her helpless husband—a wounded insurgent. The rape takes place on the rubble, in the background we see burnt buildings. The battered woman and the destroyed city are visually interrelated, the meanings of a city defeated and a nation conquered inscribed in the subjugated female body. This rape scene is included as a means of the psychological characterization of the male protagonist and the launching of the plot of the film that revolves round the man's desire to escape the trauma of loss and defeat. In the course of his journey as far away from Warsaw as possible, Tadeusz witnesses the killing of a Wehrmacht soldier by Soviet troops, and his documents and a photograph become the pretext to find his wife, the eponymous Róża.

Smarzowski's film received well-deserved praise for its depiction of the atrocities committed against the community of Masurians in East Prussia, the territory of which was incorporated into the Polish state after the defeat of the Third Reich. On the level of plot, rape is an instrument of symbolic expulsion—Róża is the "Other" both ethnically (Masurian) and nationally (she was married to a German). She is being coerced—by means of repeated rape and threats of death—to leave her house and land. The aftermath of the Second World War is a time of exodus, Germans and allegedly pro-German ethnic groups being forced out of the territories "gained" by Poland in order to make place and provide homes from the Poles evicted from the borderlands lost to the Soviet Union. It is not that the resettled Poles from the east are welcome, as indicated by the rape of Amelia, whose family traveled from afar hoping to find safety and peace in their new home, only to be subjected to violence and humiliation. On the level of historical politics, the film establishes a clear distinction between "us"—the victims of the new order (former Home Army soldiers, Masurians, Poles from the eastern borderlands) and "them"—the agents of the new order (Soviets and Polish Communists).

Róża takes Tadeusz into her home for she needs both help in un-mining the potato field and protection for herself and her daughter. Tadeusz—as a Pole—is a guarantee that the house will not be taken away from her. Though the title of the film clearly points to her as the protagonist of the film, she lacks autonomy, being consistently framed by the male gaze, and her function in the plot is to be the object of Tadeusz's love, an emotion that will bring about his psychological and emotional catharsis, and teach him empathy transcending national and ethnic boundaries. It is through his eyes that we see her fortitude. She refuses to leave her house and land, even though this will bring about her death after repeated rape and miscarriage. As the psychologically resilient victim she withstands traumatization and is a source of strength for Tadeusz, who despite all adversities (including imprisonment), will not sacrifice his principles that do not allow him to become part of this alien Polish state that has emerged in consequence of *his* Poland's defeat.

From Trauma to Tragedy: Rape Victim Typles in War Films

For James Chapman, tragedy is a category defining anti-war cinema which aims to convey a universal message on "the brutality and the indiscriminate nature of violence."[59] The concept of tragedy needs to be redefined in relation to war films which focus on historical events of a specifically national importance. Eva Hoffman's definition of tragedy in opposition to trauma is particularly useful in this context: "trauma is produced by persecution of subjects to whom all agency and principle have been denied. [...] Violent abuse can lead to a deeper penetration and fragmentation of the psychic cells, the victim's self and soul" whereas "tragedy, of course, involves a conflict—agon—between opposing principles and agents. [...] Tragic struggle may entail moral agony, but it leaves the sense of identity and dignity intact."[60] Tragedy is preferable to trauma in contexts where women and nationality/ethnicity are made to be metaphorically interchangeable, for only tragedy allows for the possibility of catharsis and the restoration of the national/ethnic self. The "translation" of trauma to tragedy is achieved through the construction of rape-victim types which I have labeled respectively the sacrificial victim—who appears in Janusz

Morgenstein's TV series *Kolumbowie/Columbuses* (1970) and Chuan Lu's *Nanjing! Nanjing!/The City of Life and Death* (2009), and the defiant victim—who is the protagonist in Max Fäberböck's *Anonyma: Eine Frau in Berlin/Anonyma—A Woman in Berlin* (2008) and Juanita Wilson's *As If I am Not There* (2010).

In the last part of *Kolumbowie/Columbuses*, a female Polish insurgent is raped by German soldiers during the Warsaw Uprising of 1944. Like Melanie in *Der Feind im Inneren/Joy Division*, the girl using the pseudonym "Niteczka" in Morgenstein's series is a typical sacrificial victim. First and foremost, the sacrificial victim is a secondary character in a plot that focuses predominantly on the male protagonist. The sacrificial victim gives her body over to the enemy so that the life of the defeated soldier may be spared. The defeated soldier is the witness of her sacrifice in a symbolically charged scene for "rape before a captive audience indicates that the invasion as a gendered process [is] not a two-, but a three-way relationship—between perpetrator, victim, and the victim's male compatriots."[61] The woman's suffering and humiliation are important only insofar as they become the conquered soldier's shame and/or trauma, and in this respect the sacrificial victim is a construct typical of representations of war rape where "women are depersonalized to the point of becoming a signifier in the power struggle between men so that wartime rape essentially targets male identity."[62] The rape of the woman is exploited as a means of characterizing the male protagonist: "While rape is used to defile and denigrate a nation, by extension, it also serves to strip a man who belongs to that nation of his honor, his masculinity, and what is seen as his exclusive right to a woman as his sole property. [...] Not only is the female body as property violated and transgressed, but the male is emasculated and allegedly confronted with his own sexual inadequacy and his failure as protector."[63]

Kolumbowie/Columbuses is an adaptation of Roman Bratny's novel under the same title. The series consists of five parts, following the actions of a group of young men, known only by their pseudonyms, working for the Polish underground during the German occupation. "Columbus" is one of the most prominent characters in the group, whereas "Niteczka" remains in the background until the last scenes set during the Warsaw Uprising. The failure of the insurgents to liberate the Old Town from the Germans means that they must evacuate themselves to another district, but "Columbus" is wounded, and "Niteczka" stays back to take care of him. She drags him out of a makeshift hospital about to be overrun by the Germans, and takes him down to a cellar. She sees through the window how SS soldiers force the wounded, doctors, nurses and a priest out of the building and shoot them. When an SS-man finds their hiding-place, "Niteczka" does not resist him. Her body is the price for the life of the Polish insurgent. "Columbus" is spared but "Niteczka" is raped and killed. He discovers her half-exposed body and covers it. The rape sequence is interrupted by a scene where another insurgent stares helplessly at a building in flames. A connection is thus established between the mutilated female body and the burning capital. The last scene shows "Columbus" swimming across the Vistula River, yet for the (Polish) viewers it is obvious what happens next. The defeat of the insurgents by the Germans will leave Warsaw defenseless against the Soviet invaders who will enter ("rape") the feminized body of the Polish capital. Yet, the sacrifice of the woman is not in vain, for the Polish soldier survives, even if defeated and powerless. He still signifies the will (if not the capability) of the nation to continue its struggle against the invaders.

In *Nanjing! Nanjing!/The City of Life and Death*, we encounter a different variant of the sacrificial victim: not one character sacrificing herself for the sake of a soldier's life, but a group of women giving their bodies and lives to save other women. The film shows the Japanese invasion of Nanking in 1937 from the combined perspective of the victorious army and the defeated community. Particular emphasis is placed in the Chinese women who cut off their hair, take off their make-up and nail polish, and put on men's clothes, all in desperate attempt to protect themselves against the Japanese soldiers who are on a rape rampage. Only Xiao Jiang refuses, and it is implied that she worked as a prostitute prior to the invasion. She is soon brutally raped on the streets. When the Japanese demand that one hundred Chinese women are to be selected from the refugee center for the pleasure of their soldiers, she is the first to volunteer, and her gesture makes other women step out from the gathered crowd. Xiao Jiang's personal sacrifice is an act of self-purification that allows her to "return", albeit symbolically, to the female and national community. The women who go with their oppressors constitute the collective sacrificial victim whose suffering and death is the only chance of survival for their mothers, sisters, daughters. The scene of the collective sacrifice is constructed through a long take on hand after hand being raised in the air. The row of female hands is the only "shield" Nanking has left, for the defeated men are no longer capable of protecting their community—in a harrowing scene with an almost a documentary feel (the film is shot in the black-and-white)—the Chinese prisoners-of-war are shown to have been rounded up the Japanese, tied together, and brutally gunned down. As in many other cinematic productions on the subject of the Nanking massacre, one can detect an indebtedness to the patterns of Chinese scar drama where "the 'body in pain' [is] symbolic of the national body in pain."[64]

Anonyma: Eine Frau in Berlin/Anonyma—A Woman in Berlin and *As If I am Not There* are war films which do not relegate female victims to a secondary role in the plot. The problem is that they rewrite the women's traumatic experiences into a tragic choice. The female protagonist in both films is the defiant rape victim type who, in contrast to the sacrificial victim, survives the atrocities. The defiant victim is exemplary of the inherent paradox of many war films, namely that "in the masculine genre of the war film, [...] women and children are the only ones who withstand the invader."[65] The defiant victim achieves a symbolic victory over the invaders by refusing to conform to the division of roles enforced by the circumstances of war, choosing to engage in a relationship with the enemy in order to discard the imposed "costume" of the defeated, and therefore passive and powerless, national body.

Anonyma: Eine Frau in Berlin/Anonyma: A Woman in Berlin depicts the fall of Berlin to the Red Army through the eyes of the unnamed female protagonist, based on a memoir under the same title. German women are raped in cellars and in the streets; many commit suicide. *As If I Am Not There*, an adaptation of Slavenka Drakulić's *S*, focuses on the inhuman treatment of Bosnian women in Serbian detention camps during the Bosnian War (1992–1995). Anonyma and Samira are comparable character constructs; they are both defiant victims who refuse to be victimized. Both decide to find a "protector" among the enemy as a means of reasserting control over their bodies. Anonyma's gesture of defiance is taking off her clothes in front of the Russian major, offering her body to the man of her choice rather than being raped by anyone and anywhere. She is no longer the German victim of Soviet violence, but a woman in relationship with a man. Samira's act of defiance is her altered appearance as she prepares for dinner with the Serbian officer-in-command, her intense make-up and extravagantly red dress signifies her choice to "be herself" as a woman instead of the raped Bosnian. Both these gestures enact a symbolic discarding of the "costume" of national victimhood and putting on the "clothes" of womanhood. The symbolism is pushed even further in the case of Samira, who becomes pregnant and must bear the child of a Serb. The last scene shows Samira taking the new-born in her arms, as the maternal instinct of love wins over the memories of who the father had been.

The difference between the sacrificial and defiant type of rape victims resides in the degree of prominence they are given in the plot. Most importantly, however, the construction of these victim types in war films serves the ideologically motivated purpose of depicting the fate of the nation and/or ethnic group as tragic and not traumatic. The sacrificial victim never survives, yet her ordeal is not in vain, for it allows for the survival of the soldier and/or members of the defeated community, thus creating hope for the future. It needs to be emphasized that the sacrificial victim type is indicative of a more general and conventional predisposition of war films to foreground the soldier as the carrier of the meaning of war, hence the viewer is forced to identify with "the male protagonist [who] is free to command the stage, a stage of spatial illusion in which he articulates the look and creates the action."[66] The defiant victim, in turn, redefines both gender and national identity: the defeated and therefore emasculated nation is no longer to be associated with the passive, helpless, humiliated, subjugated victim.

Conclusion

It would be counter-productive to launch an attack on war films as an inappropriate medium for the painful subject of war rape since it is the cinema and TV that have a much greater impact on our historical and political consciousness than historical books or documentaries. We are dealing with an impossible situation where "the erasure of rape from the narrative bears the marks of a patriarchal discourse of honour and chastity; yet showing rape [...] eroticizes it for the male gaze and purveys the victim myth."[67] Necessarily accepting that war films play an important role in bringing events to the forefront of public attention, it is nevertheless essential to put all such productions under close critical scrutiny, exposing the mechanisms governing the representations of sexual violence in this particular genre. Though much has been written on the literary and cinematic representations of rape, the realm of war film—as well as war literature—remains a largely neglected territory in academic scholarship.

The films discussed in this chapter are vivid manifestations of the manner in which war rape tends to be exploited and ideologically manipulated by filmmakers across decades and nations. There exists a film, however, that is different from all others. Interestingly, Vittorio de Sica's 1960 adaptation of Alberto Moravia's novel *La Ciociara/Two Women* is not included in Robert Davenport's *The Encyclopedia of War Movies*, even though "the rape of the two women [in a bombed-out church] is the movie's ultimate comment on the nature of war and survival."[68] This is a film predominantly about a mother and daughter, Cesira and Rosetta, who find themselves at the wrong place at the wrong time, just as an elderly man riding on bicycle, suddenly gunned down by a warplane that appears out of nowhere. Vittorio de Sica proves that it is not necessary to show rape in all its gruesome details to emotionally engage the viewer. Instead, he shows the vulnerability of the two women, the psychological impact of the rape upon Rosetta (her numbness, her need to immediately wash herself in a river, her later "brazen" behavior), and Cesira (her guilt for not having been able to protect her virgin daughter). The historical fact of the mass rapes and killings of Italian women by the French colonial troops in 1944 is shown through the trauma of two individual women. More importantly, as Cesira and Rosetta travel away from Rome to Santa Eufemia, and as they embark on their journey back home, there are many incidents indicating that the threat of rape looms everywhere because for all the men they encounter—Italians, Germans, Americans—they are objects of sexual desire. Of course, one cannot deny there is a level of political manipulation in the film. A direct threat of rape is posed by the Italian militia, and the Germans take away Cesira's lover and Rosetta's best friend Michele and kill him. In other words, the Italian fascists, the Germans and the Moroccans are all dumped into one bag as the morally despicable enemy "Other." Despite this, *La Ciociara/Two Women* must be considered an exceptional achievement in its poignant foregrounding of the rape victim's trauma.

As this chapter began with a discussion of the *Komm Frau* scandal, it seems appropriated to conclude with a memorial, testifying that trauma can be carved into stone. Located at the San Pietro fortress in Castro dei Voslci, the *Mamma Ciociara* memorial commemorates the victims of the *Marocchinate*. Designed by Fedele Andreani, the memorial was erected in 1963. It consists of two female figures. In the forefront we see a woman on her knees, grasping the hands of a girl clinging to her back. Both have their heads lifted upwards, as if seeking help from above. This is a mother desperately trying to shield her daughter, and young girl who has nowhere to escape but behind the body of her mother. We do not see the atrocity but helplessness in the face of atrocity; we see the "face" of "psychological trauma," defined decades later as "an affliction of the powerless. At the moment of trauma, the victim is rendered helpless by overwhelming force. [...] Traumatic events confront human beings with the extremities of helplessness and terror, and evoke the responses of catastrophe."[69] The artistic design of the *Mamma Ciociara* memorial transcends the specific historical context inscribed in its location and name, conveying a universal truth about the victimization of women in the time of war—any war, but—most importantly—commemorates female victims with empathy.

Notes

1. "Oświadczenie autora rzeźby *Komm Frau*" http://www.trojmiasto.pl/wiadomosci/Oswiadczenie-autora-rzezby-Komm-Frau-n73607.html (transl. M S-P).
2. Arthur C. Danto, "The Vietnam Veterans Memorial." *The Nation* (August 31, 1985), 152.
3. Mieke Bal, "Rape, Suicide, Signs and Show," in *A Mieke Bal Reader* (Chicago: Chicago University Press, 2006), 44–45.
4. Catherine N. Niarchos, "Women, War, and Rape: Challenges Facing The International Tribunal for the Former Yugoslavia," *Human Rights Quarterly*, Vol. 17, No. 4, November 1995, 650.
5. Sorcha Gunne and Zoë Brigley Thompson, "Feminism without Borders: The Potentials and Pitfalls of Re-theorizing Rape," in *Feminism, Literature and Rape Narratives: Violence and Violation*, eds. Sorcha Gunne and Zoë Brigley Thompson (New York and London: Routledge, 2010), 2.
6. "Russia Condemns Polish Artist Over Statue of Soviet Soldier Raping a Woman," *The Moscow Times* (17 October 2013) http://www.themoscowtimes.com/news/article/russia-condemns-polish-artist-over-statue-of-soviet-soldier-raping-a-woman/487979.html.
7. Joanna Bourke, "Torture as pornography." *The Guardian*, Friday 7 May 2004. http://www.guardian.co.uk/world/2004/may/07/gender.uk/print.
8. Tanya Horeck, *Public Rape: Representing Violation in Fiction and Film* (New York and London: Routledge, 2004), vi.
9. Kirby Farrell, *Post-traumatic Culture: Injury and Interpretation in the Nineties* (Baltimore and London: The John Hopkins University Press, 1998), 21.
10. Robert Davenport, *The Encyclopedia of War Movies: The Authoritative Guide to Movies about Wars of the Twentieth Century* (New York: Facts on File, 2004), vii.
11. Elie Wiesel: "A novel on Majdanek is either not a novel or not about Majdanek," qtd. by Efraim Sicher in *The Holocaust Novel* (New York and London: Routledge, 2005), x.
12. Sarah Projansky, *Watching Rape: Film and Television on Postfeminist Culture* (New York and London: New York University Press, 2001), 3.
13. Joshua S. Goldstein, *War and Gender: How Gender Shapes the War System and Vice Versa* (Cambridge: Cambridge University Pess, 2006), 363–4.

14. Dagmar Herzog, "Introduction," in *Brutality and Desire: War and Sexuality in Europe's Twentieth Century*, ed. Dagmar Herzog (New York: Palgrave Macmillan, 2011), 6.
15. Herzog, 3.
16. Rick Altman, *Film/Genre* (London: British Film Institute Publishing, 2004), 128.
17. Projansky, 116.
18. Goldstein, 356.
19. Susan Brownmiller, *Against Our Will: Men, Women and Rape* (New York: Fawcett Columbine, 1993), 32.
20. Ann Wolbert Burgess and Lynda Lytle Holmstrom , qtd by Ronald M. Doctor and Frank N. Shiromoto in *The Encyclopedia of Trauma and Traumatic Stress Disorders* (New York: Facts on File, 2010), 219.
21. Judith Lewis Herman, *Trauma and Recovery: The Aftermath of Violence—From Domestic Abuse to Political Terror* (New York: Basic Books, 1997), 32.
22. Shana Swiss and Joan E. Giller, "Rape as a Crime of War: A Medical Perspective," *The Journal of the American Medical Association*, Vol. 270, No. 5, August 4, 1993: 614.
23. Dave Grossman, *On Killing: The Psychological Cost of Learning to Kill in War and Society* (New York, Boston and London: Back Bay Books, 1996), 210.
24. Adam Jones, *Genocide: A Comprehensive Introduction* (London and New York: Routledge, 2011), 470.
25. Nicola Henry, *War and Rape: Law, Memory and Justice* (London and New York: Routledge, 2011), 3.
26. Gunne and Thompson, 3.
27. Henry, 117.
28. Laura Mulvey, "Visual pleasure and narrative cinema," in *Visual Culture: A Reader*, eds. Jessica Evans and Stuart Hall (Los Angeles: SAGE, 2009), 384.
29. Grossman, 137.
30. Joanna Bourke, *Rape: A History from 1860 to the Present* (London: Virago Press, 2008), 6.
31. Sabine Sielke, *Reading Rape: The Rhetoric of Sexual Violence in American Literature and Culture, 1790–1990* (Princeton: Princeton University Press, 2002), 5–6.
32. Dominick LaCapra, *History in Transit: Experience, identity, Critical Theory* (Ithaca: Cornell University Press 2004), 117.

33. Dori Laub, "Bearing Witness or the Vicissitudes of Listening, " in *Testimony: Crises of Witnessing in Literature, Psychoanalysis, and History*, eds. Shoshana Felman and Dori Laub (New York and London: Routledge, 1992), 57.
34. Farrell, 7.
35. Brownmiller, 35, 37–8.
36. Goldstein, 369.
37. Helke Sander (dir), *Befreier und Befreite/Liberators Take Liberties* (Bremer Institut Film & Fernsehen, 1991/1992). DVD: *Edition Der Filmemacher: Helke Sander*, Neue Visionen Medien.
38. Atina Grossmann, "A Question of Silence: The Rape of German Women by Occupation Soldiers," *October*, Vol. 72, Berlin 1945: War and Rape "Liberators Take Liberties" (Spring, 1995), 47.
39. Grossmann, 49.
40. Barbara Kosta, "Rape, Nation and Remembering History: Helke Sander's *Liberators Take Liberties*," *Modern German Studies*, Vol.4, "Gender and Germanness: Cultural Productions of a Nation," 1997, 226.
41. Grossmann, 48.
42. Peter Bradshaw, "Flandres (Flanders)," *The Guardian*, Friday 6 July 2007 http://www.theguardian.com/film/2007/jul/06/worldcin-ema.drama
43. Dora Apel, "'Heroes' and 'Whores': The Politics of Gender in Weimar Antiwar Imagery," *The Art Bulletin*, Vol. 79, No. 3, September 1997, 377.
44. Bradshaw.
45. Henry, 129.
46. These films are analyzed in detail in my article on "The Narration and Visualization of Rape and the Inadvertent Subversion of the Anti-War Message in Brian De Palma's Redacted and Casualties of War," *War, Literature and the Arts*, Vol. 24, 2012. <http://wlajournal.com/24_1/pdf/Sokolowska-Paryz.pdf>
47. Antony Beevor, *Berlin: The Downfall 1945* (London: Penguin Books, 2007), 326–7.
48. Bourke, *Rape*, 375.
49. John Horne and Alan Kramer, *German Atrocities 1914: A History of Denial* (New Haven and London: Yale University Press, 2001), 200.
50. Annette Insdorf, *Indelible Shadows: Film and the Holocaust* (Cambridge: Cambridge University Press, 2003), 30.

51. Roger Luckhurst, *The Trauma Question* (London and New York: Routledge, 2008), 180.
52. Insdorf, 28.
53. Insdorf, 30.
54. Luckhurst, 183.
55. Audoin-Rouzeau, qtd. in Horne and Kramer, 200.
56. Helen Block Lewis, qtd. by June Price Tangney and Ronda L. Dearing in *Shame and Guilt* (New York and London: The Guilford Press, 2004), 18.
57. Tangney and Dearing, 18.
58. Gerhart Piers and Milton B. Singer, *Shame and Guilt: A Psychoanalytic and a Cultural Study* (New York: W.W. Norton & Company, 1971), 35.
59. James Chapman, *War and Film* (London: Reaktion Books, 2008), 117.
60. Eva Hoffman, *After Such Knowledge: A Meditation on the Aftermath of the Holocaust* (London: Vintage, 2005), 41.
61. Horne and Kramer, 199.
62. Kosta, 221.
63. Kosta, 221.
64. Michael Berry, *A History of Pain: Trauma in Chinese Literature and Film*, New York: Columbia University Press, 2008, 18.
65. Olga Karpushina, "The Military Body: Film Representations of the Chechen and Vietnam Wars," *Studies in Slavic Cultures Issue III*: The *Russian Body*, eds. Helena Goscilo and Seth Graham, July 2002, 45.
66. Mulvey, 385.
67. Jyotika Virdi, "Reverence, Rape—and then Revenge: Popular Hindi Cinema's 'Women's Film,'" in *Killing Women: The Visual Culture of Gender and Violence*, eds. Annette Burfoot and Susan Lord (Waterloo, Ontario Canada: Wilfrid Laurier University Press, 2006), 266.
68. Brownmiller, 73.
69. Herman, 33.

CHAPTER 11

Traumatic Displacements: The Memory Films of Jonas Mekas and Robert Vas

Peter Leese

Film as Memory

For Jonas Mekas (b. 1921) and Robert Vas (1931–78), the procedures of filmmaking were also techniques to create coherence, identity, and new meanings in their migrant life stories. Looking at their lives, and exploring their work, reveals why they felt compelled to return time and again to these sense-making procedures. Speaking in a 1975 interview, towards the end of his short career, Vas reflected on editing:[1]

> I've been thinking about this [editing process] quite a lot since coming to England, that this act of putting small bits of things together stands for a great many things in my life. My life has been broken like a piece of film and all my attempts now are an enlarged version of this small act of joining it all together ... Ultimately it all comes back to joining bits of film, that I started during my childhood and which I nurture and cultivate, because it is fundamental to who I am now.

Also in a spoken statement, this time an interview from 1972, Jonas Mekas described a parallel process:

P. Leese (✉)
University of Copenhagen, Copenhagen, Denmark

P. Leese, J. Crouthamel (eds.), *Traumatic Memories of the Second World War and After*, DOI 10.1007/978-3-319-33470-7_11

> When I am filming, I am also reflecting. I was thinking that I was only reacting to the actual reality. I do not have much control over reality at all, and everything is determined by memory, my past. So that this "direct" filming becomes also a mode of reflection. Same way, I came to realize, that writing a diary is not merely reflecting, looking back. Your day, as it comes back to you during the moment of writing, is measured, sorted out, accepted, refused, and re-evaluated by what and how one is at the moment when one writes it all down.[2]

In their late teens and early 20s—around 1945—both men suffered dispiriting, life-changing experiences in the Second World War. During Europe's postwar political upheavals, each found himself stopped dead by the communist authorities of his respective birthplace resulting in forced separation from parents and homeland. Political exile left them lacking a sense of control in their lives; blind events jolted them into a new awareness of their place in the world. Giving a title to his diaries for 1944–55, Jonas Mekas (b. Semeniškiai, Lithuania) settled on *I Had Nowhere To Go*. Reflecting on his departure from Budapest following the failed Hungarian Uprising of 1956, Robert Vas (b. Budapest, Hungary) said "we had nothing to stay for".[3] Yet almost immediately after resettlement, Jonas Mekas and Robert Vas both began remarkable careers as filmmakers.

Two weeks after his arrival in New York, Mekas took possession of his first Bolex 16-mm cine camera and began work on what would later become *Lost LostLost* (Jonas Mekas, 1976). In London, Robert Vas quickly found a job at the British Film Institute and discovered the lyrical films of Humphrey Jennings. The experience transformed Vas's understanding of what documentaries could achieve. Each subsequently developed a distinctive visual language with which to express his thoughts, feelings, and life experiences after forced migration. Each cultivated a moral, aesthetic, and political sensibility in response to the particular circumstances in which they found themselves.

What I would like to do here is explore the historical origins of these two migrant "ways of seeing" in the lives of their directors, and to trace some of the central themes in the critical first phases of their mature work from the late 1960s to the mid-1970s. Wherever possible, I have used their own words, sometimes from contemporary diaries but often from interviews or articles 30 or more years later. My intention is to explore how, as members of the same generation and as historically placed actors in relatively similar circumstances, each repeatedly uses the procedure of "putting small bits of things together" in film to rethink and remake their pasts. This editing in film can be taken as an analogue of wider re-remembering procedures, which let forced migrants, among others, make powerful new interpretations of their lives, though this does not mean that all or even many were necessarily traumatized by their experiences. Later on, I will return to the possible reasons why the "bad event" of involuntary departure may or may not result in later traumatic memory. This particular comparison is fascinating in part because the two lives under consideration run in parallel. Both found innovative, truthful connections in cut celluloid, yet they worked in contrasting ways and came to interpret their lives very differently.

The difficulty for both was that while they were physically "elsewhere": historically and emotionally they belonged to a generation of Romantic nationalists who could not easily abandon the idea of a homeland. Their restrictions and border crossings were post-migratory; the borders they pushed against were as much psychically as politically patrolled.

While their views of the past remained complex and ambivalent, it was Mekas who more ably integrated past and present and who moved into a richer post migration life. Like Mekas, Vas became an accomplished, often brilliant filmmaker by using his own past and related historical stories to continuously reexamine the implications of what had befallen him. Unlike Mekas, he could not integrate his past and present selves. He tended to dwell on past traumas, both his own and others: to ruminate. These are not merely personal or temperamental differences. They indicate two shifting positions, unstable because they change across time, in a spectrum of possible forced migrant responses. What matters here, then, is that these two individuals help define a much wider field of possible memory responses.

"I touch the ground here": Jonas Mekas in Semeniškiai

Jonas Mekas was born in the small Lithuanian village of Semeniškiai, about 60 miles south of the Latvian capital Riga, in 1922.[4] His parents tended a small farm. He learned French and Latin at school, German once the Nazis arrived, and Russian during the Soviet occupation.[5] He was, in other words, part of the Eastern European borderlands world, which was erased by the Second World War.[6]

During the German occupation of 1943–44, Mekas and others in his district were involved in resistance activities. His task was to transcribe BBC radio broadcasts for a weekly underground bulletin. When the typewriter he kept hidden in his uncle's barn went missing, he was advised to flee at once because if the typeface was traced back to him he would be in immediate danger.[7] Planning to reach Vienna with forged papers, and from there to meet contacts who would guide him to Switzerland, he left Lithuania. In July 1944, he was picked up by a German patrol and sent to the forced labour camp at Elmshorn, near Hamburg. Eight months later, he escaped. After destroying his identity papers, he travelled around Germany between March and August 1945, during which time he was one among many thousands of refugees in transit.[8]

By August 1945, Mekas was in the Displaced Persons Camp at Wiesbaden and had begun studying philosophy at the University of Mainz. With the future still uncertain, except for the knowledge that he could not go back to Lithuania, he moved to Kassel in 1947 and then in 1949, not long before departing for New York, to the Schwäbisch Gmünd camp. Speaking in a 2003 interview, Mekas recalled the intellectual adventure of that time:[9]

> That's, I consider that my university was post-war Europe, was Germany and that when I came here it was already my practi- beginning to work. My childhood was in Lithuania, my university was Europe and because those four years in displaced person camps—four years—was my university where we could read. There was a lot of time, we read everything we, you can imagine that between the Soviet occupation, the German occupation, the whole war period, nothing was available from the west, from, nobody, we were so thirsty and like a dry sponge drinking everything that we could find after the war, you know, the whole American literature, the French, it was an incredible, incredible rich period for those who want, who were ready and wanted it.

Yet in a diary entry for 23 April 1948, Mekas describes his realization that the places and times of his early life were gone forever:[10]

> No, I didn't take anything with me, when I left.
>
> Ideas? Books? Ah, those found here too. But what really hurts, deep inside, it's the earth I left, that sky, those hills. It's those nights that got stuck in me, deep. They hurt, they remain painful wounds inside, those evenings, those nights.
>
> I touch the ground here—and that other soil wakes up in me. I am looking at the sky—but I see that other sky. What is there, one would think, in the objects such as wheels, rakes, plows, and dungcarts; or in cobwebs glittering in the autumn air, frost on the trees, the rain on the cabbage heads, the flax-drying season? But it all got imprinted very very deep. There is something in it, in the way the rivers bend there; there is something in that. There is

> something in the way the rain sounded there, a different sound, not like any other rain I've ever heard in my travels.
>
> And it's not those broad differentiations by line, angle, corner, bending, colour grouping—no: it's the little differences, the almost unnoticeable details ... It's in them that everything weaves together, it's there that one nation's soul separates from another.

Aged 22 when he left Lithuania, the circumstances of his departure made Mekas idealize the family, homeland, and childhood he had left behind. He cultivated his sense of the past in the hope of returning one day.

"... MAKES NO DIFFERENCE": JONAS MEKAS IN NEW YORK

In an era of mass, forced migration Jonas Mekas was one among over a million Displaced Persons who spent the early postwar years in camps, mostly in Germany, unable or unwilling to return to their prewar home.[11] Compelled by circumstances beyond their control, un-reconciled to their new lives, many felt departure more than arrival.

For Mekas too arrival and settlement felt insignificant. By good fortune a contact in Chicago found him work and got him permission to enter the USA:[12]

> There are papers for you. So, okay, what, why not? I mean, makes no difference. So, we came to New York and it was sponsored actually by the United Nations Refugee Organisation. So, we were not, we were really actually correctly speaking, we're not immigrants, we are, we were brought in here and dumped by United Nations Refugee Organisation. And you know, knowing how, the way I see it, and I, you know, have said this many times in other, on other occasions, that if one is really very much rooted in one's place like I was in, I mean, in nature, in the country, there, in that, in language, in songs in Lithuania, then once you are uprooted then it makes no difference where you are, absolutely no difference.

This overwhelming sense of departure and separation later became a defining feature in Mekas's work. Early on in his written diary entries, he notes that many other members of the Lithuanian community were, if anything, worse off. They would, he predicted, "die with homesickness in [their] eyes". Yet despite hopelessness he found himself able to resist despair, and surprisingly able to "get equally attached to new experiences, new places, new moods".[13]

Arriving in New York in late October 1949, ambitious as both a poet and filmmaker, Mekas quickly began to make plans and contacts in the New York arts scene. Responding to what he saw as the political betrayal of the Baltic States by the Allies at Yalta in 1945, one of his first ideas was for a documentary about the life of a Displaced Person in New York. He also reacted strongly against what he saw as the naiveté and sentimentality of Hollywood's portrayal of European postwar settlement in *The Search* (Fred Zinnemann, 1948). Describing his own feelings more than the content of Zinnemann's movie, he later said "[…] it made us so mad seeing that film and that anger that madness really, that's when we began to make notes for our own film, 'Lost Lost' not 'Lost Lost Lost' but 'Lost Lost' it was only two—or maybe it was four, 'Lost Lost Lost Lost'".[14]

One important discovery of the late 1940s was the lightweight, handheld Bolex which Mekas used for his earliest footage of New York. A 16-mm camera without sound recording had technical limitations, but also facilitated the film language that Mekas began to develop around this time. Although he aspired to bigger-budget films in Hollywood, it soon became clear that practically and artistically he was very far from the mainstream. The relative cheapness and mobility of the Bolex, by contrast, let the beginning director explore the city at a time when he was shy, still learning English, and felt more comfortable to observe than engage.[15]

The Bolex, as it turned out, ideally suited Mekas's developing ideas for a personal, poetic cinema. That it could film for no more than a minute continuously before the spring mechanism had to be rewound made the camera an invitation to look from many angles and distances, to cultivate a rough, unpredictable spontaneity. Breaking up scenes and moments, editing in and outside the camera, using a personal, intuitive, and observational gaze all became second nature in the director's later work. Similarly, the lack of a microphone meant that sound, commentary, and music could only be added later to supplement observation, incident, and mood.

Throughout his career, Mekas explores and expands his interest in self-documentation as an expression of wider human experience. This autobiographical impulse certainly comes to incorporate American influences, John Cage for instance, but also predates Mekas's arrival in the USA:[16]

> My first major work in Lithuanian, which to some of my Lithuanian friends is still the best thing I've done, was a cycle of twenty-odd idylls I wrote in 1946. I used long lines and an epic pace to portray my childhood in the village. I describe the people in the village and their various activities during

> the four seasons, as factually and prosaically as I could. I avoided what was accepted poetic Lithuanian language. My aim at that time—I talk about this in my written diaries—was to achieve "a documentary poetry."

"Documentary poetry" is an especially apt phrase for Mekas's written and film work. Both are as much a product of the Lithuanian landscape, folk songs, and a sense of belonging to a small nation as of chance procedures or abstract expressionism.[17]

Re-editing, Re-Remembering: Film Themes 1969–76

Mekas's notion of "documentary poetry" develops from the clash between his pre- and post-migration lives, and from his stubborn determination to make imaginative readings of his own social and psychological condition. Always a personal filmmaker, through trial and error he gradually develops narrative and aesthetic techniques to re-remember the past through the analogous procedure of re-editing film footage from his own past life. If we understand Mekas's films as interpretations of his own subjectivity, we can consider the evolution of his filmmaking as an ongoing conversation between past and present selves and as a struggle between continuously recycled loss and a fuller present- and future-mindedness. Here, I will consider the critical transition period from the late 1960s to the mid-1970s when Mekas produced three major films in his "diaries, notes and sketches" series: *Walden* (1964–69), *Reminiscences of a Journey to Lithuania* (1971–72), and *Lost Lost Lost* (1975–76).

These films have two aspects in common: they portray subjectively acts of looking and listening, and they reevaluate sequentially the recent and distant past. Throughout, the camera eye judders and flits across scenes and moments. The sound track captures mood in a speech phrase or music. Intertitle cards flash up like random thoughts. Scratchy gramophone tunes hark back to a particular time and place of hearing. The camera continuously mimics the mind in simultaneously observing the present and interpreting it as the past. Such recollective mechanisms are never stable or decisive in their portrayal of the past, but across these three films the viewer sees a change as Mekas gradually faces his memories and puts them into the perspective of his current life. He looks at everyday events and their relationship to what and how he remembers. He explores not just the slow abandonment of a painful, persistent memory world, but the stages, methods, and consequences of his transition from past- to present-mindedness.

Critical to this process of integrating memories is Mekas's idea of the diary film. In the early 1960s, he had already begun to take apart his earlier, less autobiographical work and to re-edit the first footage from his New York years. He now began to incorporate it into his first fully realized diary film, originally titled *Diaries, Notes and Sketches, also known as Walden.*[18] *Walden* uses diary footage mostly from 1964 to 1969. It is at one level a chronicle of street life in the mid-1960s New York, but its title also draws attention to Henry David Thoreau's 1854 journal of transcendentalism, spiritual discovery, and reclusive self-reliance. All themes which matter as the viewer are caught up in Mekas's seemingly spontaneous flood of screen images. Through these flashes and blurs, the director makes his own Thoreau-like study of solitude, sounds, and above all traces of nature and seasons. Like many of Mekas's later works, *Walden* is divided into numbered sections, in this case each about 30 minutes long, referred to by the director as chapters. Within each chapter, various moods and events are recounted in roughly chronological order. Since Mekas was so active on the New York avant-garde arts scene heroes of the counterculture—Lennon, Warhol, Ginsberg—appear in passing, acting themselves.

Commenting on Mekas's *Walden,* the French critic Jean-Jacques Lebel has described the way in which the director's "anything and everything" filming is filtered through a precise emotional gaze. The film also develops a particular visual grammar: still shots for babies and children, close-ups for plants and wine glasses, "by accident" flashes of sky, lights, and groups of people.[19] We can supplement Lebel's observation by noting how the spontaneous, immediate "now" character of the images is simultaneously a lens through which to view the past. Without knowing it at first, Mekas looks constantly for traces of his Lithuanian life in the American city. He seeks out the trees, sky, and frost which will remind him of his rural beginnings. "When I started looking at my film diaries again", the director later said, "I noticed they contained everything that New York *didn't have* [...] In truth I am filming my childhood, not New York".[20]

Reminiscences of a Journey to Lithuania returns physically to the past as the director manages to engineer a trip back to his home village while on a visit to the Soviet Union. The central section of the film is a series of a hundred or so short scenes, call them "memory images", which go back to the landscape of childhood, and which document a seemingly unchanged past. Yet, the film must also confront change: the death of Mekas's father, the ageing of his mother, and his distance from the new Soviet Lithuania. He commented in 1989 "You don't see how Lithuania is today; you see it only through the memories of a Displaced Person back home for the first time in twenty-five years".[21]Within this landscape of memory, Mekas seems to become fully aware for the first time that it is impossible to "go back". So, while the physical location for much of the film is Semeniškiai in 1971, in the director's mind the film is also set on the path back to his pre-Second World War childhood. The creative tension of the account is generated by Mekas's attempt to locate and articulate his past in light of the in-between years in New York.

To better understand the difficulty of this articulation, we can consider the term "reminiscence", which stresses the resemblance between diary film and oral history. In both cases, the subject searches for ways to express a past through language, here the visual language of celluloid. He revises according to his circumstances at the moment of telling, not least according to the presumed audience. He appropriates and re-works genres of storytelling—tragedy, nostalgia, or romantic quest—to his own ends. Within the wider body of Mekas's work, this act of reminiscence, of seeing past "memory images" superimposed onto the present, becomes a critical turning point. In this new iteration, the inability to reach his past changes the way Mekas sees himself, the places he comes from, and the life he might have subsequently led. Commenting not long after he made the film, speaking in the third person, he said "You think about your old home, you romanticise it, it swells and swells. You have to see it again, to actually go back there and start it all from the beginning. You have to leave your home for a second time. Then it begins to change."[22]

In *Lost Lost Lost,* Mekas goes back once again to his first footage in New York, which he has already edited and re-edited at least twice since the early 1960s. He works again through the years since 1949 towards the present, this time exploring more fully, as he puts it "the mood of a Displaced Person who hasn't yet forgotten his native country, but hasn't yet gained a new one".[23] Yet after confronting his past in 1970s Lithuania, he can transform his reminiscences into the new narrative arc of a forward journey. Awareness of the present arises. Mekas no longer spends quite so long looking towards the snow and trees of *Walden.* Instead, the physicality of the film as the medium within which memory functions comes further to the fore. Fragmented, imagined, and half-glimpsed scenes stress the fragility and disintegration of the past at the moment it comes into focus. Variable speeds, jump cuts from close-up to long shot, highlight the act of recording and projecting, editing and viewing a personal history. The imaginative procedures by which we continually make sense of the past in each successive present are scrutinized anew because they change constantly.

The sense of "re-editing as re-remembering" becomes richer and deeper in *Lost Lost Lost* because it is the film which most systematically reviews Mekas's origins, movement, and resettlement. Stephen MacDonald, one of Mekas's critical supporters, puts it as follows:[24]

> In order to edit the film to produce the final, complex form we've been exploring, Mekas had to take himself back to those painful times—or at least to the one enduring record of them—for many months, and with enough intensity to construct this complex and coherent personal interpretation of them.

Repetitions also matter. The title signals three kinds of lostness, but also three versions of a single story about being lost. The intensity and varieties of loss—disorientation, helplessness, frustration—also imply its opposite, which is being found or finding. So, if by this stage in the "diaries, notes and sketches" series we understand any given telling of the past to be one of many, we also see that it is possible for the director to find himself and a sense of his own future.

"A WHOLE WORLD TURNED UPSIDE DOWN": ROBERT VAS IN HUNGARY

Jonas Mekas achieves nothing so simple as a definitive version of his forced migrant journey or its consequences. What he does make is a set of artistic procedures which allow him to explore the past and come closer to a sense of new possibilities. For Robert Vas, the past grows in intensity until it seems to eclipse his present, but from his prescient gaze comes a passionately original moral and artistic vision.

A Hungarian Jew born in Budapest in 1931, Vas was 13 at the time of the 1944 German occupation. His parents managed to obtain "Schutzpasses". Created by Swedish diplomat and businessman Raul Wallenberg, the pass helped shield thousands of Hungarian Jews, if only temporarily, from persecution. It granted designated buildings as Swedish territory and prevented deportation.[25] The Vas family left the "official" Budapest ghetto, then, for another more "privileged" ghetto district close to the Danube. There, they felt in less immediate danger, but eventually the German occupiers refused any remaining pretence of safety. Vas observed as many of his neighbours were rounded up, taken to the embankment to be shot, then dumped into the river.[26] Soon after the war ended, his mother died and his father fled to Australia. He was now 17.

Companionship and purpose came from the postwar Communist Youth movement. Reviewing *The Confrontation* (1968) by fellow Hungarian Miklós Janscó, Vas praises the film's powerful dissection of political idealism. The opening scenes of revolutionary fervour were so affecting because they echoed Vas's youthful experiences:[27]

> There they stand, a group of young boys and girls, with their newly acquired freedom, pressing their flushed faces against the old-fashioned wrought-iron gate of a church school, convinced about their own truth, holding a piece of red cloth which stands for their flag, their eyes shining, singing with fervour: 'Tomorrow we'll see the whole world turned upside down!' The picture expresses what we all felt in those days, twenty to twenty-five years ago: not only were we happy to be young, but to our exuberant youth we were given, without having to work out something for ourselves, a view of life, an ideology to believe in.

His father was abroad though, in a capitalist country. Robert was consequently treated with suspicion, then disdain, by the state communist authorities. Following conscription and attacks by political officers, he spent time in an army psychiatric hospital. Increasingly, like many of his generation, he became aware of "a devastating gap between the things we were told and the things that happened to us".[28]

In writing and interviews, Vas did not speak much about his involvement in the Uprising of 1956, but he does describe three vivid scenes which stuck in his mind and shaped his later work. The first was early on when thousands stood in front of the Parliament building:[29]

> One of my most precious memories of '56 is standing in the huge square in front of the Parliament shouting together with thousands of people in the crowd "Switch off the lights! Switch off the lights!" What we meant was the red star on the top of the Parliament building. And the regime replied by switching off all the street lights in the square itself. We were standing there in darkness, our anger mounting. Without a moment's hesitation torches started to burn and I saw there were two cameramen from the State newsreel company starting to roll, and people were shouting to them "*This* is what you should have been filming all the time."

In the same interview, Vas describes a collective euphoria over several days as he worked with students and friends frantically to print and deliver leaflets. He felt "The unbelievable had happened: the revolution was victorious. We had the incredible experience of a few days of democratic socialism."[30] Yet, in an earlier description, three years after 1956, Vas stresses his despair before the Soviet tanks arrived. Speaking of himself in the third person, he describes volunteering to listen to a United Nations debate in the vain hope he could report some sign of intervention. By this stage his fellow activists were sheltering in a tenement basement, there was gunfire in the streets, and a profound sense of helplessness among the rebels. "It was a faint hope. In the streets there was bloodshed; something had to be done, we could not tell what, but something concrete and definite to stop violence. But what they said was just generalities." So that after the Uprising was crushed "there was nothing to stay for".[31] Indeed, there was every reason to leave.

"A Self-Appointed Survivor": Robert Vas in London

In his directorial debut *Refuge England* (Robert Vas, 1959), Vas creates a semi-fictionalized account of a Hungarian refugee's first day in London. Lászlo Cs. Szabó's epigraph, written by a Hungarian exile of an earlier generation, expresses Vas's feeling too: "Restore to me, last rock of refuge, England / Dignity that befits me as a man". A nameless narrator looks back to his first day in a new country:

> I want to tell you about my first day in London. Many years have passed since, but I can still remember clearly what I saw and felt on the first day I arrived from the camp.
>
> It was a misty autumn morning. Rush hour. It was the terminus of the town where from then on I had to live [...] They asked me 'where do you want to live? Choose a place.' Well, I have chosen. Here I am.

He spends the day wandering the streets, looking at people, and asking himself how he can be connected to them or if they will begin to understand him. He describes loneliness, feeling out of place, and reluctance. "'I didn't want to come. We were fighting, we had lost, I had to come. That's all. It wasn't my fault [...] Are we the ones who form our own history? Or do we just go where we have to go?"

Soon Vas discovered an artistic milieu with which he could identify. *Refuge England* was financed by the British Film Institute, where he found work as a cataloguer and archivist. Initially without much English, he spent his days detailing movie times and titles. During lunch breaks he watched the films of Eisenstein and of the great 1930s documentarists. Humphrey Jennings, who so brilliantly observed and reported Britain's Home Front during the Second World War, was above all the artist who helped Vas understand both England and the idea of "a particular sort of subjective poetic documentary".[32] "To a film maker from another country", Vas said in *Heart of Britain. Humphrey Jennings, Filmmaker* (1970) "he was able to put into pictures and sound the spirit of an era, and of a nation [...] He invented a particular kind of film language, a visual thought process, complex and essentially humane, that is unique in the history of cinema".

More immediate influences were Karel Reisz and Lindsay Anderson, leaders of the then emerging Free Cinema movement, itself part of the revival of British arts and society in the later 1950s. Both supported Vas; both became close friends and admirers of his work. They encouraged too his next tentative step into film-making and England. *The Vanishing Street* (Robert Vas, 1962) observes the music, food, conversations and market sellers of a predominantly Jewish district, Hessel Street in East London, which was then about to be demolished to make way for high rise apartment blocks. The subject echoes Vas's own disappeared Jewish childhood in interwar Budapest.

In these early films, the beginning director chooses subjects that bridge past to present, which connect Budapest to London, but he also quickly expands his range of subjects and techniques. Distinctive themes and the beginnings of a new film language emerge as he concentrates on putting disconnected images side by side to spark unusual visual metaphor. Even at the beginning of his career, the act of seeing has a brooding, meditative quality for Vas. Like his best work from the 1970s, these first films provoke questions as well as understanding. They bear singular witness. Vas described what he saw as his own moral obligation to testify:[33]

> I see myself as a self-appointed survivor. I was scarred by two shattering events: the Nazis and 1956—and that baggage, the message that nobody asked me to speak about, is absolutely central to me; I can't exist without it. I must talk about it. And I must talk about it to an *English* audience, which never experienced these things directly.

Refuge England, for example, expresses the necessity to leave the past behind in a matter-of-fact unemotional language. Returning to forced departure seems too difficult, too raw, even in thought. Yet it is also clear, as in Mekas's work, that no matter how troubled, the refugee has also survived. Observing a communal rather than a personal past, *The Vanishing Street* remains ambivalent. The prospects for survival are not at all secure. The protagonist is the street itself found in snatches of conversation and song, but endings, departures, and echoes of a rich, vibrant past are all around in Hessel Street.

Testifying, Ruminating: Film Themes 1969–76

With his early films as a calling card, Vas approached the BBC and began work as a professional, freelance documentarist. He found in his first contacts with the Corporation a refreshing openness to ideas, willingness to encourage personal statements, and like-minded enthusiasm from colleagues. Later on, he described how "that personal kind of film was not only tolerated but promoted. Television was the only showcase for that kind of film and gradually one was educating the viewer to understand, to read between the lines, and *see*".[34]

Vas encouraged his audience to "see" in three particular ways. First, by his engagement with subjectivity: by considering the inner feelings and mental processes of his own experience, as well as those of others caught in a particular historical situation. Second, by his search for testimony: looking for and engaging with people who were "there", searching out alternative archives if there are no direct witness statements. Third, by his sensitivity to the surreal: editing for visual and spoken contrast, metaphor, and contradiction to portray what he called "the *spiritual* story of the event". (37) Here, I will consider some of the other films leading up to it—particularly *The Issue Should Be Avoided* (Robert Vas, 1971), and *Nine Days in '26* (Robert Vas, 1974)—but will concentrate mostly on one of the finest expressions of the director's working practices, *My Homeland* (Robert Vas, 1976).

Before doing so, it is important to note that Vas did not want his viewers to "*see*" only his personal past. His films are statements against personal oblivion, but equally oppose the collective amnesia of societies and vested interest groups. Like Jonas Mekas, Vas was a highly skilled, intuitive filmmaker; unlike Mekas, he was always politically minded both in subject matter and in his intention. Until his untimely death at the age of 47, Vas created subtle, eloquent exposés in which every creative act or personal statement by an interviewee had wider social implications. Hence, his choice of subjects included particular events during the Second World War, 1956, and its aftermath, but also analogous moments such as the British General Strike of 1926. Vas's work explores, then, the inseparability of the personal and the political. More importantly, it describes how they are intimately, fruitfully connected.

The Issue Should Be Avoided, for example, uses Winston Churchill's words as its title to stress the silence that surrounded the 1940 Katyń Forest massacre during and after the Second World War. Noting the non-acknowledgement of these events from either the Soviet Union or Germany, the film attempts a "documentary" investigation into the mass murder of 22,000 members of the Polish Officer class in 1940. An assembly of BBC actors gathers in a forest clearing near London and are filmed as they sit around a table and out, loud read manuscript extracts and reports from Polish, Soviet, German, and Western Allied sources. The Polish Major Adam Solski was among those murdered by the Narodnyi Komissariat Vnutrennikh Del (NKVD) in 1940. The diary, found on Solski's body three years later, provides an eyewitness account for the film.

Detailing events up to the massacre, investigating evidence to uncover who committed the crime, and coming to a tentative verdict of Soviet guilt, *The Issue Should Be Avoided* is one of Vas's most powerful films. Like much of his best work, it addresses a particular anniversary, but also reminds the viewer of recent similar events. In this case, the massacres at Sharpeville (South Africa, 1960), and Mai Lai (Vietnam, 1968), which had taken place little more than two years earlier. By staging an investigation, the director puts his faith in the search for evidence and the possibility of uncovering hidden truths. By confronting events and communicating human experience, he argues for the continuing relevance of the past and the importance of communicating with a broad audience.

Testimony was critical to Vas in his willingness to confront what his colleague and friend Barry Gavin called "subjects which others might prefer to avoid or be terrified to touch on".[35] For fellow director Karel Reisz, Vas "had this gift for making his films speak through the experiences of honourable, decent people", whose voices he would set against newsreel library shots to "fuse them with the feelings of people who had been part of that history".[36] This willingness to confront painful histories sometimes caused difficulties in screening and distribution. His film about the survivors of Hiroshima was only promoted and shown with difficulty in the USA. Vas was especially dismayed to face censure from the BBC over his film about the British General Strike of 1926.

Nine Days in '26 emerged, characteristically for Vas, from his realization that "this particular segment of British social history, with which I socially and humanly felt such an affinity, was constantly and repeatedly seen from *one* viewpoint".[37] For Vas, this "cosy [middle class] consensus" ignored "the real price of human suffering". The film appeared at a partisan, topical moment. The original broadcast date was 11 January 1974, but as *Sight and Sound* noted a few months later "to have shown it then, when the miners were supposed to have been holding the country to ransom, would have made it political dynamite".[38] The first BBC screening of the film was delayed until after the strike and finally took place on 19 April 1974. Much to Vas's disappointment, it was relegated to a late night spot, and not repeated on the 50th anniversary of the General Strike in 1976.

Nine Days in '26 is a remarkable film. It expands the documentary form by its innovative use of collage, stills, newsreels, cartoons, and newspaper headlines. It incorporated footage from *Today We Live* (Paul Rotha, 1936), *A Day in the Life of a Coal Miner* (1910), and *Royal Cavalcade* (1935). It examines the roots and consequences of the strike and used sources, as Vas put it "not only for what they show, but for *how* they show it".[39] The director talked at length to participants and observers on all sides, including a footballer who took part in the strike and who describes his shock finding hungry, shoeless children on a visit to Merthyr Tydfil. It is hard to imagine how Vas's nuanced, partisan interpretation, which upended a well-established mythology, could have avoided trouble. His attempt to contribute to a discussion tripped across invisible class boundaries, but was rejected also for reasons of politics. Assimilated and accepted in many ways, he well understood the nuances of English society, yet in some respects he remained distinctly "foreign". His passionate expressions of political engagement, his moral seriousness, his highly attuned sense of irony and tragedy, even his accent continued to set him apart. Sometimes, he felt out of place in English society; doubtless he felt the refusal to show *Nine Days in '26* as personal rejection by his adopted homeland.[40]

By 1976, Vas was ready to confront his own past head on in his startling, original, and deeply felt *My Homeland* (1976). After circling around parallel and analogous events (Katyń, the rise of Stalin, the General Strike), after considering intellectual frameworks and creative techniques (Claude Levi-Strauss, Humphrey Jennings), and after making several early films around the themes of displacement and exile (*Ernst Niesvestny*, *The Border*), Vas finally had the film language and distance to address Hungary, 1956, and his own displacement. He asks in his film "Who are we as a people? What is the nation really about? What does my homeland, that so attracts and so repels me, really mean to me after so many years?"

To answer these questions, Vas turns again to the work of Humphrey Jennings, for reasons both intellectual and aesthetic. Jennings and Vas both understood the social world ethnographically. Jennings's films emerged from the Mass Observation movement of the 1930s; Vas's film *The Savage Mind* was effectively a collaboration with influential French anthropologist Claude Levi-Strauss. So, both directors saw "true" nationalism as organically expressed in everyday behaviour and artefacts, especially in literature, music, and the visual arts. Aesthetically, Vas found in Jennings anthology film of passages from Shakespeare, Milton, and Churchill, *Words for Battle* (1941), a way to evoke national values and traditions. In his 1970 film on Jennings, Vas noted too the usefulness of "concrete, true-to-life images [...] Disjointed, but stand back and they begin to relate to one another. Their juxtapositions add up and fuse into the image" (*Heart of Britain*, 1970). Bringing together and creatively re-working these ideas, *My Homeland* expresses Vas's sense of Hungarian history, and especially of 1956.

The director also turns to personal testimony. *My Homeland* was first broadcast on the November 4, 1976, exactly 20 years after the tanks arrived in Budapest to reassert Soviet control. Vas begins with elegy: "Year after year, on this day, on the 4th of November, I remember you. I walk past your graves one by one [...]. In the morning, there was a deep ominous silence. And by this time of night, twenty years ago today, we knew we had lost; that the miracle, our victory, was condemned to be a nine days wonder" (*My Homeland*, 1976). The commentary is accompanied by Hungarian tourist promotion clips, shots of supposed consumer affluence, cabaret dinner dances, and by the grief-stricken faces of mothers and wives at a funeral for 84 victims of a secret police massacre during the Uprising. Through these surreal contrasts, by gesturing towards the uncanny moment, the eerie atmosphere hardly believable even to those who were there, Vas expresses his own memory of "twenty years ago today". Where Jennings shot and sometimes staged his own material, Vas literally scours the cutting room floor for leftover newsreel footage and discarded still photographs. In this way, he re-invents, transposes, and transforms Jennings's surrealist sensibility to his own ends.

Finally, Vas conceptualizes the nation by turning to the inner voice of poetry which, he argues, transfers the experience of life and of collective recollection 'in spite of differences of language, custom and social system'. *My Homeland* incorporates substantial passages by Sándor Petőfi (1823–49), Attila József (1905–37), and Miklós Radnóti (1909–44). The film's long final section is a reading, by actors Michael Bryant and Judy Dench, of Gyula Illyés' "A Sentence on Tyranny". Vas said that it was always his intention to end the documentary with this piece, and that in doing so he sought to express the meaning of 1956, to consider "what my country, Hungary, meant to me", but also to make a wider statement against the very idea of political oppression.[41]

Considering Vas's wider body of work, my contention is that by making films on his distinctive set of subjects, the director sought to make sense of his own past, sometimes directly, often obliquely by analogy. Yet, he was also trapped by the need to explain; unable to move beyond rumination. Each attempt, each film, was only satisfactory for as long as the reexamination lasted. The impossibility of finding a real answer to his political exile, and the impossibility of return, meant that the whole procedure of re-witnessing had to be replayed time and again.

Memory as Film

The American psychiatrist Robert Jay Lifton, who became his collaborator and friend in the 1970s, was acutely aware that Robert Vas's intense moral conviction and artistic vision grew from personal experience. Because of his insistence that atrocity degraded perpetrator as well as victim, and because of his fertile, imaginative political conscience, Lifton compared Vas to Primo Levi. Both had "survivor wisdom".[42] Likewise in her eye-opening essay on Jonas Mekas, Maureen Turim notes how *Reminiscences of a Journey to Lithuania* "suggests in its gaps and processes a poetics of our dispossessed and conflicted selves; at its best it expresses more than it knows".[43]

Mekas more readily, obsessively even, re-runs his personal past not just in film but also in his diaries, writings, and interviews. His displacement and arrival story is repeated over and over again so that it becomes an artistic credo, a founding myth, and an expression of personal identity. Yet, by working so consistently with his own life as subject matter, as Turim suggests, he makes a much wider existential statement on every individual. Mekas's greatest achievement is to reveal the full difficulty of adapting and resettling after forced migration. He is gripped by feelings of regret, abandonment, and uprootedness for many years. Only very gradually and after constant, struggling attempts to understand the past does he manage to achieve a kind of equilibrium. As a creative artist in his "Notes, Diaries and Sketches" series, and too as a human being, he eventually achieves sufficient reconciliation with the past to live more fully in the present.

Robert Vas's life is not very different in its outline, except that he was never able to return physically to his homeland, and rather than gradual acceptance and integration he found himself increasingly at odds with his life in Britain. For these reasons, he was never fully able to reconcile himself to the political and personal losses of 1956. For these reasons too, Vas expresses a distinctly different kind of traumatic memory processing in his film work and personal statements. Where Mekas integrated his difficult past into the living present, Vas's sense of the past remained overwhelming. He found it particularly difficult to move beyond his own and others' troubled experiences and feelings. Robert Jay Lifton sums this up well when he notes how shaken Vas was by the Hiroshima footage he saw in the Washington archives while researching *To Die—To Live. The Survivors of Hiroshima* (Robert Vas, 1975), and kept "a piece of burned stone from the A-bomb dome on his desk, never out of sight".[44] Yet, one of Vas's most remarkable achievements is to transform rumination into creative vision by unsentimental observation and moral clarity.

Speaking historically, both filmmakers suggest the imaginative possibilities and time-bound restrictions that were present for political refugees and forced migrants in the aftermath of the Second World War. By historical accident, both men were young enough to adapt when they lost their families and their homelands, but adult enough to be deeply disturbed by the experience. Members of a generation that witnessed and took part in profound political upheaval, both struggled throughout their lives with the intellectual, psychological, and moral implications of forced departure. The extent to which they were able to integrate themselves and overcome their traumatic memories depended in large part on the circumstances of their later lives. In their work, Jonas Mekas and Robert Vas suggest procedures of creative re-interpretation for the displaced, for the traumatized. Accompanied or not by a camera, the reworking of memory across the course of a lifetime becomes an agent through which rich new interpretations and meanings for life experiences are potentially created.

Notes

1. Robert Vas and Alan Rosenthal '*My Homeland* and *Nine Days in '26*', in: Alan Rosenthal, *The Documentary Conscience. A Casebook of Film Making* (Berkeley, Los Angeles and London: University of California Press, 1980), 262–3.
2. Jonas Mekas, 'The Diary Film (A Lecture on *Reminiscences of a Journey to Lithuania*)' in: P.A. Sitney, ed., *The Avant-Garde Film. A Reader of Theory and Criticism* (New York: Anthology Film Archives 1987), 191–2.
3. Jonas Mekas, *I Had Nowhere To Go*, (New York: Black Thistle Press, 1991); Vas and Rosenthal, 264.
4. Mekas, J. Interview with Any Taubin (2003), seg.1. [Accessed: 01.03.13] http://www.webofstories.com/play/jonas.mekas/1
5. Taubin, 2003, seg.8; Mekas, 1991, 18.
6. Omer Bartov and E.D. Weitz, eds., *Shatterzone of Empires: Coexistence and Violence in the German, Habsburg, Russian, and Ottoman Borderlands* (Bloomington: Indiana University Press, 2012).
7. Mekas, 1991, 8–19.
8. Taubin, 2003, seg.23–25.
9. Taubin, 2003, seg.25.
10. Mekas, 1991, 162–3.
11. Ben Shephard, *The Long Road Home. The Aftermath of the Second World War* (London: Vintage, 2011) 360.
12. Taubin, 2003, seg.26.
13. Mekas, 1991, 287; 328.
14. Taubin, 2003, seg.30; Jonas Mekas and MacDonald, S. "Interview with Jonas Mekas" *October* (29, 1984), 84–5.
15. Mekas and MacDonald, 1984, 87–8; 95.
16. Turim, M. "Reminiscences, Subjectivities and Truths" in: David E. James, ed., *To Free Cinema. Jonas Mekas& the New York Underground* (Princeton, NJ: Princeton University Press, 1992, 198; Mekas and MacDonald, 1984, 93.
17. Mekas and MacDonald, 1984, 96; Taubin, 2003, seg.46.
18. Taubin, 2003, seg.88.
19. Jean-Jacques Lebel, "Jonas Mekas celebrates what he sees: The Moebius Strip. Jonas Mekas. Walden."(Paris: Potemkine Films DVD boxed set booklet, 2012). 16.
20. Mekas, 1987, 191.

21. Turim, 1992, 207.
22. Mekas, 1987, 197.
23. Mekas and MacDonald, 1984, 82.
24. Stephen MacDonald, "Lost Lost Lost over 'Lost Lost Lost'", *Cinema Journal* 25 (2) (1986), 32.
25. Paul A. Levine, *Raoul Wallenberg in Budapest: Myth, History and Holocaust* (London: Valentine Mitchell, 2010).
26. Vas and Rosenthal, 1980, 262.
27. Robert Vas, "The Confrontation", *Sight and Sound* 39 (3) (1970), 157.
28. Vas and Rosenthal, 1980, 264.
29. Vas and Rosenthal, 1980, 268.
30. Vas and Rosenthal, 1980, 264.
31. Vas, R., "Power Among Men", *Sight and Sound* 28 (3/4)(1959), p. 175; Vas and Rosenthal, 1980, 264.
32. Vas and Rosenthal, 1980, 265.
33. Vas and Rosenthal, 1980, 265–6.
34. Vas and Rosenthal, 1980, 267.
35. Gavin and Rosenthal, 1978, 187.
36. *Robert Vas Filmmaker 1931–1978.* (Written, directed and presented by Karel Reisz. First BBC broadcast 03.05.1978.)
37. Vas and Rosenthal, 1980, 273.
38. David Wilson and Jerome Kuehl, "The Truth of Film History", *Sight and Sound* 42 (4)(1974), 241.
39. Wilson and Kuehl, 1974, 242.
40. Robert J. Lifton, *Witness to an Extreme Century* (London and New York: Free Press, 2011), 156; Alan Rosenthal (2013) private communication with the author; John Berger (2013) private communication with the author.
41. Vas and Rosenthal, 1980, 268–9.
42. Lifton, 2011, 161.
43. Turim, 1992, 211.
44. Lifton, 2011, 161.

PART VI

A Coda on Trauma

CHAPTER 12

Why History Hurts

Joanna Bourke

When invited to write an epilogue to this volume of essays, my thoughts went immediately to a poem written by R.L. Barth, former US Marine. Entitled "Epilogue", Barth reflected on his war service, observing that

> Twenty years later, the poor sons of bitches
> Learn jungle rot, decaying flesh, still itches
> And, spreading body part to body part,
> Even corrupts the chambers of the heart.[1]

Less poetically: history hurts. Twenty or more years after perpetrating, suffering, and witnessing massacres and other atrocities, military violence still irritates, disturbs, and torments survivors. Why do individual and collective experiences of violence continue to cause distress long after the hostilities are over? This is the question that preoccupies many of the authors in this book.

Why does history hurt? Of course, the "history" in this question does not refer to some reified essence. There is no capitalized "Past". Rather, "history" is an active process in which individuals construct a sense of self and other through language, material objects, bodily movements, and other practices of symbolization. Historians often claim to possess a

J. Bourke (✉)
Birkbeck, University of London, London, UK

P. Leese, J. Crouthamel (eds.), *Traumatic Memories of the Second World War and After*, DOI 10.1007/978-3-319-33470-7_12

particular expertise in the practices of creating and re-creating historical narratives but, in fact, it is a joint enterprise. Individual memory both contributes to history and takes some of its knowledge from history. Memory not only assails history, demanding that it "pays attention" to agents and eyewitnesses, but history also assails individual and collective memory, providing (albeit partial) scripts and priorities.[2] That is partly why the practice of telling stories about the past is so messy.

History-making is never more fractured than in the context of war. Since the 1970s, attempts to make sense of the confusion of tongues associated with extremes of violence—including massacres, mass rapes, torture, and rites of humiliation—have turned time and again to one concept: trauma. It is not an exaggeration to state that commentators in the affluent West have become obsessed with "trauma narratives".

The Invention of Psychological Trauma

However, in its psychological manifestation, the concept of trauma is relatively young. As late as 1887, philosopher Friedrich Nietzsche could bluntly state that

> I consider even "psychological pain" to be not a fact but only an interpretation—a causal interpretation—of facts that have hitherto defied exact formulation—too vague to be scientifically serious.

In his memorable words, the notion of psychic trauma is nothing more than "a fat word replacing a very thin question mark". Nietzsche went on to argue that

> When someone cannot get over a "psychological pain" that is <u>not</u> the fault of his "psyche" but, to speak crudely, more probably even that of his belly.... A strong and well-constituted man digests his experiences (his deeds and misdeeds included) as he digests his meals, even when he has to swallow some tough morsels.[3]

Today, very few people would support Nietzsche in questioning the existence of emotional trauma, although many agree with his contention that modern people are a bit too delicate for the rough and tumble of life. Such people need to manfully gulp down the "tough morsels" thrown at them by fate.

When Nietzsche claimed that psychological distress was the fault of a person's "belly", he was of course being clever. However, for millennia, trauma was physiological rather than psychological. The word "trauma" comes from the Greek word *τραυμα*, referring to a *physiological* wound. In other words, for most of human history, to "*have* a trauma" meant to suffer a bodily wound. It could also refer to the act of bodily wounding, that is, to *inflict* a physiological wound.[4]

The shift from the external (physiological) wound to the internal (psychological) rupture only occurred in the mid-1860s. John Eric Erichsen, professor of surgery at the University College Hospital in London, was largely responsible for this redefinition of trauma. In 1866, Erichsen coined the term "railway spine" in his attempt to make sense of the nervous disarrangement suffered by victims of railway accidents. In the 1860s, railways were new. Culturally, they were not only an exhilarating proof of the dawn of modernity but also terrifying evidence that the world was changing too rapidly for people to properly grasp. New explanations were therefore needed to explain the effects that an industrialized, fast-moving society was having on ordinary men and women. In *On Railway and Other Injuries of the Nervous System* (1866), Erichsen concluded that railway accidents caused a psychic "shock" that was unlike any "ordinary accident". This was because

> The rapidity of the movement, the momentum of the person injured, the suddenness of its arrest, the helplessness of the sufferers, and the natural perturbation of mind that must disturb the bravest, are all circumstances that of a necessity greatly increases the severity of the resulting injury to the nervous system.[5]

In other words, Erichsen added a psychological dimension to the understanding of "trauma" as a physiological injury to the spinal cord.

Nearly a decade later, Erichsen was even more convinced that psychological trauma played an independent role to organic lesions in causing nervous disorders. In *On Concussion of the Spine, Nervous Shock, and Other Obscure Injuries of the Nervous System in Their Clinical and Medico-Legal Aspects* (1875), he explained that

> The mental or moral unconsciousness may occur without the infliction of any physical injury, blow, or direct violence to the head or spine. It is commonly met with in persons who have been exposed to comparatively trifling degrees of violence, who have suffered nothing more than a general shock or concussion of the system.[6]

The existence of an inner, psychological self that could be traumatized by "bad events" (such as a railway accident) gradually morphed into something much broader, thanks to the work of psychologists and neurologists such as Pierre Janet, Jean-Martin Charcot, and Hermann Oppenheim. The work of Sigmund Freud was particularly important, especially his 1895 book with Josef Breuer (*Studies on Hysteria*), his article "The Aetiology of Hysteria" (1896), and his "Introduction to Psycho-Analysis and the War Neuroses" (1919). For Freud, the "human ego" defends itself "from a danger which threatens from without" or from within by developing a traumatic neurosis.[7] Over the entire corpus of his writings, Freud posited different ways of thinking about trauma. In *Studies in Hysteria* (1893), for instance, trauma was inaccessible to the consciousness; therefore, it returns time and again in the form of compulsive, repetitive behaviors. By contrast, in *Beyond the Pleasure Principle*, he placed more emphasis on the "death drive". Other historians have elucidated these shifts in his thinking.

Wartime experiences were also crucial in the development and spread of the concept of psychological trauma. Although wartime emotional disturbances had been observed in every conflict since ancient times, debates about shell shock during the First World War and combat neuroses during the 1939–45 war were decisive in shaping the modern understanding of trauma.[8] In 1941, Abram Kardiner first invented the term "post-traumatic stress disorder (PTSD)". He observed that the traumatized person

> acts as if the original traumatic situation were still in existence and engages in protective devices which failed on the original occasion. This means in effect that his conception of the outer world and his conception of himself have been permanently altered.[9]

It was not until the aftermath of the war in Vietnam that PTSD was admitted into the American Psychiatric Association's third edition of their *Diagnostic and Statistic Manual of Mental Disorders* (DSM III: 1980). The diagnosis proved popular. PTSD moved rapidly from wartime ordeals to the full range of other "bad events", including the trauma of being hijacked,[10] working as an attorney[11] or an animal activist,[12] abduction by aliens,[13] and being abused as a nonhuman animal.[14] In other words, the notion of trauma catapulted into mainstream understandings of the self, quickly being applied to every "bad event". It became commonplace to recognize that "the poor sons of bitches" (as Barth put it) returning war-scarred from the battlefields or after any other "bad event" would continue to hurt "twenty years later".

Defining Trauma

Given the vast range of events and practices subsumed under the trauma label, it is not surprising that there is no common understanding of either the ontology or etiology of the concept. For instance, it is difficult to reconcile Erichsen's understanding of nervous shock (a "bad event" model) with Freud's notion of the traumatic neuroses (with its emphasis on *thanatos* and *eros*). When Kardiner first invented the term "post-traumatic stress disorder" in 1941, he did not intend it to apply outside of war contexts, yet that is exactly what happened.[15] In more recent years, trauma theorists such as Bessel van der Kolk have complicated definitions even further by locating trauma within the brain. He conceives of PTSD as a physioneurosis, or a kind of neurological activity that can be revealed in brain scans.[16]

In commonplace as well as scientific debate, there is also a bewildering swing between mimetic and anti-mimetic theories of trauma. Although they often appear side by side, the two theories are in fact incompatible.[17] The mimetic theory is the more psychoanalytical one. It presents the person as traumatized by unconscious forces. Because trauma does not enter into any cognitive or perceptual framework, the traumatized person cannot have direct access to it. She often ends up mirroring or imitating it. In this volume, the essay by Sophie Delaporte ("Making Trauma Visible") best represents this tradition. Indeed, Delaporte suggests that the French tradition of trauma has remained closer to Freud's original framework of the neuroses and she laments the decision of DSM III to move toward a more descriptive, "stress-based" nosology. Maria Kobielska's chapter on the memory of the Katyń massacre in Polish culture also contains elements of mimetic theory. She argues that Poles cannot come to terms with the trauma of Katyń because suffering "cannot be fully experienced". Representations of the massacre can never "confront the traumatic": films such as Andrzej Wajda's *Katyń* (2007), she argues, "smoothes the trauma, familiarizes it, relates to it lucidly" but "cancels its horror and uniqueness".

By contrast, the anti-mimetic model is favored by most of the other essays in this volume. It posits trauma as an external event that the traumatized person struggles to manage. Such an approach encourages an analysis of the specificities of human experiences, including meticulous evaluations of variations according to ideological and political adherence, class, gender, age, generation, sexuality, marital status, geographical location, type of "bad event", and so on. An exemplary example of this approach can be found in Hazel Croft's chapter. Entitled "Rethinking Civilian Neuroses in the Second World War", Croft emphasizes the constructed nature of war neuroses among civilians in the UK, including the "political context in which government ministers, and their psychiatric advisors, decided and limited what disorders were counted as psychiatric casualties caused by the war". Through an ingenious use of Raymond Williams' concept of "structures of feelings", Croft is able to show how the "myth of psychological resilience" in the face of aerial bombardment was "constantly in the process of being shaped, reshaped, reiterated and resisted". This "bad event" model of trauma (and resistance to it) has been particularly productive in research focusing on armed conflicts.

Nevertheless, the proliferation of definitions and approaches to psychological trauma poses difficulties for anyone attempting to illuminate the diverse and shifting ways people in the past negotiated and gave meaning to events as harrowing as war and its disruptive aftermaths. In analyses that seek to illuminate trauma through historical exegesis, it is tempting to fall back on the favorite methodological sleight of hand of the social historian: trauma is whatever people say is traumatic. In other words, for the purposes of historical analysis, so long as someone says that they have been traumatized by an event, that claim is accepted.

In practical terms, there are many advantages of this approach. It avoids putting words into other peoples' mouths. It neither pretends that the historian can psychoanalyze dead people nor does it treat people in the past as analysands on our couches. It is courteous to the way people in the past have sought to make sense of their lives. It is respectfully neutral about which specific approach to trauma is being employed by people in the past, allowing for multitude, even conflicting, characterizations of trauma. In other words, the historian does not have to choose between mimetic or non-mimetic approaches, but is simply required to observe which approach historical actors (within their specific contexts) grasped when attempting to communicate to others. Crucially, the approach allows historians to explore how the label "trauma" changes over time. The chief question becomes: what does the *content* of any historically specific and geographically situated ontology tell us about the way people in the past have understood trauma? By what mechanisms do these understandings change?

However, defining trauma as "whatever people says is trauma" is also problematic. Might the definition be all-encompassing? "Trauma-speech" has become so ubiquitous in many contemporary societies since the mid-twentieth century that it can include everything from surviving a murderous siege, to witnessing an acrimonious divorce on reality television, to burying a pet goldfish. A history of "trauma" turns out to be a history of human experience *en tout*.

There is also the opposite risk. Might Nietzsche be right when he claimed that psychological pain was a "fat word replacing a very thin question mark"? As we have already seen, "trauma" is a very recent, Anglo-European concept. This was what Frantz Fanon argued in *Wretched of the Earth* (1963). He criticized the concept of trauma for being a western artifact, assembled out of American and European experiences: it was hardly appropriate for colonized peoples.[18] Equally, people can be traumatized without possessing the word "trauma". Do we want to exclude worlds of suffering that occurred in previous centuries and in other localities around the globe?

More to the point, how do we know what people are "actually feeling"? It has become commonplace to cite Freud's assertion that "Psychical trauma—or more precisely the memory of the trauma—acts like a foreign body, which long after its entry must continue to be regarded as an agent that is still at work".[19] Trauma theorist Cathy Caruth has also popularized the idea of trauma as a "crying wound".[20] But trauma conceived of as a wound is metaphorical. It is an ontological fallacy to confuse metaphor for materiality. Trauma is a subjective experience that lacks a visible scar. True, witnesses may observe bodily reactions (trembling, sweating, panting, crying) but—like all subjective experiences—are reliant on the person herself to confirm or otherwise whether these reactions are due to psychological trauma or something else (appendicitis or even sexual jouissance, for instance).

How to avoid these problems? Other theorists have approached the question of subjective (or inner) feelings through "private language" debates. I discuss this approach in detail in my book *The Story of Pain: From Prayer to Painkillers* (2014) but the basic point is that it does not fundamentally matter if everyone is "feeling" something different when they say they are traumatized, so long as there is a shared language for the sensation. The most helpful exposition of this point can be found in Ludwig Wittgenstein's *Philosophical Investigations.* He observes that people learn how to attach words to sensations. To have any meaning, Wittgenstein notes, words for feeling states such as pain must be intersubjective and, therefore, shareable. In other words, the naming of a "trauma" always occurs in public realms and can never be wholly private.

In order to clarify his argument, Wittgenstein asks his readers to imagine a world in which everyone possesses a box that contains a beetle. People only know the "beetle" by looking into their own box since they are unable to open anyone else's box. It is possible, in other words, that each person's "beetle" is completely different. But if everyone believes that they possess a "beetle in a box", then the word "beetle" is useful in communication. In terms of language, in other words, the "actual content" of the box does not actually matter. What is important is the role of the "beetle in the box" in terms of public communication.

If we substitute the word "trauma" for "beetle", it no longer matters that one person has no direct access to another person's subjective consciousness, so long as they have a shared language to discuss their various "traumas". As Wittgenstein succinctly put it, "mental language is rendered significant not by virtue of its capacity to reveal, mark, or describe mental states, but by its function in social interaction".[21] For the historian, then, the task is to interrogate the *different* language games that people in the past have played, in order to make educated guesses about the diverse and distinctive ways people have packaged their subjective "traumas". An event is called "traumatic" if it is identified as such by the person claiming that kind of consciousness. The concept "trauma" requires an individual to give significance to this particular being-in-the-world.

The advantages of this approach are many, but not least is the fact that it allows trauma to be explored in all its variability, fluidity, and unpredictability. Furthermore, the traumatized person is given agency. This is frequently overlooked in analyses of trauma that start from a "bad event". Commentators worry that they might be accused of "blaming the victim". It is no judgment on the traumatized person to observe that trauma is not an inevitable outcome for survivors of a "bad event". To reiterate: this does not place responsibility on victims, but is simply an admission that victims are embedded in social, interpersonal, cognitive, emotional, and other networks of being, all of which impinge on their lived experience in the world. "Trauma" does not have agency; people do. "Bad events" do not intrude upon a person independent of context.

At the most brutal level, not all "bad events" have victims because there are no survivors. As Barth put it in "Epitaph"

> Tell them quite simply that we died
>   Thirsty, betrayed, and terrified.[22]

The dead no longer hurt. Trauma is the suffering of survival.

The second point can be stated just as bluntly: not all traumatized people are victims. As we saw in Susan Derwin's chapter, perpetrators can be victims. She argues that the introduction of the term "moral injury" enables people sympathetic to veterans returning from the wars in Iraq and Afghanistan to identify a kind of ethical suffering arising from participating (or witnessing ones' comrade participating) in atrocities. In American-led wars, there is a formidable asymmetry between the armaments of the opposing sides. The risk to (US) troops of being killed is significantly lower than the risk of injury or death to innocent (Iraqi) civilians, meaning that it is no longer fear that causes trauma to US troops but shame, survivor's guilt, and a recognition of moral transgression. Indeed, Derwin could have gone a lot further: the moral injury of perpetration can actually trump the brutal physiological and psychological trauma of their victims.

One possible outcome of this distortion is the creation of a pornography of pain. In this volume, Sokołowska-Paryż is particularly insightful when she shows how naturalistic rape scenes in cinema actually exonerate perpetrators and revictimize violated women. By foregrounding perpetrators and "metonymically equat[ing] the victims with their nations", the films that Sokołowska-Paryż analyses make rape universal and inevitable. Filmic rape scenes focus attention not on the victims but on the traumatized perpetrators who struggle to act honorably in brutalizing environments. In Sokołowska-Paryż's words,

> These films create a gender-based hierarchy of suffering where the female victim is relegated to the function of the instigating factor of the man's trauma. The woman is downgraded to a fleeting character.... In these cinematic representations of war rapes the violation of the female body is of lesser importance than the violation of the male psyche.

Worse, as I argue elsewhere, *victims* can even be portrayed as perpetrators since it was their suffering that caused the armed troops such pain.[23] The effacing or "wiping out" of the real victims of war (the mutilated, tortured, and killed civilians) is a particularly strong theme in the context of the war in Vietnam where, for the first time, widespread and institutionalized dismay over American involvement in the war enabled servicemen to deflect blame onto the state. Furthermore, for all my sympathy and immense respect for the Winter Soldier Investigation of 1974 (an event run by Vietnam Veterans Against the War, which set out to expose American-led atrocities), it was structured like a press conference in which the perpetrator's pain trumped that of the victims. Its politics was not restorative, but simply ameliorative: remove Americans from Vietnam and the atrocity, the trauma, ends. Such perpetration narratives are "about" healing, with the incumbent reaffirmation of traditional power structures afterwards. Empathy is accorded to the perpetrators who made the "wrong choice" (but who can blame them given an impressive list of environmental and military "stressors", including racism, harsh conditions, fear of an "invisible enemy", and peer pressure).

In other words, the problem with the concept of "moral injury" is that healing and forgiveness might not be appropriate. Primo Levi recognized this in his chapter "The Memory of the Offense" (1986), which struggled with how we should write about the "memory of a trauma... *inflicted*". Levi concluded that,

> Here, as with other phenomenon, we are dealing with a paradoxical analogy between victim and oppressor, and we are anxious to be clear: both are in the same trap, but it is the oppressor, and he alone, who has prepared it and activated it, and if he suffers from this, it is right that he should suffer.[24]

If not all traumatized people are victims, so, too, not all terrible events are perceived as traumatic to survivors. As Peter Leese expressed it in "Traumatic Displacements: The Memory Films of Jonas Mekas and Robert Vas", the "bad event" of forced exile "may or may not result in later traumatic memory". Depending on the presence or absence of friends, family, or members of one's own community, a person might be "traumatized" or simply "stressed". Victims may not even respond to a "bad event" in a way that they register as "traumatic". Freud observed this in *Civilization and its Discontents* when he stated that "on occasions when the most extreme form of suffering have to be endured special protective devices come into operation".[25] Leese even suggests that people who undergo traumatic events might even be able to use them for "creative re-interpretation".

Cultural rules play an important role in providing such "protective devices". This theme is strongly argued in Sandra Kessler's contribution to this volume. The political nature of remembrance of the Korean War is strikingly revealed in the name given to the conflict—"yug-i-o" or "six-two-five", meaning 25 June 1950. This name communicates the belief that the war was the result of communist belligerence from the North. In interviewing Korean veterans about their war experience, Kessler was conscious of the cross-cultural differences in the way Korean veterans narrated their war experiences compared with veterans elsewhere. She also recognized the importance of interpersonal dynamics in the interview situation, which altered the content of the rules for reciting memories of traumatic events.

An equally striking example of the influence of culture can be observed in explorations of Soviet responses to war. In *Night of Stone: Death and Memory in Russia* (2000), historian Catherine Merridale argues that, despite exceptional suffering during the Great Patriotic War and in its aftermath, veterans did not respond by developing traumatic neuroses. Their watchword was stoicism.[26] Her arguments are elaborated in Robert Dale's chapter, entitled "'No Longer Normal': Traumatized Red Army Veterans in Postwar Leningrad". Dale points out that "bad events" might increase the *risk* of trauma but do not make it inevitable. Russian veterans proved remarkably resilient. He admits that it was "not that Leningrad's veterans did not suffer psychological pain". Rather, their pain was "rarely recognized as trauma and rarely resulted in mental breakdown". Above all, their mental stoicism was bolstered by ideological adherence to the idea that they had contributed to the "supreme collective sacrifice and national rebirth".

There is another way of explaining the lack of a direct relationship between the "bad event" and "trauma", and it returns us to the point made earlier about the agency of victims. It is not the case that a person "experiences" a "bad event", *after which* affective, cognitive, and motivational processes "kick in", enabling the person to respond and interpret the event. People perceive what is happening around them through the prism of the entirety of their lived experiences, including their sensual physiologies, emotional states, cognitive beliefs, and relational standing in various communities. This is not to deny that surviving a massacre will make most people feel very unwell indeed. But not necessarily. Different emotional reactions can adhere to even "*very* bad events". Depending on the presence of other objects and people, "bad events" can elicit feelings of exhilaration, surprise, or even pride for having survived. It makes a difference whether the "bad event" is anticipated or if it is believed to be "natural". It makes a difference if the psychological or physiological "wound" is inflicted by a spouse, former friend, or neighbor. Trauma that is followed by financial or other forms of compensation "feels" different to trauma that is rudely shunted aside or stigmatized. In other words, trauma is a way of perceiving an experience. Trauma is not the "bad event" as such but the way we *evaluate* what has happened to us.

This way of thinking about trauma places less emphasis on innate, biological responses ("fight or flee"), and more on performativity. This is why the clarity (or otherwise) of a social script for dealing with "bad events" is important. There are social expectations to the way people express their trauma, and these norms differ according to gender, class, occupation, life stage, generation, ethnicity, sexuality, and so on. They change dramatically over time as people creatively perform trauma. Subtle messages communicated though language, facial expressions, and gestures inform traumatized people how they *ought to* comport themselves.

Unfortunately, this also means that people who fail to "perform trauma" according to the prescribed script will often fail to have their suffering acknowledged. This comes sharply into focus in relation to the Holocaust. In the chapter "Testimonies of Trauma: Surviving Auschwitz-Birkenau", Lisa Pine asks the most important question for trauma scholars: "whose traumatic experiences gain attention and why, and whose have been ignored?" She convincingly argues that gender is crucial: in the camps, men and women responded to the horrific abuse in very different ways. Unfortunately, male experiences have been noticed and prioritized by scholars, at least until recently.

In the early 1990s, the artist Judy Chicago responded to this problem of the invisibility of gendered suffering in her work "Double Jeopardy" (which was part of her "Holocaust Project"). Chicago's chief aim was to portray how women during the Holocaust were doubly traumatized. They were persecuted because they were Jews; they were raped because they were women. Her artistic challenge was to establish women's unique encounter with trauma. She observed that victims of the Holocaust were usually represented through photographs and films, both of which routinely excluded female suffering. Her solution was to combine photography and painting. In "Double Jeopardy", therefore, the lower half of the work shows a widely circulated photograph of male inmates in Buchenwald during liberation while, in the top half, she "paints in" women's very different experience of liberation: they were raped by German, Soviet, and American soldiers. This is gender-specific trauma.[27]

Women are not the only group whose trauma can become invisible: class also matters. As Croft shows in her chapter, working-class Britons during the bombing of British cities were severely disadvantaged when they contemplated going to their doctors with emotional complaints. Their failure to adhere to the propagandist "stoical" model and their unfamiliarity with medical models made it difficult for them to confront the class superiority of physicians.

However, the tyranny of emotional comportment is important for all victims, who are only acknowledged *as victims* through acting in particular ways. "Mistakes" in following the script enable the harm to be minimized. In Western societies, this often requires confessional speech. This is what feminists Linda Alcoff and Laura Gray argue in "Survivor Discourse: Transgression or Recuperation?" (1993). They observe that victims of rape are expected to "break [...] the silence", which is conceived of as "the necessary route to recovery or as a privileged political tactic". However, this risks becoming "a coercive imperative on survivors to confess, to recount our assaults, to give details, and even to do so publicly. Our refusal to comply might then be read as weakness of will or as re-enacted victimization". Might it not also be the case, they continued, that "survival itself sometimes necessitates a refusal to recount or even a refusal to disclose and deal with the assault or abuse"? Disclosure could be more emotionally, financially, and physically damning to victims of atrocity than silence.[28] In other words, confessional discourse requires the adoption and framing of the traumatic experience along rigid lines shaped by Anglo-American legal doctrines and moralistic codes, which may not be in keeping with an individual's process of self-creation.

Clearly, the concept of "trauma" does a formidable amount of political and ideological work. Trauma is always practiced within interpersonal, historical, and environmental contexts. This is yet another way of insisting that there is no decontextual trauma event: trauma is always infused with politics of power. This can be seen in two distinctive ways. The first involves individualizing suffering. This is often the approach of those working within the mimetic tradition, where trauma recedes into a very personal ego in its encounter with *thanatos*. As a result, violence is privatized; material violence, thrusted aside. It shifts attention from the external wound to the inner one. The political becomes personal.

The second tendency is precisely the opposite—that is, a focus on the political. For example, second-wave feminists pressed for rape to be admitted into the pantheon of "traumatic events". This culminated in the introduction of "rape trauma syndrome"—defined as an "acute stress reaction to a life-threatening situation"—in 1974.[29] Other groups used the trauma label to *validate* violence, as did the Bush administration after 9/11. Still others used trauma counseling as a form of therapeutic governance or cultural imperialism. This is exactly what happened in Kosovo, argues Vanessa Pupavac. She rails against the assumption of humanitarian groups from Western nations after the war in Kosovo that refugee populations would be traumatized. When they intervened to help displaced persons, they imposed a PTSD model based on the American experience of defeat in the Vietnam War. The result was disastrous.[30]

Some of the best work about the political aspects of trauma has been done in the German context. As Mikkel Dack cogently argues in his article on postwar Germany, "victim status" was used for economic and social advantage. This occurred at a personal level, as Dack shows through an examination of the denazification questionnaire or "Fragebogen". However, it also occurred at a communal level, as when emphasis was placed on the expulsion of 11 million Germans from eastern and central Europe and on the many thousands of German Prisoners of War who died in Soviet hands. According to Volker Heins and Andreas Langenohl in a chapter they published in a book entitled *Narrating Trauma. On the Impact of Collective Suffering* (2011), postwar Germans could not commemorate the air raids as a trauma because their country had been occupied by the perpetrators of those raids. Instead, the memory of the war revolved around the Holocaust and war-guilt. Perpetrator trauma overrode victim trauma.[31]

This point has been made by many historians. As Alon Confino dryly observed, "The often-made contention that the past is constructed not as fact but as myth to serve the interest of a particular community may still sound radical to some, but it cannot (and should not) stupefy most historians".[32] Wulf Kansteiner echoed this point when he pointed out that although "specific versions of the past may originate in traumatic experiences, they do not retain that quality if they become successful collective memories". He concluded that

> The concept of trauma, as well as the concept of repression, neither captures nor illuminates the forces that contribute to the making and unmaking of collective memories. Even in cases of so-called delayed collective memory (as in the case of the Holocaust or Vietnam), the delayed onset of public debates about the meaning of negative pasts has more to do with political interest and opportunities than the persistence of trauma or any "leakage" in the collective unconscious.

People who experienced traumas such as war will only see their narratives enter the public realm "if their vision meets with compatible social or political objectives and inclinations among other important social groups".[33] Why is it important that some "bad events" are rated higher than others and that some people who experience "bad events" are viewed as more traumatized than others? It leads to an unequal distribution of sympathy. In the words of Slavoj Zizek in *The Fragile Absolute, or, Why is the Christian Legacy Worth Fighting For?* (2000),

> the Other to be protected is good in so far as it remains a victim (which is why we were bombarded with pictures of helpless Kosova mothers, children, and old people telling moving stories of their suffering); the moment it no longer behaves like a victim, but wants to strike back on its own, it magically turns all of a sudden into a terrorist/fundamentalist/drug-trafficking Other.[34]

Clearly, trauma is a normative concept. It distinguishes "normal" violence from what is excessive and therefore "traumatizing". For example, "trauma" is not assigned to children starving in the Third World or to any other kinds of systemic violence. It usually requires a sudden event—a violent fissure. It allows for instrumental, dispassionate, state violence while castigating zealous cruelty by non-state or illegitimate actors. Furthermore, it is not only the fact that many underprivileged people have to fight to have their trauma noticed: it is also the case that many people might *themselves* not register an occurrence as distressing simply because it is so typical. Nightmares, excessive sweating, trembling, flashbacks, and suchlike may be interpreted as part of everyday experiences. In other words, the language of psychological trauma might not make much sense to many people for whom "bad events" are endemic and related to issues such as poverty, patriarchy, and racial prejudice. The idea that there is an "after", a "post-", to abuse is based on an assumption that there is a non-assaultive "before". It assumes that violence is an event limited in time and different from everyday life. After all, it is interesting to observe that "rape trauma syndrome" was invented in the context of *middle-class* young women. Thus, one of the first academic attempts to formulate the idea of rape trauma was published by Sandra Sutherland and Donald J. Scherl in 1970. They formulated the "three stages" of trauma in the context of middle-class volunteers (each of whom "had a background consistent with accomplishment, independence, and apparent psychological health") who had been sexually assaulted while working in "low-income neighborhoods". The suffering of these middle-class women allowed the harm of sexual violation to be recognized for the first time.[35] By contrast, for working-class, black girls and women who lived in these areas, violence was seen as "natural"—for both victims and perpetrators.

Critique

What is the way forward in writing "history that hurts"? The editors to this volume have rightly suggested that there is an "urgent need… for a broader cultural and historical analysis of trauma which takes account of social dynamics, politics and medical conceptualization, but which is not confined to them". In this volume, they emphasize the diversity and instability of different constructions of trauma, approached from a range of methodological and theoretical standpoints. The volume has been exemplary in showing that "it is not the 'bad event' which makes trauma, but the material, emotional and communal context within which it is remembered". They call for more rigorous and nuanced analysis of the ideology, practice, and performance of "trauma" across historical time and geographical space. Implicit in their analysis is the need for greater self-reflexivity and self-critique.

In the spirit of critical solidarity, I might add that the ambivalence of trauma scholars toward perpetrators of violence remains problematic. It remains too easy for perpetrators to be turned into traumatized victims, conflating the differences between victim/perpetrator suffering. Ruth Leys pointed this out as long ago as 2000 in her trenchant critique of Caruth's *Unclaimed Experience*.[36]

This ambivalence is exacerbated by a tendency to give too much agency to the perpetrator and too little to the victim. As Marzena Sokołowska-Paryż cogently argues in her chapter entitled "War Rape: Trauma and the Ethics of Representation", this was the problem with Jerzy Bohdan Szumczyk's memorial to Polish women raped by Red Army soldiers during the Second World War. In the sculpture, the woman's trauma was "visually subjugated by male aggression. The victim was completely dominated by the towering soldier figure".

The problem is twofold. On the one hand, there is a risk that perpetrators of "bad events" are overburdened with power. Trauma studies should not be based on fear of perpetrators, but disgust of them. This continued genuflecting toward the perpetrator is worrying. Perpetrators become omnipotent demons, scarcely human. Of course, such representations of violent men and women accurately reflect the all-too-human terror of death. But it is bad politics. On the other hand, traumatized victims risk becoming single-dimensional, cardboard cut-outs. They are relentlessly innocent, never violent themselves, and not consumed with vengeance. Their totalizing innocence is damning. They are not "real". Perhaps, this also relieves us of the anxiety that we, too, might become victims.

Excessive emphasis on the harm done by psychological trauma can obscure three facts. The first is that psychological trauma belongs to those who are not killed outright. The second is that the emphasis can eradicate the victim in a different way—that is, by defining that individual solely in terms of her trauma. This risks trapping them forever in the "bad event". The traumatized person steps out of her own history and becomes defined by "it", the "bad event".

As I argue elsewhere, this was one of the risks when second-wave feminists responded furiously to the systematic disregard of the harm of sexual and domestic violence against girls and women.[37] In their struggles to counter contempt for women, some feminist therapists went so far as to argue that *all* women were suffering from post-traumatic stress disorder or "insidious trauma". As one feminist argued, "No one has yet beaten or raped me, or torn me from my home or taken my job or threatened my life. That is not to say that no one even will". Every woman is a PTSD sufferer brought on by the stress of knowing that "they may be raped at any time and by anyone".[38] As a result, however, femininity *itself* becomes defined as traumatic. Feminist theorist Sharon Marcus perceptively argues that this risks taking

> male violence or female vulnerability as the first and last instances in any explanation of rape is to make the identities of rapist and raped pre-exist the rape itself.[39]

In addition, trauma studies have been dogged by its adherence to an outdated Cartesian distinction between mind and body. It is widely acknowledged that what we call "physical pain" does not exist without a mental component, but too many analyses of psychological trauma ignore its physiological (neurochemical, muscular, nervous, etc.) aspects. The challenge will be to invent a language that goes beyond the physiological/psychological dualism.

Ignoring the visceral body is particularly worrying in trauma accounts that conflate personal trauma and secondary witnessing. The corporeal and the imaginary are not the same. Implying that they are similar effaces the horror of the encounter with dismemberment and death.

Finally, it may be useful to reassess what it meant by saying that something is "unspeakable". As Jacque Derrida wrote in his essay "How To Avoid Speaking", the trope of unspeakability is usually followed by a great deal of talk.[40] The trope of unspeakability is always negated the moment it is uttered. In other words, the statement exists in historical time and the moment something it is said to be "unspeakable", it no longer is. By naming "trauma", it is represented. Death and major psychoses may be beyond the reach of language. But the vast majority of traumatized people still exist in the world. Their world may be imprisoned within a *different* frame, but it is nevertheless one that they own and one that scholars of trauma have a duty to explore.

Indeed, there may even be an argument that the traumatized people are those who truly reside in the world. This was acknowledged after the terrible wars of the twentieth century. In 1919, for instance, G. Elliott Smith and T.H. Pear wrote *Shell Shock and its Lessons.* In it, they pointed out that it was common to describe shell-shocked men as losing their reason when, actually, the opposite was the case. The senses of traumatized servicemen from the war were "usually not lost but functioning with painful efficiency". It was insane *not* to be driven mad by what had taken place between 1914 and 1918. The war poet Herbert Read put it like this:

> It must have been the experience of many men, when the war was over and they came back with minds seared with the things they had seen, to find a civilian public weary and indifferent, and positively unwilling to listen. The public was, indeed, suffering from a war-neurosis far worse than any the active soldier had contracted.

Traumatized people might not lack a language to communicate their suffering; instead, witnesses to their trauma may be refusing to listen.

Conclusion

As we have seen in this book, trauma is an essentially contested category. It has become a master narrative, fuelling fascination with wounds and abject bodies. As critical scholar Susannah Radstone explained as long ago as 2001, trauma has become a "popular cultural script", which needs "contextualization and analysis in its own right—a symptom, the cause of which needs to be sought elsewhere".[41] In other words, the trauma trope performs a vast amount of political, ideological, rhetorical, and personal labor. It is collective, material, historical, and spatial, rather than individual, linguistic, universal, and free floating. In the words of Barth's poem, trauma "corrupts the chambers of the heart".[42] It hurts.

Notes

1. R.L. Barth, "Epilogue", in his, *Deeply Dug In* (Albuquerque: University of New Mexico, 2003), 22.
2. For an interesting discussion, see Yael Zerubauel, "The Death of Memory and the Memory of Death: Masada and the Holocaust as Historical Metaphors", *Representations*, 45 (winter 1994), 73.

3. Friedrich Nietzsche, *On the Genealogy of Morals*, 1st pub 1887, ed. Walter Kaufmann (New York: Random House, 1989), 128.
4. David D. Phillips, "'Trauma ek pronoias' in Athenian Law", *The Journal of Hellenic Studies*, 127 (2007), 75–105.
5. John Eric Erichsen, *On Railway and Other Injuries of the Nervous System* (London: Walton and Maberly, 1866), 9.
6. John Eric Erichsen, *On Concussion of the Spine, Nervous Shock, and Other Obscure Injuries of the Nervous System in Their Clinical and Medico-Legal Aspects* (London: Longman, Green and Co., 1875), 195.
7. Sigmund Freud, "Introduction to Psycho-Analysis and the War Neuroses", in James Strachey (ed.), *The Standard Edition of the Complete Psychological Works of Sigmund Freud*, xvi, 1st pub. 1919 (London: Hogarth Press, 1953), 210.
8. Note that there was a vast array of names for shell shock and combat neuroses (both terms commonly used in the British and American contexts). Other terms, all of which contain subtly different meanings, include "choc traumatique" (France), "kriegshysterie" (Germany), and "voennaiakontuziia" (the Soviet Union). I am emphasizing British and American contexts here simply because they are the histories I am most familiar with. These are also the countries with the richest historiography.
9. Adam Kardiner, *The Traumatic Neuroses of War* (New York: Paul B. Hoeber, 1941), 82.
10. Karen M. von Campbell, "The Emotional Trauma of Hijacking: Who Pays?", *Kentucky Law Journal*, 74 (1985), 599–22.
11. Andrew P. Levin and Scott Greisberg, "Vicarious Trauma in Attorneys", *Pace Law Review*, 24.1 (Fall 2003), 245–52.
12. Taimie L. Bryant, "Trauma, Law, and Advocacy for Animals", *Journal of Animal Law and Ethics*, 1 (2006), 63–138.
13. Bridget Brown, *They Know Us Better Than We Know Ourselves* (New York: New York University Press, 2007); Edith Fiore, *Abductions: Encounters with Extraterrestrials* (London: Sidgwick and Jackson, 1989).
14. For instance, see "ISIS: A Collection and Showing of Captive Animal Statistics", *The Journal of Zoo Animal Medicine*, 7.1 (March 1976), 4–7.
15. Abram Kardiner, *The Traumatic Neuroses of War* (New York: Paul B. Hoeber, 1941).
16. Bessel van der Kolk, "Posttraumatic Stress Disorder and the Nature of Trauma", *Dialogues in Clinical Neuroscience*, 2:1 (2000), 12–3.
17. For the best critical discussion, see Ruth Leys *Trauma: A Genealogy* (Chicago: University of Chicago Press, 2000).

18. Frantz Fanon, *Wretched of the Earth* (Harmondsworth: Penguin, 1967).
19. Joseph Breuer and Sigmund Freud, "On the Psychical Mechanism of Hysterical Phenomena: Preliminary Communication", in *Studies in Hysteria*, trans. and ed. James Strachey with collaboration of Anna Freud, 1st pub. 1893 (New York: Basic Books, 2000), 6.
20. Cathy Caruth, *Unclaimed Experience: Trauma, Narrative, and History* (Baltimore: The Johns Hopkins University Press, 1996), 8.
21. Ludwig Wittgenstein, *Philosophical Investigations*, trans. by G.E.M. Anscombe (Oxford: Basil Blackwell, 1953), 188.
22. R.L. Barth, "Epitaph", in his *Deeply Dug In* (Albuquerque: University of New Mexico, 2003), 20.
23. See my *Rape: A History from 1860s to the Present* (London: Virago, 2007).
24. Primo Levi, *The Drowned and the Saved*, trans. Raymond Rosenthal (New York: Simon and Schuster, 1988), 24.
25. Sigmund Freud, *Civilization and its Discontents* (New York: Dover, 1994), 22.
26. Catherine Merridale, *Night of Stone: Death and Memory in Russia* (London: Granta Books, 2000).
27. Rochelle G. Saidel and Sonja M. Hedgepeth, "July Chicago Led the Way Artistically Portraying Sexual Violence against Women During the Holocaust", *Forward. The Jewish Daily* (22 October 2010), at http://forward.com/articles/132148/judy-chicago-led-the-way-in-artistically-portrayin/. Also see Judy Chicago, *Holocaust Project. From Darkness into Light*, with photography by David Woodman (New York: Viking, 1993), 126.
28. Linda Alcoff and Laura Gray, "Survivor Discourse: Transgression or Recuperation?", *Signs: Journal of Women in Culture and Society*, 18:2 (winter 1993), 281.
29. Ann Wolbert Burgess and Lynda Lytle Holmstrom, "Rape Trauma Syndrome", *American Journal of Psychiatry*, 981 (1974), 981. For a detailed analysis, see my "Sexual Violence, Bodily Pain, and Trauma: A History", *Theory, Culture and Society*, 29.3 (May 2012), 25–51, open access at PMC 4001210.
30. Vanessa Pupavac, "Pathologizing Populations and Colonizing Minds: International Psychosocial Programs in Kosovo", *Alternatives: Global, Local, Political*, 27:4 (October–December 2002), 489–511.

31. Volker Heins and Andreas Langenohl, "A Fire that Doesn't Burn? The Allied Bombing of Germany and the Cultural Politics of Trauma", in Ron Eyerman, Jeffrey C. Alexander, and Elizabeth Butler Breese (eds.), *Narrating Trauma. On the Impact of Collective Suffering* (Boulder: Paradigm Publishers, 2011), 3–26.
32. Alon Confino, "Collective Memory and Cultural History: Problems of Method", *The American Historical Review*, 102:5 (December 1997), 1387.
33. Wulf Kansteiner, "Finding Meaning in Memory: A Methodological Critique of Collective Memory Studies", *History and Theory*, 41 (May 2002), 187–88.
34. Slavoj Zizek, *The Fragile Absolute, or, Why is the Christian Legacy Worth Fighting For?*(London: Verso, 2000), 60.
35. Sandra Sutherland, and Donald J. Scherl, "Patterns of Response Among Victims of Rape", *American Journal of Orthopsychiatry*, 40:3 (April 1970), 503–11.
36. Ruth Leys *Trauma: A Genealogy* (Chicago: University of Chicago Press, 2000), 297.
37. See my "Sexual Violence, Bodily Pain, and Trauma: A History", *Theory, Culture and Society*, 29.3 (May 2012), 25–51, open access at PMC 4001210.
38. Laura S. Brown, "Not Outside the Range: One Feminist Perspective on Psychic Trauma", in Cathy Caruth (ed.), *Trauma: Explorations in Memory* (Baltimore, MD: John Hopkins University Press, 1995), 107.
39. Sharon Marcus, "Fighting Bodies, Fighting Words: A Theory and Politics of Rape Prevention", in Judith Butler and Joan W. Scott (eds.), *Feminists Theorize the Political* (London: Routledge, 1992), 391.
40. Jacques Derrida, "How to Avoid Speaking", in Sanford Budick and Wolfgang Iser (eds.), *Languages of the Unsayable: The Play of Negativity in Literature and Literary Theory*, (New York: Columbia University Press, 1989), 3–70.
41. Susannah Radstone, "Trauma and Screen Studies: Opening the Debate", *Screen*, 42:2 (2001), 189.
42. R.L. Barth, "Epilogue", in his, *Deeply Dug In* (Albuquerque: University of New Mexico, 2003), 22.

Bibliography

Alcoff, Linda, and Laura Gray. 1993. Survivor Discourse: Transgression or Recuperation? *Signs: Journal of Women in Culture and Society* 18(2): 260–290.

Allen, A. 1997. The Holocaust and the Modernization of Gender: A Historiographical Essay. *Central European History* 30(3): 349–364.

American Psychiatric Association. 1980. *The Diagnostic and Statistical Manual of Mental Disorders*, 3rd edn. Washington, DC: American Psychiatric Association.

———. 2013. *The Diagnostic and Statistical Manual of Mental Disorders*, 5th edn. Washington, DC: American Psychiatric Association.

Ashplant, T.G., Graham Dawson, and Michael Roper. 2009. The Politics of War Memory and Commemoration: Contexts, Structures and Dynamics. In *The Politics of Memory: Commemorating War*, eds. T.G. Ashplant, Graham Dawson, and Michael Roper, 3–85. New Brunswick, NJ: Transaction.

Assmann, Aleida. 2006. *Der lange Schatten der Vergangenheit. Erinnerungskultur und Geschichtspolitik*. Munich: Beck.

———. 2011a. *Cultural Memory and Western Civilization: Functions, Media, Archives*. Cambridge: University Press.

———. 2011b. From Collective Violence to a Common Future: Four Models for Dealing with a Traumatic Past. In *Other People's Pain. Narratives of Trauma and the Question of Ethics*, eds. Martin Modlinger and Philipp Sonntag. Bern: Peter Lang.

Apel, Dora. 1997. 'Heroes' and 'Whores': The Politics of Gender in Weimar Antiwar Imagery. *The Art Bulletin* 79(3): 366–384.

Bal, Mieke. 2006. Rape, Suicide, Signs and Show. In *A Mieke Bal Reader*. Chicago: Chicago University Press.

Barham, Peter. 2007. *Forgotten Lunatics of the Great War*. New Haven: Yale University Press.

P. Leese, J. Crouthamel (eds.), *Traumatic Memories of the Second World War and After*, DOI 10.1007/978-3-319-33470-7

Baron, Nancy, Soeren B. Jensen, and Joop de Jong. 2002. Mental Health of Refugees and Internally Displaced People. In *Guidelines For Psychosocial Policy and Practice in Social and Humanitarian Crises*, eds. John A. Fairbank et al., 243–270. New York: Report to the United Nations.

Barth, R. L. 2003. Epilogue. In *Deeply Dug In*. Albuquerque: University of New Mexico.

Bartrop, P. 2000. *Surviving the Camps: Unity in Adversity During the Holocaust*. New York: University Press of America.

Bartov, Omer. 2001. *The Eastern Front, 1941–45, German Troops and the Barbarisation of Warfare*, second edn. Basingstoke: Palgrave Macmillan.

Bartov, Omer, and Eric D. Weitz, eds. 2012. *Shatterzone of Empires: Coexistence and Violence in the German, Habsburg, Russian, and Ottoman Borderlands*. Bloomington: Indiana University Press.

Baskin, J., ed. 1994. *Women of the Word: Jewish Women and Jewish Writing*. Detroit: Wayne State University Press.

Bauer, Y. 2001. *Rethinking the Holocaust*. New Haven: Yale University Press.

Baumeister, Roy F., and Leonard S. Newman. 1994. How Stories Make Sense of Personal Experiences: Motives that Shape Autobiographical Narratives. *Personality and Social Psychology Bulletin* 20: 676–690.

Beevor, Antony. 2007. *Berlin: The Downfall 1945*. London: Penguin Books.

Bell, Amy Helen. 2011. *London Was Ours: Diaries and Memoirs of the London Blitz*. London: I. B. Tauris.

Berger, M., B. Wallis, and S. Watson, eds. 1995. *Constructing Masculinity*. New York: Routledge.

Berry, Michael. 2008. *A History of Pain: Trauma in Chinese Literature and Film*. New York: Columbia University Press.

Bessel, Richard. 2005. Hatred after War: Emotion and the Postwar History of East Germany. *History & Memory* 17(1/2): 195–216.

Bessel, Richard, and Dirk Schumann. 2003. Introduction: Violence, Normality and the Construction of Postwar Europe. In *Life After Death. Approaches to a Cultural and Social History of Europe During the 1940s and 1950s*, eds. Richard Bessell and Dirk Schumann, 1–13. Cambridge/Washington, DC: Cambridge University Press/the German Historical Institute.

Bettelheim, B. 1986. *Surviving the Holocaust*. London: Fontana.

Bhattacharjee, Y. 2008. Shell Shock Revisited: Solving the Puzzle of Blast Trauma. *Science* 319: 406–408.

Bielik-Robson, Agata. 2004. Słowo i trauma: czas, narracja, tożsamość. *Teksty Drugie* 5(89): 23–34.

Biess, Frank. 2010. Feelings in the Aftermath. In *Histories of the Aftermath: The Legacies of the Second World War*, eds. Frank Biess and Robert G. Moeller. New York: Berghahn.

Bigley, James D., et al. August 2010. Motivations for War-related Tourism: A Case of DMZ Visitors in Korea. *Tourism Geographies* 12(3): 371–394.

Bitton-Jackson, L. 1999. *I Have Lived a Thousand Years*. London: Simon and Schuster.

Boudreau, Tyler. Autumn/Winter 2011. The Morally Injured. *The Massachusetts Review* 52(2/3): 746–754.

Bourke, Joanna. January 2000. Effeminacy, Ethnicity, and the End of Trauma: The Sufferings of 'Shell-shocked' Men in Great Britain and Ireland, 1914–39. *Journal of Contemporary History* 35(1): 57–69.

———. 2008. *Rape: A History from 1860 to the Present*. London: Virago Press.

———. 2012. Sexual Violence, Bodily Pain, and Trauma: A History. *Theory, Culture and Society* 29(3): 25–51.

Bos, P. 2003. Women and the Holocaust: Analysing Gender Difference. In *Experience and Expression: Women, the Nazis, and the Holocaust*, eds. E. Baer and M. Goldenberg, 23–50. Detroit: Wayne State University Press.

Brockmeier, Jens, and Donal Carbaugh, eds. 2001. *Narrative and Identity: Studies in Autobiography, Self, and Culture*. Amsterdam: John Benjamins.

Brown, Bridget. 2007. *They Know Us Better Than We Know Ourselves The History and Politics of Alien Abduction*. New York: New York University Press.

Brown, Julie V. 1994. Heroes and Non-Heroes. Recurring Themes in the Historiography of Russian-Soviet Psychiatry. In *Discovering the History of Psychiatry*, eds. Mark S. Micale and Roy Porter, 297–307. Oxford: Oxford University Press.

Brown, Laura S. 1995. Not Outside the Range: One Feminist Perspective on Psychic Trauma. In *Trauma: Explorations in Memory*, ed. Cathy Caruth. Baltimore, MD: John Hopkins University Press.

Brownmiller, Susan. 1993. *Against Our Will: Men Women and Rape*. Fawcett Columbine: New York.

Bryant, Taimie L. 2006. Trauma, Law, and Advocacy for Animals". *Journal of Animal Law and Ethics* 1: 63–138.

Burgess, Ann Wolbert and Lynda Lytle Holmstrom. 1974. Rape Trauma Syndrome. *American Journal of Psychiatry*, 981.

Caplan, E. Ann. 2005. *Trauma Culture. The Politics of Terror and Loss in Media and Literature*. London: Rutgers University Press.

Caruth, Cathy, ed. 1995. *Trauma: Explorations in Memory*. Baltimore, MD: Johns Hopkins University.

———. 1996. *Unclaimed Experience: Trauma, Narrative and History*. Baltimore, MD: Johns Hopkins University.

Chapman, James. 2008. *War and Film*. London: Reaktion Books.

Cherepenina, Nadezhda, "The Demographic Situation and Healthcare on the Eve of War", in *Life and Death in Besieged Leningrad, 1941–44*. John Barber and Andrei Dzeniskevich (London: Palgrave Macmillan, 2005).

Chicago, Judy, and Holocaust Project. 1993. *From Darkness into Light, with photography by David Woodman*. New York: Viking.

Choko, I., F. Irwin, L. Kahana-Aufleger, M. Kalina, and J. Lipski. 2005. *Stolen Youth: Five Women's Survival in the Holocaust*. Yad Vashem: New York.

Confino, Alon. December 1997. Collective Memory and Cultural History: Problems of Method. *The American Historical Review* 102(5): 1386–1403.

Connell, R. 1995. *Masculinities*. Cambridge: Polity Press.

Crocq, Louis. 2012. *16 leçons sur le trauma, 10e leçon, « Trauma et sommeil »*. Paris: Odile Jacob.

Crouthamel, Jason. 2009. *The Great War and German Memory: Society, Politics and Psychological Trauma, 1914–1945*. Liverpool: Liverpool University Press.

Cumings, Bruce. 2007. The Korean War. What Is It that We Are Remembering to Forget? In *Ruptured Histories. War, Memory, and the Post-Cold War in Asia*, eds. Sheila Miyoshi Jager and Rana Mitter. Cambridge, MA: Harvard UP.

Dale, Robert. April 2013. The Valaam Myth and the Fate of Leningrad's Disabled Veterans. *Russian Review* 72(2): 260–284.

Davenport, Robert. 2004. *The Encyclopedia of War Movies: The Authoritative Guide to Movies about Wars of the Twentieth Century*. New York: Facts on File.

Dawson, Graham. 2007. *Making peace with the past? Memory, trauma and the Irish Troubles*. Manchester: Manchester University Press.

Derwin, Susan. 2014. The Warrior's Subjectivity. *MLN* 129(3, German Issue): 504–513.

Delbo, C. 1995. *Auschwitz and After*. New York: Yale University Press.

de Silva, C., ed. 1996. *In Memory's Kitchen: Recipes from Terezin, Introduction by Michael Berenbaum*. Northvale: Rowman and Littlefield.

Des Pres, T. 1976. *The Survivor: An Anatomy of Life in the Death Camps*. New York: Oxford University Press.

de Wijze, L. 1997. *Only My Life: A Survivor's Story*. New York: St. Martin's Press.

Doctor, Ronald M., and Frank N. Shiromoto. 2010. *The Encyclopedia of Trauma and Traumatic Stress Disorders*. New York: Facts on File.

Dokoupil, Tony. 2012. A New Theory of PTSD and Veterans: Moral Injury. *Newsweek*, December 3. http://www.newsweek.com/new-theory-ptsd-and-veterans-moral-injury-63539.

Douglas, Ray M. 2012. *Orderly and Humane: The Expulsion of the Germans after the Second World War*. New Haven: Yale University Press.

Edkins, Jenny. 2010. *Trauma and the Memory of Politics*. Cambridge: Cambridge University Press.

Erikson, Kai T. 1971. *Everything in its Path: Destruction of Community in the Buffalo Creek Flood*. New York: Simon and Schuster.

Etkind, Alexander, et al. 2012. *Remembering Katyn*. Cambridge: Polity Press.

Eyerman, Ron, Jeffrey C. Alexander, and Elizabeth Butler Breese, eds. 2011. *Narrating Trauma: On the Impact of Collective Suffering*. Boulder, CO: Praeger.

Fairbairn, W.R. D. 1990. The Repression and the Return of Bad Objects (with Special Reference to the 'War Neuroses'). In *Psychoanalytic Studies of the Personality*, 59–81. Routledge: London.

Fanon, Frantz. 1967. *Wretched of the Earth.* Harmondsworth: Penguin.

Farley, Lisa. 2012. 'Operation Pied Piper': A Psychoanalytic Narrative of Authority in a Time of War. *Psychoanalysis and History* 14: 29–52.

Farrell, Kirby. 1998. *Post-Traumatic Culture: Injury and Interpretation in the Nineties.* London: Johns Hopkins University Press.

Felman, S., and D. Laub. 1992. *Testimony: Crises of Witnessing in Literature, Psychoanalysis, and History.* New York: Routledge.

Field, Geoffrey. 2011. *Blood, Sweat and Toil: Remaking the British Working Class.* Oxford: Oxford University Press.

Fiore, Edith. 1989. *Abductions: Encounters with Extraterrestrials.* London: Sidgwick and Jackson.

Fivush, Robyn, and Catherine A. Haden, eds. 2003. *Autobiographical Memory and the Construction of a Narrative Self: Developmental and Cultural Perspectives.* Mahwah, NJ: L. Erlbaum.

Foley, James A. 2003. *Korea's Divided Families. Fifty Years of Separation.* London: Routledge.

Förster, Alice, and Birgit Beck. 2003. Post-Traumatic Stress Disorder and World War Two: Can a Psychiatric Concept Help Us Understand Postwar Society? In *Life After Death. Approaches to a Cultural and Social History of Europe During the 1940s and 1950s*, eds. Richard Bessell and Dirk Schumann, 15–35. Cambridge/Washington, DC: Cambridge University Press/the German Historical Institute.

Frankl, V. 2004. *Man's Search for Meaning.* London: Simon and Schuster.

Freeman, Mark. 2009. *Hindsight: The Promise and Peril of Looking Backward.* Oxford: Oxford University Press.

———. 2003. Rethinking the Fictive, Reclaiming the Real: Autobiography, Narrative Time, and the Burden of Truth. In *Narrative and Consciousness: Literature, Psychology and the Brain*, eds. Gary D. Fireman, Ted E. McVay, and Owen J. Flanagan. Oxford: Oxford University Press.

Fuchs, E., ed. 1999. *Women and the Holocaust: Narrative and Representation.* Oxford: University of America Press.

Fulbrook, Mary. 1999. *German National Identity after the Holocaust.* Cambridge: Blackwell Publishers.

Gabriel, Richard A. 1986. *Soviet Military Psychiatry. The Theory and Practice of Coping with Battle Stress.* New York: Greenwood.

Gardiner, Juliet. 2010. *The Blitz: The British Under Attack.* London: Harper Press.

Gelissen, R. 1996. *Rena's Promise: A Story of Sisters in Auschwitz.* London: Weidenfeld and Nicolson.

Gellately, Robert. 1997. Denunciations in Twentieth-century Germany. In *Accusatory Practices: Denunciation in Modern European History, 1789-1989*, eds. Sheila Fitzpatrick and Robert Gellately. Chicago: University of Chicago Press.

Goeschel, Christian. 2009. *Suicide in Nazi Germany.* Oxford: Oxford University Press.

Goldenberg, M. 1990. Different Horrors, Same Hell: Women Remembering the Holocaust. In *Thinking the Unthinkable: Meanings of the Holocaust*, ed. R. Gottlieb, 150–166. New York: Paulist Press.

Goldstein, Joshua S. 2006. *War and Gender: How Gender Shapes the War System and Vice Versa*. Cambridge: Cambridge University Pess.

Grossman, Dave. 1996. *On Killing: The Psychological Cost of Learning to Kill in War and Society*. New York: Back Bay Books.

Grossmann, Atina. Spring, 1995. "A Question of Silence: The Rape of German Women by Occupation Soldiers, *October*, Vol. 72, Berlin 1945: War and Rape "Liberators Take Liberties".

Healey, Dan. 2001. *Homosexual Desire in Revolutionary Russia: The Regulation of Sexual and Gender Dissent*. Chicago, IL: University of Chicago Press.

Gottesfeld Heller, F. 2005. *Love in a World of Sorrow: A Teenage Girl's Holocaust Memoirs*. New York: Devora Publishing Company.

Greenspan, H. 1998. *On Listening to Holocaust Survivors: Beyond Testimony*. Westport: Praeger.

Grinker, Roy Richard. 1998. *Korea and its Futures. Unification and the Unfinished War*. New York: St. Martin's Press.

Gunne, Sorcha, and Zoë Brigley Thompson. 2010. Feminism without Borders: The Potentials and Pitfalls of Re-theorizing Rape. In *Feminism, Literature and Rape Narratives: Violence and Violation*, eds. Sorcha Gunne and Zoë Brigley Thompson. New York: Routledge.

Gurewitsch, B., ed. 1998. *Mothers, Sisters, Resisters: Oral Histories of Women Who Survived the Holocaust*. Tuscaloosa: University of Alabama Press.

Hardmann, A. 2000. Women and the Holocaust. In *Holocaust Educational Trust, Research Papers*, vol. 1, no. 3. London.

Hass, Kristin. 2009. Remembering the 'Forgotten War' and Containing the 'Remembered War': Insistent Nationalism and the Transnational Memory of the Korean War. In *Transnational American Memory*, ed. Udo J. Hebel. Berlin: Walter de Gruyter.

Heinemann, M. 1986. *Gender and Destiny: Women Writers and the Holocaust*. London: Greenwood Press.

Heins, Volker, and Andreas Langenohl. 2011. A Fire that Doesn't Burn? The Allied Bombing of Germany and the Cultural Politics of Trauma. In *Narrating Trauma. On the Impact of Collective Suffering*, eds. Ron Eyerman, Jeffrey C. Alexander, and Elizabeth Butler Breese, 3–26. Boulder: Paradigm Publishers.

Henry, Nicola. 2011. *War and Rape: Law Memory and Justice*. London: Routledge.

Herbert, Zbigniew. 2007. *The Complete Poems: 1956–1998*. New York: Ecco Press.

Herman, Judith. 1992. *Trauma and Recovery: From Domestic Abuse to Political Terror*. New York: Basic Books.

Herzog, Dagmar. 2011. Introduction. In *Brutality and Desire: War and Sexuality in Europe's Twentieth Century*, ed. Dagmar Herzog. Palgrave Macmillan: New York.

———. 2005. *Sex after Fascism: Memory and Morality in Twentieth Century Germany*. Princeton: Princeton University Press.

———, ed. 2005. *Sexuality and German Fascism*. New York: Berghahn.

Hoffman, Eva. 2005. *After Such Knowledge: A Meditation on the Aftermath of the Holocaust*. London: Vintage.

Hoge, C.W., C.A. Castro, and S.C. Messer. 2004. Combat duty in Iraq and Afghanistan, mental health problems, and barriers to care. *New England Journal of Medicine* 1: 13–22.

Hoge, C.W., A. Terhakopian, C.A. Castro, and S.C. Messer. 2007. Association of post-traumatic stress disorder with somatic symptoms, health care visits, and absenteeism among Iraq, War Veterans. *American Journal of Psychiatry* 164: 150–153.

Horeck, Tanya. 2004. *Public Rape: Representing Violation in Fiction and Film*. New York: Routledge.

Horne, John, and Alan Kramer. 2001. *German Atrocities 1914: A History of Denial*. New Haven: Yale University Press.

Horowitz, S. 2000. Gender, Genocide and Jewish Memory. *Prooftexts: A Journal of Jewish Literary History* 20(1): 158–190.

——— 1994. Memory and Testimony of Women Survivors of Nazi Germany. In *Women of the Word: Jewish Women and Jewish Writing*, ed. J. Baskin. Detroit: Wayne State University Press.

Hunt, Nigel. 2010. *Memory, War and Trauma*. Cambridge: Cambridge University Press.

Hydén, Lars-Christer, and Jens Brockmeier, eds. 2008. *Health, Illness and Culture*. New York: Routledge.

Insdorf, Annette. 2003. *Indelible Shadows: Film and the Holocaust*. Cambridge: Cambridge University Press.

Inter-Agency Standing Committee. 2007. *IASC Guidelines on Mental Health and Psychosocial Support in Emergency Settings*. Geneva: IASC.

Isaacson, J. 1991. *Seed of Sarah*. Chicago: Univerity of Illinois Press.

Konrad Jarausch. 1945 and the Continuities of German History: Reflections on Memory, Historiography, and Politics, in *Stunde Null: The End and the Beginning Fifty Years Ago*, ed. Geoffrey Giles (Washington, Washington, DC: German Historical Institute, 1997).

Johnstone, Barbara. 2006. *The Linguistic Individual: Self-Expression in Language and Linguistics*. New York: Oxford University Press.

Jones, Adam. 2011. *Genocide: A Comprehensive Introduction*. London: Routledge.

Jones, Edgar, and Simon Wessely. 2006. *Shell Shock to PTSD: Military Psychiatry from 1900 to the Gulf War*. Abingdon: Psychology Press.

———. 2005. War Syndromes: The Impact of Culture on Medically Unexplained Symptoms. *Medical History* 49: 55–78.

Jones, Edgar, Robin Woolven, Bill Durodie, and Simon Wessely. 2004. Civilian Morale During the Second World War: Responses to Air-Raids Re-examined. *Social History of Medicine* 17: 463–479.

———. 2006. Public Panic and Morale: Second World War Civilian Responses Re-examined in the Light of the Current Anti-Terrorist Campaign. *Journal of Risk Research* 9: 57–73.

Gen James Jones and Dan Goldenberg. 2013. Put Veterans To Work. *Los Angeles Times*, Opinion/Op-Ed, November 11. http://www.latimes.com/opinion/op-ed/la-oe-jones-employ-veterans-20131111-story.html#axzz2kMCYJGVO

Jordanova, Ludmilla. 2012. *The Look of the Past. Visual and Material Evidence in Historical Practice*. Cambridge: Cambridge University Press.

Judt, Tony. 2006. *Postwar: A History of Europe Since 1945*. New York: Penguin Books.

Kaes, Anton. 2009. *Shell Shock Cinema. Weimar Culture and the Wounds of War*. Princeton, NJ: Princeton University Press.

Kal, Hong. 2011. *Aesthetic Constructions of Korean Nationalism. Spectacle, politics and history*. London: Routledge.

———. 2008. Commemoration and the Construction of Nationalism: War Memorial Museums in Korea and Japan. *The Asia-Pacific Journal* 6: 1–25.

Kansteiner, Wulf. 2002. Finding Meaning in Memory: A Methodological Critique of Collective Memory Studies. *History and Theory* 41: 179–197.

Karpushina, Olga. 2002. The Military Body: Film Representations of the Chechen and Vietnam Wars. In *Studies in Slavic Cultures, special issue on: The Russian Body* (3, July 2002): 33–52.

Kemp, Janet and Robert Bossarte. 2012. Suicide Data Report. Department of Veterans Affairs Mental Health Services Suicide Prevention Program. http://www.va.gov/opa/docs/Suicide-Data-Report-2012-final.pdf

Kim, Dong-Choon. 2010. The Truth and Reconciliation Commission of Korea: Uncovering the Hidden Korean War. *The Asia-Pacific Journal*, 1.

Kim, Hunjoon. 2009. Seeking Truth after 50 Years: The National Committee for Investigation of the Truth about the Jeju 4.3 Events. *The International Journal of Transitional Justice*, 3

Kim, Suk-Young. 2011. Staging the 'Cartography of Paradox': The DMZ Special Exhibition at the Korean War Memorial, Seoul. *Theatre Journal* 63(3): 381–402.

———. 2013. Documenting the 'Flower of Reunification': Lim Su-gyeong and the memories of Korean border crossing. *Memory Studies* 6(2): 204–217.

Kohlhaas, Elisabeth. 2003. Die Mitarbeiter der regionalen Staatspolizeistellen: Quantitative und qualitative Befunde zur Personalausstattung der Gestapo. In *Die Gestapo: Mythos und Realität*, eds. Gerhard Paul and Klaus-Michael Mallmann, 220–235. Darmstadt: Wissenschaftliche Buchgesellschaft.

Kolinsky, E. 2004. *After the Holocaust: Jewish Survivors in Germany after 1945*. London: Pimlico.

Korzeniewski, Bartosz. 2007/3. Medializacja i mediatyzacja pamięci—nośniki pamięci i ich rola w kształtowaniu pamięci przeszłości. *Kultura Współczesna*.

Kosta, Barbara. 1997. Rape, Nation and Remembering History: Helke Sander's *Liberators Take Liberties, Modern German Studies*, Vol. 4, "Gender and Germanness: Cultural Productions of a Nation.

Kowalczyk, Izabela. 2010. *Podróż do przeszłości. Interpretacje najnowszej historii w polskiej sztuce krytycznej.* Warszawa: SWPS Academica.

Kwon, Heonik. 2010. Korean War Traumas. *The Asia-Pacific Journal.*

———. 2013. Legacies of the Korean War: Transforming Ancestral Rituals in South Korea. *Memory Studies* 6(2): 161–173.

Kremer, S. Lillian. 1999. *Women's Holocaust Writing: Memory and Imagination.* University of Nebraska Press: Lincoln.

Krylova, Anna, "'Healers of Wounded Souls': The Crisis of Private Life in Soviet Literature, 1944–1946," *The Journal of Modern History*, 73:2, 2001, 307-331.

LaCapra, Dominick. 2004. *History in Transit: Experience, identity, Critical Theory.* Ithaca, NY: Cornell University Press.

———. 2001. *Writing History, Writing Trauma.* Baltimore, MD: Johns Hopkins University.

Lagerway, M. 1998. *Reading Auschwitz.* London: Sage.

Landau, Judith, and Jack Saul. 2004. Facilitating Family and Community Resilience in Response to Major Disaster. In *Living Beyond Loss: Death in the Family, ed*, 285–309. Froma Walsh and Monica McGoldrick. New York: Norton.

Langer, L. 1982. *Versions of Survival: The Holocaust and the Human Spirit.* Albany: Suny Press.

——— 1988. Interpreting Survivor Testimony. In *Writing and the Holocaust*, ed. B. Lang. New York: Holmes and Meier.

——— 1991. *Holocaust Testimonies: The Ruin of Memory.* New Haven: Yale University Press.

Laub, Dori. 1992. Bearing Witness or the Vicissitudes of Listening. In *Testimony: Crises of Witnessing in Literature, Psychoanalysis, and History*, eds. Shoshana Felman and Dori Laub. New York: Routledge.

Lebel, Jean-Jacques. 2012. *Jonas Mekas celebrates what he sees: The Moebius Strip. Jonas Mekas. Walden.* Paris: Potemkine Films DVD Boxed Set Booklet.

Leese, Peter. 2014. *Shell Shock: Traumatic Neurosis and the British Soldiers of the First World War.* Basingstoke: Palgrave Macmillan.

Leitner, I. 1978. *Fragments of Isabella: A Memoir of Auschwitz.* New York: Dell Publishing Company.

Lengyel, O. 1995. *Five Chimneys: The Story of Auschwitz.* Chicago: Academy Chicago Publishers.

Levi, Primo. 1988. *The Drowned and the Saved.* . Trans. Raymond Rosenthal. New York: Simon and Schuster.

———. 2000. *If this is a Man.* London: Abacus Books.

Levin, Andrew P., and Scott Greisberg. 2003. Vicarious Trauma in Attorneys. *Pace Law Review* 24(1): 245–252.

Levine, Paul A. 2010. *Raoul Wallenberg in Budapest: Myth, History and Holocaust.* London: Valentine Mitchell.

Levinson, Nan. 2012. Mad-Bad-Sad: What's Really Happened to America's Soldiers. *Huffington Post*, June 28. http://www.huffingtonpost.com/nan-levinson/mad-bad-sad-whats-really-_b_1633856.html

Leys, Ruth. 2000. *Trauma: A Genealogy.* Chicago: University of Chicago Press.

Lieblich, Amia, Dan P. McAdams, and Ruthellen Josselson, eds. 2006. *Identity and Story: Creating Self in Narrative.* Washington, DC: American Psychological Association Press.

Lifton, Robert Jay. 1986. *The Nazi Doctors: Medical Killing and the Psychology of Genocide.* London: Macmillan.

———. 2011. *Witness to an Extreme Century.* London: Free Press.

Linden, R. 1993. *Making Stories, Making Selves: Feminist Reflections on the Holocaust.* Columbus: Ohio State University Press.

Litz, Brett T., et al. 2009. Moral Injury and Moral Repair in War Veterans: A Preliminary Model and Intervention Strategy. *Clinical Psychological Review* 29: 695–706.

Loughran, Tracey. January 2012. Shell Shock, Trauma, and the First World War: The Making of a Diagnosis and Its Histories. *Journal of the History of Medicine and Allied Sciences* 67(1): 94–119.

Lubelski, Tadeusz. 2006. *Wajda.* Wrocław: Wydawnictwo Dolnośląskie.

Luckhurst, Roger. 2008. *The Trauma Question.* New York: Routledge.

MacDonald, Stephen. 1986. Lost Lost Lost over 'Lost Lost Lost'. *Cinema Journal* 25(2).

Mackay, Robert. 2002. *Half the Battle: Civilian Morale During the Second World War.* Manchester: Manchester University Press.

Małczyński, Jacek. 2009. Drzewa—żywe pomniki w Muzeum-Miejscu Pamięci w Bełżcu. *Teksty Drugie* 1-2: 208–214.

Marcus, Sharon. 1992. Fighting Bodies, Fighting Words: A Theory and Politics of Rape Prevention. In *Feminists Theorize the Political*, eds. Judith Butler and Joan W. Scott. London: Routledge.

Marlantes, Karl. 2011. *What It Is Like To Go To War.* New York: Grove Press.

Matthias, J., ed. 2009. *Approaching an Auschwitz Survivor: Holocaust Testimony and its Transformation.* Oxford: Oxford University Press.

Mekas, Jonas. 1987. The Diary Film (A Lecture on *Reminiscences of a Journey to Lithuania*). In *The Avant-Garde Film. A Reader of Theory and Criticism*, ed. P.A. Sitney. New York: Anthology Film Archives.

———. 1991. *I Had Nowhere To Go.* New York: Black Thistle Press.

Mekas, J. 2003. Interview with Any Taubin. http://www.webofstories.com/play/jonas.mekas. Accessed 01 March 2013

Merridale, Catherine. 2000. The Collective Mind: Trauma and Shell-shock in Twentieth-century Russia. *Journal of Contemporary History*, 35(1).

———. 2001. *Night of Stone. Death and Memory in Russia*. London: Granta.

———. 2006. *Night of Stone. Death—. Ivan's War. The Red Army 1939–45*. London: Faber and Faber.

Micale, Mark S., and Paul Lerner. 2001. Trauma, Psychiatry, and History: A Conceptual and Historiographical Introduction. In *Traumatic Pasts. History, Psychiatry, and Trauma in the Modern Age, 1870–1930*, eds. Mark S. Micale and Paul Lerner, 1–28. Cambridge: Cambridge University Press.

Millu, L. 1997. *Smoke over Birkenau*. Evanston: Northwestern University Press.

Jager, Sheila Miyoshi. 2003. *Narratives of Nation Building. A Genealogy of Patriotism*. Armonk: M. E. Sharpe.

———. 2013. *Brothers at War. The Unending Conflict in Korea*. London: Profile Books.

Jager, Sheila Miyoshi, and Jiyul Kim. 2007. The Korean War after the Cold War. Commemorating the Armistice Agreement in South Korea. In *Ruptured Histories. War, Memory, and the Post-Cold War in Asia*, eds. Sheila Miyoshi Jager and Rana Mitter. Cambridge, MA: Harvard UP.

Moeller, Robert, and War Stories. 2001. *The Search for a Usable Past in the Federal Republic of Germany*. Berkley: University of California Press.

Moeller, Robert G. 2010. Winning the Peace at the Movies: Suffering, Loss, and Redemption in Postwar German Cinema. In *Histories of the Aftermath: The Legacies of the Second World War*, eds. Frank Biess and Robert G. Moeller. New York: Berghahn.

Morris, David J. 2015. *The Evil Hours: A Biography of Post-Traumatic Stress Disorder*. New York: Eamon Dolan/Houghton Mifflin Harcourt.

Morris-Suzuki, Tessa. 2013. Remembering the Unfinished Conflict. Museums and the contested memory of the Korean War. In *East Asia Beyond the History Wars. Confronting the Ghosts of Violence*, eds. Morris-Suzuki et al. London: Routledge.

Morrison, Toni. 2012. *Home*. New York: Alfred A. Knopf.

Mosse, Georg L. 1990. *Fallen Soldiers: Reshaping the Memory of the World Wars*. New York: Oxford University Press.

Mrozek, Witold. 2009. *Film pamięci narodowej. Najnowsze kino polskie w dyskursie polityki historycznej*. In *Kino polskie jako kino narodowe*, eds. Tadeusz Lubelski and Maciej Stroiński. Kraków: Korporacja Ha!art.

Niarchos, Catherine N. 1995. Women, War, and Rape: Challenges Facing The International Tribunal for the Former Yugoslavia. *Human Rights Quarterly* 17(4): 640–690.

Nijakowski, Lech. 2008. *Polskie polityki pamięci. Esej socjologiczny*. Warszawa: WAiP.

Nakashima Brock, Rita and Herman Keizer, Jr. 2013. Helping Veterans Suffering Moral Injury After War (PDF). Accessed December 10. http://network.crcna.org/sites/network.crcna.org/files/Slides_HelpingVeteransSufferingMoralInjuryAfterWar.pdf

Niven, Bill, ed. 2006. *Germans as Victims: Remembering the Past in Contemporary Germany*. New York: Palgrave Macmillan.

NPR Books. 2013. Interview: Roy Scranton, "In 'Fire And Forget,' Vets Turned Writers Tell Their War Stories," Terry Gross, host, November 11. http://www.npr.org/2013/11/11/244520706/in-fire-and-forget-vets-turned-writers-tell-their-war-stories

Oh, Yoo-Seok. 2008. Formen südkoreanischer Erinnerung an Krieg und Nachkrieg. In *Der Koreakrieg. Wahrnehmung—Wirkung—Erinnerung*, eds. Christoph Kleßmann and Bernd Stöver. Cologne: Böhlau.

Olick, Jeffrey K. 2007. *The Politics of Regret. On Collective Memory and Historical Responsibility*. New York: Routledge.

Ostolski, Adam. 2011. *Trauma i pamięć publiczna. Spuścizna II wojny światowej w pamięci zbiorowej współczesnej Polski* (unpublished manuscript of doctoral thesis, University of Warsaw, Faculty of Philosophy and Sociology.

Park, Insook Han and Cho, Lee-Jay. 1995. Confucianism and the Korean family," *Journal of Comparative Family Studies* 26(1).

Paul, C. 1995. *Zwangsprostitution: Staatlich errichtete Bordelle im Nationalsozialismus*. Berlin: Hentrich.

Petrone, Karen. 2011. *The Great War in Russian Memory*. Bloomington, IN: Indiana University Press.

Phillips, David D. 2007. 'Trauma ek Pronoias' in Athenian Law. *The Journal of Hellenic Studies* 127: 75–105.

Phillips, Laura L. 2007. Gendered Dis/ability: Perspectives from the Treatment of Psychiatric Casualties in Russia's Early Twentieth Century Wars. *Social History of Medicine* 20: 2.

Piers, Gerhart, and Milton B. Singer. 1971. *Shame and Guilt: A Psychoanalytic and a Cultural Study*. New York: W.W. Norton & Company.

Pine, L. 1997. *Nazi Family Policy, 1933–1945*. Oxford: Berg.

——— 2004. Gender and the Family. In *The Historiography of the Holocaust*, ed. D. Stone. Basingstoke: Palgrave Macmillan.

Pinnow, Kenneth. 2007. Lives Out of Balance: The 'Possible World' of Soviet Suicide during the 1920s. In *Madness and the Mad in Russian Culture*, eds. Angela Britlinger and Ilya Vinitsky, 130–149. Toronto: Toronto University Press.

Plamper, Jan. Summer 2009. Fear: Soldiers and Emotion in Early Twentieth-Century Russian Military Psychology. *Slavic Review* 68(2): 259–283.

Projansky, Sarah. 2001. *Watching Rape: Film and Television on Postfeminist Culture*. New York: New York University Press.

Przewoźnik, Andrzej, and Jolanta Adamska. 2010. *Katyń. Zbrodnia—prawda—pamięć*. Warszawa: Świat Książki.

Pupavac, Vanessa. October-December 2002. Pathologizing Populations and Colonizing Minds: International Psychosocial Programs in Kosovo. *Alternatives: Global, Local, Political* 27(4): 489–511.

Radstone, Susannah. 2001. Trauma and Screen Studies: Opening the Debate. *Screen* 42(2): 188–192.

Reading, A. 2002. *The Social Inheritance of the Holocaust: Gender, Culture and Memory.* Palgrave Macmillan: Basingstoke.

Reid, Anna. 2011. *Leningrad. Tragedy of a City Under Siege, 1941–44.* London: Bloomsbury.

Reid, Fiona, and Broken Men. 2011. *Shell Shock, Treatment and Recovery in Britain, 1914–1930.* London: Bloomsbury.

Ringelheim, J. 1985. Women and the Holocaust: A Reconsideration of Research. *Signs: Journal of Women in Culture and Society* 10.

Rittner, C., and J. Roth, eds. 1993. *Different Voices: Women and the Holocaust.* New York: Paragon House.

Roper, Michael. 2009. *The Secret Battle: Emotional Survival in the Great War.* Manchester: Manchester University Press.

Rose, Gillian. 2011. *Visual Methodologies: An Introduction to Researching with Visual Materials.* London: Sage.

Rose, Sonya O. 2003. *Which People's War? National Identity and Citizenship in Wartime Britain 1939–1945.* Oxford: Oxford University Press.

Rothberg, Michael. 2009. *Multidirectional Memory: Remembering the Holocaust in the Age of Decolonization.* Stanford: Stanford University Press.

Rubin, A., and H. Greenspan. 2006. *Reflections: Auschwitz, Memory, and a Life Recreated.* Paragon House: St. Paul.

Salisbury, Harrison E. 1969. *The 900 Days. The Siege of Leningrad.* Secker & Warburg: London.

Sarbin, Theodore R. 1998. Believed-In Imaginings: A Narrative Approach. In *Believed–In Imaginings: The Narrative Construction of Reality*, eds. Theodore Sarbin and Joseph de Rivera. Washington, DC: American Psychological Association.

———, ed. 1986. *Narrative Psychology: The Storied Nature of Human Conduct.* New York: Praeger.

Schloss, E. 2013. *After Auschwitz.* London: Hodder and Stoughton.

Schmitz, Helmut, ed. 2008. *A Nation of Victims? Representations of German Wartime Suffering 1945 to the Present.* Amsterdam: Rodopi.

Schmitz, Helmut, and Annette Seidel-Arpac, eds. 2011. *Narratives of Trauma: Discourses of German Wartime Suffering in National and International Perspective.* Amsterdam: Rodopi.

Sebald, W.G. 2009. Contemporary Trauma Theory and Dieter Forte's Air Raid Epic. In *Germans as Victims: In the Literary Fiction of the Berlin Republic*, eds. Stuart Taberner and Karina Berger. Rochester, NY: Camden House.

Sendyka, Roma, "Pryzma – zrozumieć nie-miejsce pamięci," *Teksty Drugie* 2013/1-2.

Shane, Leo III. 2014. Report: Suicide rate spikes among young veterans. *Stars and Stripes* 09. http://www.stripes.com/report-suicide-rate-spikes-among-young-veterans-1.261283

Shapira, Michal. 2013. *The War Inside: Psychoanalysis, Total War, and the Making of the Democratic Self in Postwar Britain*. Cambridge: Cambridge University Press.

Shay, Jonathan. 2002. *Odysseus in America: Combat Trauma and the trials of Homecoming*. New York: Scribner.

Shephard, Ben. 2011. *The Long Road Home. The Aftermath of the Second World War*. London: Vintage.

———. 2000. *A War of Nerves: Soldiers and Psychiatrists in the Twentieth Century*. London: Jonathan Cape.

Shik, N. 2009. Sexual Abuse of Jewish Women in Auschwitz-Birkenau. In *Brutality and Desire: War and Sexuality in Europe's Twentieth Century*, ed. D. Herzog, 221–246. Basingstoke: Palgrave Macmillan.

Sielke, Sabine. 2002. *Reading Rape: The Rhetoric of Sexual Violence in American Literature and Culture, 1790–1990*. Princeton: Princeton University Press.

Sirotkina, Irina. 2002. *Diagnosing Literary Genius. A Cultural History of Psychiatry in Russia, 1880–1930*. Baltimore, MD: John Hopkins University Press.

Smith, Malcolm. 2000. *Britain and 1940: History, Myth and Popular Memory*. Abingdon: Routledge.

Sokołowska-Paryż, Marzena. 2012. The Narration and Visualization of Rape and the Inadvertent Subversion of the Anti-War Message in Brian De Palma's Redacted and Casualties of War. *War, Literature and the Arts* 24.

Stansky, Peter. 2007. *The First Day of the Blitz: September 7, 1940*. New Haven: Yale University Press.

Steele, Robert S. 1986. Deconstructing Histories: Toward a Systematic Criticism of Psychological Narrative. In *Narrative Psychology: The Storied Nature of Human Conduct*, ed. Theodore R. Sarbin, 268–271. New York: Praeger.

Summerfield, Penny. 1998. *Reconstructing Women's Wartime Lives: Discourse and Subjectivity in Oral Histories of the Second World War*. Manchester: Manchester University Press.

Sutherland, Sandra, and Donald J. Scherl. 1970. Patterns of Response Among Victims of Rape. *American Journal of Orthopsychiatry* 40(3): 503–511.

Shana Swiss and Joan E. Giller. 1993. Rape as a Crime of War: A Medical Perspective. *The Journal of the American Medical Association* 270(5).

Taberner, Stuart, and Karina Berger, eds. 2009. *Germans as Victims: In the Literary Fiction of the Berlin Republic*. Rochester, NY: Camden House.

Tec, N. 2003. *Resilience and Courage: Women, Men and the Holocaust*. New Haven: Yale University Press.

Thomas, Gregory M. 2009. *Treating the Trauma of the Great War: Soldiers, Civilians, and Psychiatry in France, 1914–1940*. Baton Rouge: Louisiana State University Press.

Thompson, Mark. 2011. The Other 1%. *Time Magazine*. November 21. http://www.time.com/time/magazine/article/0,9171,2099152,00.html

Thomson, Mathew. 2013. *Lost Freedom: the Landscape of the Child and the British Post War Settlement*. Oxford: Oxford University Press.

Timm, A. 2005. Sex with a Purpose: Prostitution, Venereal Disease, and Militarised Masculinity in the Third Reich. In *Sexuality and German Fascism*, ed. D. Herzog, 223–255. New York: Berghahn.

Turim, Maureen. 1992. *Reminiscences*, Subjectivities and Truths. In *To Free Cinema. Jonas Mekas & the New York Underground*, ed. D.E. James, 193–212. Princeton, NJ: Princeton University Press.

van der Kolk, Bessel. 2000. Posttraumatic Stress Disorder and the Nature of Trauma. *Dialogues in Clinical Neuroscience* 2(1).

Vas, Robert. 1970. The Confrontation. *Sight and Sound* 39(3).

———. 1959. Power Among Men. *Sight and Sound* 28(3/4).

Vas, Robert and Alan Rosenthal. *My Homeland* and *Nine Days in '26*. In Alan Rosenthal, *The Documentary Conscience. A Casebook of Film Making* (Berkeley, LA: University of California Press, 1980) 261-275.

Vees-Gulani, Susanne. 2003. *Trauma and Guilt: Literature of Wartime Bombing in Germany*. Berlin: Walter de Gruyter.

Virdi, Jyotika. 2006. Reverence, Rape—and then Revenge: Popular Hindi Cinema's 'Women's Film. In *Killing Women: The Visual Culture of Gender and Violence*, eds. Annette Burfoot and Susan Lord. Waterloo, ON: Wilfrid Laurier University Press.

von Campbell, Karen M. 1985. The Emotional Trauma of Hijacking: Who Pays? *Kentucky Law Journal* 74: 599–622.

Wachter, Alexandra. The Last Heroes of Leningrad. Coping Strategies of Siege Survivors in Soviet and Post-Soviet Society (Ph.D Dissertation, Queen Mary, University of London, In Progress).

Walsh, Froma. 2007. Traumatic Loss and Major Disasters: Strengthening Family and Community Resilience. *Family Process* 46(2): 207–227.

Wanke, Paul. 2005. *Russian/Soviet Military Psychiatry, 1904–1945*. London: Frank Cass.

Waxman, Z. 2006. *Writing the Holocaust: Identity, Testimony, Representation*. Oxford: Oxford University Press.

——— 2000. Unheard Stories: Reading Women's Holocaust Testimonies. *The Jewish Quarterly* 47(177).

Weine, Stevan M., et al. 2002. Guidelines for International Training in Mental Health and Psychosocial Interventions for Trauma Exposed Populations in Clinical and Community Settings. *Psychiatry* 65(2): 156–164.

Weitzman, L., and D. Ofer. 1998. The Role of Gender in the Holocaust. In *Women in the Holocaust*, eds. D. Ofer and L. Weitzman. New Haven: Yale University Press.

Welzer, Harald, Sabine Moller, and Karoline Tschuggnall. 2002. *Opa war kein Nazi: Nationalsozialismus und Holocaust im Familiengedächtnis*. Frankfurt am Main: Fischer.

Wermuth, H. 1993. *Breathe Deeply My Son*. London: Vallentine Mitchell.

Weyneken, JonDavid. 2007. Driving Out the Demons: Denazification, German Churches, and Allied Policies in Occupied Germany, 1945–1949 (PhD dissertation, Ohio University).

Wiesel, E. 1988. *Night: with Connections*. London: Holt, Rinehart and Winston.

Williams, Timothy. 2012. Suicides Outpacing War Deaths for Troops. *New York Times*. June 08. http://www.nytimes.com/2012/06/09/us/suicides-eclipse-war-deaths-for-us-troops.html?r=0.

Wilson, David and Jerome Kuehl. 1974. The Truth of Film History", *Sight and Sound* 42(4).

Withuis, Jolande. 2010. Introduction: The Politics of War Trauma. In *The Politics of War Trauma: The Aftermath of World War II in Eleven European Countries*, eds. J. Withuis and A. Mooij, 1–11. Amsterdam: Askant.

Wood, David. 2014. The Grunts: Damned If They Kill; Damned If they Don't. *Huffington Post*, March 18. http://projects.huffingtonpost.com/moral-injury/the-grunts

Wyatt, Frederick. 1986. The Narrative in Psychoanalysis: Psychoanalytic Notes on Storytelling, Listening, and Interpreting. In *Narrative Psychology: The Storied Nature of Human Conduct*, ed. Theodore R. Sarbin. New York: Praeger.

Yang, Sungeun and Paul C. Rosenblatt. 2001. Shame in Korean families. *Journal of Comparative Family Studies* 32(3).

Young, Allan. 1997. *The Harmony of Illusions*. Princeton: Princeton University Press.

———. 2014. Resilience for All by the Year 20-. In *Stress, Shock and Adaptation in the Twentieth Century*, eds. D. Cantor and E. Ramsden, 73–95. Rochester: Rochester University Press.

Young, James. 1990. *Writing and Rewriting the Holocaust: Narrative and the Consequences of Interpretation*. Bloomington: Indiana University Press.

Zajicek, Benjamin. 2009. *Scientific Psychiatric in Stalin's Soviet Union: The Politics of Modern Medicine and the Struggle to Define 'Pavlovian' Psychiatry, 1939–1953*. Ph.D diss., University of Chicago.

Zerubauel, Yael. 1994. The Death of Memory and the Memory of Death: Masada and the Holocaust as Historical Metaphors. *Representations*, 45.

Zubkova, Elena. 1998. *Russia After the War. Hopes, Illusions and Disappointments, 1945–1957*. Trans. Hugh Ragsdale. Armonk, NY: M.E. Sharpe.

Index

P. Leese, J. Crouthamel (eds.), *Traumatic Memories of the Second World War and After*, DOI 10.1007/978-3-319-33470-7

The manufacturer's authorised representative in the EU is Springer Nature Customer Service Centre GmbH, Europaplatz 3, 69115 Heidelberg, Germany. If you have any concerns regarding our products, please contact ProductSafety@springernature.com

Printed and bound by CPI Group (UK) Ltd, Croydon, CR0 4YY
30/09/2026
02225649-0012